karl h. pribram

stanford university

languages
of the brain

experimental paradoxes
and principles
in neuropsychology

prentice-hall, inc.

englewood cliffs, new jersey

Prentice-Hall Series in Experimental Psychology
James J. Jenkins, Editor

13-522730-5

Library of Congress Catalog Card Number 73-163862

Printed in the United States of America
Current printing (last digit):
10   9   8   7   6   5   4   3   2

PRENTICE-HALL INTERNATIONAL, INC., *London*
PRENTICE-HALL OF AUSTRALIA, PTY. LTD., *Sydney*
PRENTICE-HALL OF CANADA, LTD., *Toronto*
PRENTICE-HALL OF INDIA PRIVATE LIMITED, *New Delhi*
PRENTICE-HALL OF JAPAN, INC., *Tokyo*

contents

iii

preface

Languages of the Brain speaks to several needs. There is, first, the professional urge to express to myself and to my colleagues the beliefs which have grown out of, and now guide, my work. Thus, the manuscript, while primarily a theoretical statement, consists of formulations arising from paradoxes and puzzles which emerged unexpectedly from experimental results. At the time the research was conducted these results defied explanation within the theoretical framework held by most investigators. Because such personal encounters with paradox have provided a good deal of the spice of the brain-behavior laboratory fare, I have tried to retain this flavor.

But the professional problems per se would not have produced the book in its present form. Over the years larger audiences have become excited by the richness of yield and importance of the work on the relation of the brain to behavior and to subjective experience. These audiences are *not* ordinarily made up of trained behaviorists or experts in neurological science; rather, they are composed of intellectually alive undergraduates, engineers and physicists, biologists and biochemists, social scientists and psychiatrists, philosophers and humanists. Such audiences demand more than "the latest data on the basolateral nucleus of the amygdala" or "the difference between active and passive avoidance tasks." With considerable insight, they know that what is being discovered in the brain-behavior endeavor is important not just to "science" but *to them.* This book, therefore, attempts to grapple with the many questions raised by the audiences who shared my encounters with paradox.

Thus, this book tries to chart a middle course between professional detail and general interest. The focus of my laboratory work provides an ideal preparation for following this course: my experiments, to a large extent, deal with determining by behavioral analysis the function of various systems of neural structures that make up the brain. This "systems" neuropsychology furnishes a halfway house between neurophysiology—the electrical and chemical study of the functions of nerve cells (and their parts)—and experimental psychology—the behavioral analysis of functions of the organism-as-a-whole. And in recent years, a third dimension in the form of the computer has aided this enterprise. Computers help control experiments, aid in analyzing data, and furnish a new way to inaugurate investigations; biological resources can often be conserved if an approach can be given a "dry run" to test its feasibility and to portray in detail consequences which are implicit but not apparent in the initial formulation. Enactment by computer thus functions for the biobehavioral scientist as the in vitro (in-glass, test tube) experiment performs for the biochemist. For both, the in vitro simulations provide the opportunity to construct powerful tools of precise concepts, coherent languages, with which to analyze the living process.

The systems neuropsychologist perforce, therefore, listens to—and relates his investigations to—disciplines that have encountered their own sets of problems and have developed their own concepts and styles to deal with these problems. In short, the systems neuropsychologist becomes conversant in several distinct languages.

The substantive results of my research have reinforced this attention to variety in language. The brain apparently organizes perceptual, motor, and memory processes by repeatedly restructuring its own activity. Sensory excitations are transformed into patterns of neural activity without undue loss of information. Further transformations into other neural patterns, other neural "codes," take place as "information processing" continues and behavioral acts become organized. Much of my work, therefore, entails the identification of the set of brain codes, the brain's languages that are involved in one or another phase of psychological processing. What brain codes make visual pattern recognition possible? What brain codes coordinate the building of a nest or the skillful rendering of a piano sonata? What brain codes do I interpret as feeling hungry, sleepy, sexy, apathetic, or interested? And what are the brain's coding operations that allow it to communicate with another brain? What are the "Languages of the Brain"?

This book endeavors to determine principles common to the brain's coding mechanisms and the transformations involved in recoding. Here paradox was encountered in experimental results that puzzled because they departed from those predicted and thus made suspect the predictive value of currently held views about how the brain was supposed to work. So new theories and theses were developed.

Languages of the Brain uses the biological language of chemistry, physiology, and neurology, the behavioral language of psychology, and the engineering language of computers. But, by the necessity of its reach for an audience that encompasses several disciplines or none, the concepts and words in these languages are kept basic. Also, the contents are organized into four separate parts each of which is, to a considerable degree, sufficiently independent of the others to provide an introduction to the remainder—relevance to particular interests or groups of readers might dictate different order.

Languages of the Brain thus delineates principles of brain coding. Its four parts address distinct sets of problems. The first part deals directly with basic *brain function* and the logic of neural wetware which enable codes to be formed in the brain. The second part concerns the role played by brain in *psychological* processes. Coding involved in the organization of perception, motivation, and emotion is analyzed. The third part of the book focuses on the *neural control and modification of behavior.* The final part is devoted to the *structure of communication* between brains in terms of signs and symbols, and of the thoughtful talk that regulates the affairs of man.

These parts thus portray the brain's compulsion to generate languages. This compulsion both creates the disparate tongues that make of the intellectual community a present-day Tower of Babel and provides the means to transcend it. Among these tongues are the various dichotomies that today still universally plague discussions of the qualities that make man human—mind-body, mind-machine, mind-brain, and mind-behavior. The following pages are devoted to coming to terms with these dichotomies through the realizations that (these) are "Languages of the Brain."

My initial thanks go to those authors who have recently written texts in physiological psychology. Their success freed me to pursue the personal form of *Languages of the Brain,* thus making it complementary to a more standard treatment of brain-behavior relationships. Several such texts are now available—Richard Thompson's *Foundations,* Peter Grossman's and Peter Milner's *Physiological Psychology,* and Charles Butter's *Neuropsychology* are examples. The availability of detailed and comprehensive treatments of individual topics in the *Handbook of Physiology* and the two volumes of *The Neurosciences* also greatly helped me decide what need *not* be included because it could be found better stated elsewhere. In addition *The Neurosciences* provided a feast of superb illustrations.

Many individuals participated. Those who formed my laboratory over the years are quoted in the text when their work is pertinent. Many others sharpened my conceptions through discussion and when they do not find themselves represented are asked to be patient—the next book I undertake will cover the results of the laboratory's work specifically.

Some of the crucial working through of ideas was achieved in two centers devoted to creative thinking: The Center for Theoretical Psychology at the University of Alberta and the Salk Institute. The director of the Canadian center, Joe Royce, and its leading constituents, Bill Rozeboom, Kelly Wilson, and Herman Tennessen had much to do with formulating and enacting the semifinal drafts of the book; Part IV was launched at the Salk Institute at La Jolla to which Bruno Bronowski invited Roman Jakobson, Peter Reynolds, and me to join Ed Klima and his wife, Ursula Bellugi-Klima, for several linguistic feasts.

The manuscript was solicited and obtained for Prentice-Hall by a superb critique by Ed Stanford who has shepherded it since. In the almost a year that has elapsed, the text has accrued one sixth of its present volume and become considerably better documented. The revisions resulted in large part from detailed criticisms by Audrey Konow which necessitated clarification and expansion, especially of material in Part II; and through additions to Part III which came about when I was alerted by Stephen Glickman to evidence in support of my theoretical statements that had accrued during the past few years while I was too busy writing to read properly. Glickman also offered pertinent suggestions for some rearrangements of subject matter in the entire first half of the book that were gratefully accepted. During this period of final revision, the editorial comments of Jim Jenkins and Hew Crain (who stood in as representative of the engineering community) also aided the manuscript's clarity a great deal. Specific suggestions made by Bob Isaacson, Marjorie Grene, and Michael Scriven rescued the manuscript from unnecessary errors, omissions, and ambiguities. And so many others helped: Carolyn Csongradi's suggestion about the introduction, her and Carol Christiansen's careful reading of the initial chapters to be sure one thought led clearly into another; Bob Phelps, Stan Smerin, and Bruce Bridgeman bringing up topics and figures for consideration just in the nick of time, etc. James Dewson's reading of the entire manuscript for an overall appraisal (which did lead to some important changes) was reminiscent of his last minute help in editing my Penguin Brain and Behaviour Series—he was at the time half a world closer to London than I, so had been then, as now, pressed into service. And the volunteering of Dr. Walter Tubbs, my sole editor of the Penguin volumes, to help carry out the indexing of *Languages,* proved a welcome opportunity for renewing a cherished relationship. So many things go on behind the scenes in the final stages of such a manuscript that an author can become aware of only some of them and then only momentarily.

The final form of *Languages of the Brain* resulted from the efforts of a small team of talented book makers. Mrs. Phyllis Ellis typed and typed and typed as she had not since the last book we did together: *Plans and the Structure of Behavior.* All this she did while serenely running my laboratory, answering telephones, handling budgets, people, and me. In addition Mrs. Ellis collated the entire bibliography and saw to it that titles, references, and index were correctly entered. These items alone would have kept me from finishing this or any other book.

The book's editor, Joan Brooks, also performed an heroic job: putting the manuscript into good English. George Miller once remarked that in order to understand my writing he had to read each paragraph backward and then wipe the blood off it. *Languages of the Brain* still has some upside down paragraphs and I refused to have it other than a bloody book, but it is more readable than it would have been without Joan's keen and carefully guided green pen.

Jim Beggs calmly composited the pages and supervised the art work while all else around the book reached a stage of chaos this winter. He patiently redid pages when the author changed what was left of his mind; or when gobs of obvious errors were missed in galley. Artwork for a book with biological content can do much to make it clear and beautiful. After some worrisome weeks our art problems were brought to rest in the person of Jill Leland. I waved my hand over pieces of paper and she produced the figures I had intended. Sometimes she waited patiently while I decided where an arrowhead should point; sometimes she would snatch a nearly completed figure from me lest I spoil it with over detail. To these persons and the unnamed others, thank you for joining me in the joy and travail that now has become a real book, not just the manuscript of *Languages of the Brain.*

But most of the hard writing occurred over weekends. This and many other problems associated with the intense involvement demanded by an enterprise such as this caused Amy, my wife, much suffering though I hope moments of pleasure were not altogether lacking as when she suggested where the chapter synopses ought to go and when she insisted that no book could properly be complete with only nineteen chapters—which brought forth the penultimate twentieth. Her suffering never shook an unflagging faith in the worth of *Languages of the Brain* and for this and much else, thank you.

(15 March 1971)
Stanford, California

languages
of the brain

"*When Clerk-Maxwell was a child it is written that he had a mania for having everything explained to him, and that when people put him off with vague verbal accounts of any phenomenon he would interrupt them impatiently by saying, 'Yes; but I want you to tell me the* particular go *of it!' Had his question been about truth, only a pragmatist could have told him the particular go of it. . . . Truths emerge from facts; but they dip forward into facts again and add to them; which facts again create or reveal new truth. . . and so on indefinitely. The 'facts' themselves meanwhile are not* true. *They simply* are. *Truth is the function of the beliefs that start and terminate among them.*"

William James, 1931, pp. 197, 225

part 1

a two process
mechanism
of
brain function

"That language in which information is communicated [in the brain]. . . neither needs to be nor is apt to be built on the plan of those languages men use toward one another."

Pitts & McCulloch,
in McCulloch, Embodiments of Mind, *1965, p. 56.*

states and operators

introduction

"I love you." It was spring in Paris, and the words held the delightful flavor of a Scandinavian accent. The occasion was a UNESCO meeting on the problems of research on Brain and Human Behavior. The fateful words were not spoken by a curvaceous blonde beauty, however, but generated by a small shiny metal device in the hands of a famous psycholinguist.

The device impressed all of us with the simplicity of its design. The loudspeaker was controlled by only two knobs. One altered the state of an electronic circuit that represented the tension of the vocal cords; the other regulated the pulses generated by a circuit that simulated the plosions of air puffs striking the cords.

Could this simple device be relevant to man's study of himself? Might not all behavior be generated and controlled by a neural mechanism equally simple? Is the nervous system a "two knob" dual process mechanism in which one process is expressed in terms of neuroelectric states, the other in terms of distinct pulsatile operators

3

on those states? That the nervous system does, in fact, operate by impulses has been well documented. The existence of neuroelectric states in the brain has also been established, but this evidence and its significance to the study of psychology has been slow to gain

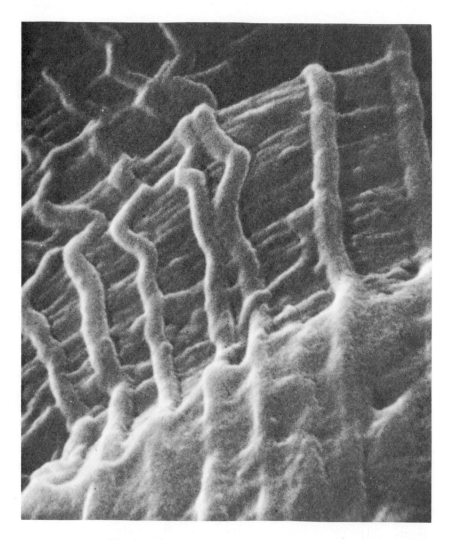

Fig. 1-1. Scanning electron micrograph showing the arrangement of nerve fibers in the retina of Necturus. Fibers (dendrites) arise in the inner segment and course over the outer segment of a cone. Note that points of contact do not necessarily take place at nerve endings. From Lewis, 1970.

acceptance even in neurophysiology. This first chapter therefore examines the evidence which makes a two-process model of brain function plausible.

To understand brain function we must first understand the units of organization that make up the nervous system. The classic analysis identifies these units as neurons—cells completely and functionally separated from one another by membranous barriers. However, this oversimplified view of the neuron in isolation as the sole organizer of brain processes becomes cumbersome when we attempt to characterize the neuroelectric states part of the dual mechanism. This and the next section sketch the background of the neuron doctrine and the reasons it must presently be amended.

In the last part of the nineteenth century a great controversy raged in neurobiology about whether brain tissue is made up of units— cells—as are all other tissues of the body. The controversy has been settled so conclusively that the neuron and its capacity to act as a unit by discharging an electrical potential in an all-or-none fashion, is no longer considered theoretical. Yet no one has ever "seen" a neuron in brain tissue, i.e., traced its entire extent and shown it to be truly separate from its neighbors (See Fig. 1-1.). How then did neuron doctrine become so universally accepted? And why should we reexamine the topic now?

Controversy concerning the neuron doctrine reached a climax toward the end of the nineteenth century. On the side of the essential continuity of neural tissue were such notable neuro-anatomists as Bielschowsky and Golgi; taking the part of the neuron as an independent but contiguous unit were Waldeyer and Ramon y Cajal. The convincing analysis was given not by these neuroanatomists, however, but by Sir Charles Sherrington in his Silliman lectures at Yale University (published as the classic volume, *The Integrative Action of the Nervous System, 1947).* Sherrington had earlier coined with Foster the term *synapses* to describe the discontinuities presumed to occur between nerve cells. He now made a remarkable theoretical contribution by contrasting neuro-*physiological* data based largely on electrical studies of nerve trunks with neuro*behavioral* data based on the study of reflex action (con-ceptualized in terms of reflex-arc, see Chapter 5) in the "spinal" animal. He pointed out that paradoxical discrepancies between the results of the neurophysiological and the behavioral studies could be resolved by recourse to the neuro*anatomically* derived synapse. The crucial discrepancies were that (1) signal conduction in the isolated nerve trunk stimulated anywhere along its extent is bidirectional while signal conduction in the spinal reflex is unidirectional, and (2)

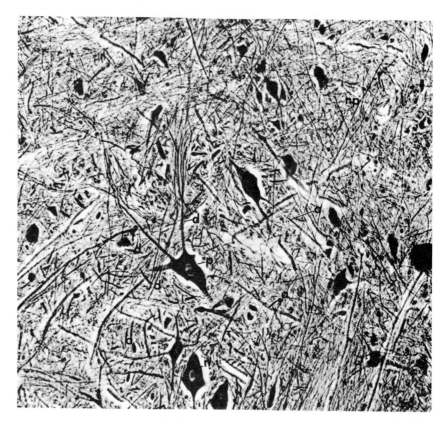

Fig. 1-2. Cluster of neurons in the gray matter of the spinal cord of the monkey, illustrating a common arrangement of neuron cell bodies and their axon and dendrite processes. Much of the space between cell bodies is occupied by a feltwork consisting of these processes and a large number of incoming, branched axon terminals. The feltwork of axons and dendrites, within which neuron-to-neuron communication largely occurs, is known as the "neuropil." p—perikaryon. a-axon. d-dendrite. np—neuropil. n—nucleus of large neuron, probably a motoneuron. Paraffin section, 15 μ. Bodian silver stain. X150. (The apparent space around the neuron cell bodies is a shrinkage artifact.) From Bodian, 1967.

impulse conduction within a nerve trunk is considerably more rapid than the response obtained when a reflex is initiated. Nine additional discrepancies were noted. Most of these were concerned with the closeness of correspondence between the stimulus applied and the response obtained: correspondence was always closer for the neural than for the behavioral response. Inferred functions such as spatial convergence and temporal summation, fatigability, facilitation, and inhibition were attributed to the synapse as explaining the discrepancies. The following summary statement by Sherrington gives the flavor of his thinking:

> Salient among the characteristic differences between conduction in nerve-trunks and in reflex-arcs respectively are the following:
>
> Conduction in reflex-arcs exhibits: (1) slower speed as measured by the latent period between application of stimulus and appearance of end-effects, this difference being greater for weak stimuli than for strong; (2) less close correspondence between the moment of cessation of stimulus and the moment of cessation of end-effect, i.e., there is a marked "after discharge"; (3) the less close correspondence between rhythm of stimulus and rhythm of end-effect; (4) less close correspondence between the grading of intensity of the stimulus and the grading of intensity of the end-effect; (5) considerable resistance to passage of a single nerve-impulse, but a resistance easily forced by a succession of impulses (temporal summation); (6) irreversibility of direction instead of reversibility as in nerve-trunks; (7) fatigability in contrast with the comparative indefatigability of nerve-trunks; (8) much greater variability of the threshold value of stimulus than in nerve-trunks; (9) refractory period, 'bahnung,' inhibition, and shock, in degrees unknown for nervetrunks; (10) much greater dependence on blood-circulation, oxygen (Verwor, Winterstein, v. Baeyer, etc.); (11) much greater susceptibility to various drugs—anaesthetics. [Sherrington, 1947, pp. 13–14]

In short, the results of electrophysiological study of nerve trunks and the results of behavioral investigation of the reflex did not coincide. Nerves seemed to be simple conductive wires for impulses; the reflex showed a complexity of organization that could not be accounted for by a simple "wire" model. Sherrington therefore adopted the "neuron doctrine" that the "wires" making up the nervous system, instead of forming a continuous network, were slightly separated from each other and joined by a structure that he baptized the *synapse*. He then endowed the synapse with all of the complexity necessary to account for the behavior of the reflex. Thus the properties of the observed behavior became attributed to the properties of the junctions between neurons and not to its conducting "wire" part. (See Figs. 1-2 and 1-3.)

Sherrington's theoretical insight has been largely ignored by neurophysiological and neurobehavioral scientists. Attention has been focused on the existence and the properties of the synapse and these have been amply documented by electron microscopy and by

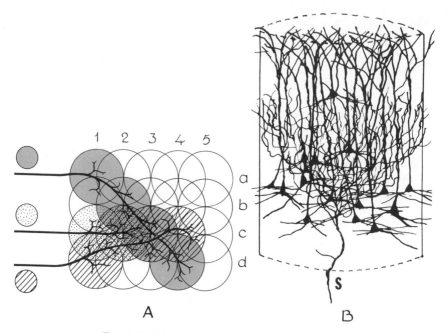

Fig. 1-3. Diagram of microstructure of synaptic domains in cortex. The ensemble of overlapping circles represents the junctions between branches of input axons and cortical dendrites. Redrawn after Scheibel and Scheibel in Chow and Leiman, 1970.

recordings of junctional electrical and chemical activities. But interpretation of these results has almost invariably been within the framework of the question "How does the conduction of nerve impulses pass the *barrier* of the synapse?" Reference restricted to cell discharge of impulses and the conducting properties of synaptic pathways is so often viewed as adequate and sufficient.

Few scientists have followed Sherrington's thesis that the complexity of behavior (and of psychological processes) must be accounted for in terms of the complexity of organization of the junctional (synaptic) mechanisms in the central nervous system. The chapters of this book aim to remedy this neglected opportunity. They flow from a thesis modelled on Sherrington's in an attempt to come to terms with the problems of the relationship between brain, mind, and behavior, much as Sherrington handled the relationship between spinal cord and reflex. The problems involving brain are more subtle and complicated than those involving spinal cord; nonetheless, considerable headway in understanding these problems can be made even today by cautiously applying Sherrington's classical neurobiological approach. The alternatives held by neurologists, physiologists, and psychologists range from despair to empty pronouncement of undefined hopes—if the existence of the problem is admitted at all. But the brain-mind-behavior issue can be productive when restricted problems are posed. What are some of these problems?

some neuropsychological facts

Although neuron theory has been the framework underlying neurophysiological experiment, a prominent group of psychologists has repeatedly claimed that a nervous system which functions exclusively as a set of discrete conducting units does not handle their experimental data. These investigators have explained their observations by one or another kind of field model rather than by quantal, discrete, probabilistic neuron theory. The issue is succinctly stated as follows:

> The physiologist holds to the faith that the brain, being made up of neurons, is capable only of that excitation which is the sum of the excitations of many neurons, and that these central neurons obey the same laws and are excited under the same limitations as apply to the peripheral neurons which have been experimentally studied. To this article of faith the psychologist sometimes opposes another belief, that the organization of cerebral excitation corresponds to the organization of phenomenal experience. [Boring, 1932, p. 32]

Specifically, the problem arises when neurobehavioral experiments involving brain are undertaken. Two opposing views have been advocated. One view maintains that each cortical point, each cell or cell aggregate, is specialized for a unique function. The integration necessary to account for behavioral and psychological processes is, according to this view, accomplished by the inborn presence of, or by the establishment through experience of, permanent associative connections between neurons.

The alternative view, espoused in these chapters, holds that certain interactions important to the organization of behavior and the psychological process occur in brain tissue, and that these interactions cannot be specified solely in terms of permanent associative connections among neurons. Karl Lashley, a pioneer proponent of this alternative, bases his argument on three lines of evidence: (1) equivalence in receptor function; (2) spontaneous reorganization of motor reactions; and (3) the survival of behavior after destruction of any *part* of a system in the brain when total destruction of the system abolishes that behavior. Let us pursue these lines for a moment.

Concerning the equivalence of receptor function, experiments show that "within very wide limits, the absolute properties of the stimulus are relatively unimportant for behavior and that the reactions are determined by ratios of excitation which are equally effective when applied to any group of receptor cells within the system." For instance, an "animal trained to choose the largest of three circles may immediately react positively to the widest lines when confronted with three fields with different widths of stripes" (Lashley, 1960, p. 238–39). The details of such evidence makes up Part II of this book; it is sufficient now to point out that the problem exists.

Regarding spontaneous motor reorganization, "the results indicate that when habitually used motor organs are rendered nonfunctional by removal or paralysis, there is an immediate spontaneous use of other motor systems which had not previously been associated with or used in the performance of the activity" (Lashley, 1960, p. 239). For instance, the essential patterns imposed on muscles in the act of writing are preserved when a person shifts from writing with a pencil held with his fingers to writing with a pencil held between the teeth. How the brain can accomplish this feat makes up the substance of the initial chapters of Part III.

The evidence for substitutability among parts of the organism's functional systems in the organization of behavior and of psychological processes extends also to central stations in the brain. This evidence introduces Part II. Again we need here only to note that extremely large holes can be made in the brain with very little effect on just that highly complex behavior which one would expect to be especially sensitive to disruption if integration depended entirely on the presence of permanent associative connections.

Lashley (in Beach, et al., 1960) summarizes the problem succinctly:

These three lines of evidence indicate that certain coordinated activities, known to be dependent upon definite cortical areas, can be carried out by any part (within undefined limits) of the whole area. Such a condition might arise from the presence of many duplicate reflex pathways through the areas and such an explanation will perhaps account for all of the reported cases of survival of functions after partial destruction of their special areas, but it is inadequate for the facts of sensory and motor equivalence. These facts establish the principle that once an associated reaction has been established (e.g., a positive reaction to a visual pattern), the same reaction will be elicited by the excitation of sensory cells which were never stimulated in that way during the course of training. Similarly, motor acts (e.g., opening a latch box), once acquired, may be executed immediately with motor organs which were not associated with the act during training. [pp. 237–40]

At least two issues are admixed in Lashley's statement: substitutability among parts of the organism and transfer of training, which encompasses the problem of reactions of familiarity and novelty. Nevertheless, these passages indicate the need for reconciling the data of psychology with those of neurophysiology. Such reconciliation must make a wider use of brain facts than is now possible under the commonly held restricted interpretation of neuron theory. The resulting view of brain function would nonetheless have to be firmly based in classical neurophysiological data. Let us therefore look at those recent advances in neurophysiological techniques which suggest that such reconciliation is indeed possible (e.g., Bullock, 1959). These techniques enable a differentiation between primarily *intra*neuronal nerve impulse patterns, and primarily *inter*neuronal junctional patterns of activity—a distinction which widens the range of applicable approaches considerably.

the junctional microstructure

The significance of neuroelectric processes occurring at and beyond the synapse became apparent to neurophysiologists from specific evidence. For many years the electrical activity recorded from the scalp was thought to reflect the aggregate of nerve impulses generated by the neurons of the brain lying somewhere beneath the recording site. When it became possible to record simultaneously the electrical activity from local sites in brain tissue and from aggregates, the supposition became suspect (Purpura, 1958). Intracellular recordings show that *even in the absence of propagated nerve impulses,* rhythmic slow potential changes occur and when these are compared to the rhythms recorded simultaneously from aggregates of neurons in the same location, they coincide (Creutzfeld, et al. 1966; Fugita and Sato, 1964; Elul and Adey, 1966; Morrell, 1967). When the membrane of the nerve cell is arbitrarily polarized by imposing an electrical potential across it, the amplitude of the intracellular rhythms is altered and this alteration is reflected in the gross recording (Eccles, 1964; see Fig. 1-4). Thus strong evidence was produced for a major contribution by the slowly

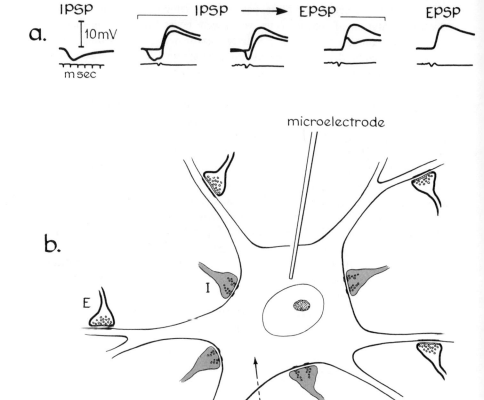

Fig. 1-4. Diagram of neuron (b) with excitatory (E) and inhibitory (I) synapses and intracellular records (a) of slow postsynaptic potentials (EPSP and IPSP) above. Note ·that impulse generated at origin of axon is well over 50 mV while intracellular records range around 5 mV. Only the axonal nerve impulse is propagated. Redrawn after Eccles, 1967.

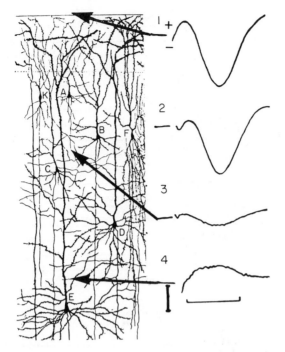

Fig. 1-5. Records of dendritic slow potentials (right side of figure) showing approximate level of recording in cortex. Calibration 0.2 mv; 10 msec. From Purpura, 1967.

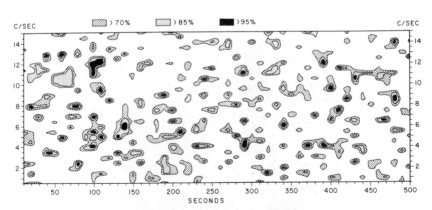

COHERENCE (LINEAR PREDICTABILITY RELATIONSHIP)
BETWEEN NEURONAL WAVES AND EEG

Fig. 1-6. Plot of coherence over a 500 second time period between intracellular slow potential records and the EEG from the cortical surface in the same domain of tissue. From Adey, 1967

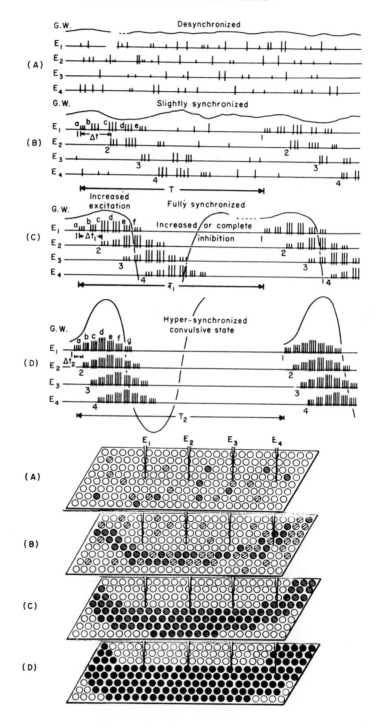

Figs. 1-7 and 1-8. Relations between neuronal discharge, circulation of neuronal activity, and synchronization of the gross waves, as they appear when recorded simultaneously with four microelectrodes with tips separated by 100 to 150μ. Bot.: Diagrammatic two-dimensional representation of neuronal fields, showing the neuronal activity corresponding to each successive state. From Verzeano, et al., 1970.

occurring fluctuations of potentials of neural membranes to the electrical activity recorded grossly as the electroencephalogram, the EEG (See Fig. 1-5). Only when the activity of a large number of units is synchronized—as when their discharge is evoked by a flash of light or a click of sound—are the gross recordings and unit nerve impulse discharges alike (Figs. 1-7, 1-8). In one such study (Fox and O'Brien, 1965) many light flashes (3000 to 5000) were presented. When unit impulse discharges were averaged over this number of presentations, the probability of discharge of a single visual cortical cell during the time following the flash (immediately to 1 second) approximates the wave form of the gross potential recorded simultaneously. The gross potential thus provides an estimate of the probability that a unit will fire after the presentation of an abrupt stimulus which is able to synchronize neuronal aggregates. However, when no such dramatic synchronization is elicited, the gross record reflects the electrical potential changes occurring in the feltwork of nerve fibers which disposes the neural tissue towards, but does not actually trigger unit discharges. (Li, Cullen, and Jasper, 1956; Creutzfeld, 1961; Verzeano and Negishi, 1960; See Figs. 1-5, 1-6.).

Experimental results such as these have made it practical to distinguish between two types of neuroelectric activity: nerve impulse unit discharges on the one hand, and graded slow potential changes on the other. Only nerve impulses are propagated; graded changes wax and wane locally in the brain tissue and are sensitive to a variety of influences, such as the local chemical environment, which are not strictly neuronal.

The distinction between graded slow potentials and nerve impulses depends in part on the fact that the amplitude and speed of conduction of a nerve impulse is proportional to the diameter of the nerve trunk in which the impulse is generated. Thus in sizable nerve fibers impulses tend to be of considerable magnitude and to travel rapidly. In small nerve fibers the electrical potential which characterizes an impulse is lower in amplitude (at least when recorded extracellularly) and conduction speed is slower. As nerve fibers extend away from their cell body of origin, they tend to narrow and branch—as a result impulses become smaller and slower, especially at the terminals of the fibers (Fig. 1-9). Thus chemical mediators are necessary to amplify the potential change occurring at nerve endings so that the electrical signal can exert an influence across the structural junctions between neurons. Despite the chemical booster, the potentials that are generated beyond the synapse (called postsynaptic potentials) are initially rudimentary, slow, graded electrical changes readily influenced by the chemical medium created by the vascular supply and the nonneural (glial) cells which surround the fibers. Further, finer nerve fibers lack an insulating fatty coating (the myelin sheath) which in large fibers prevents interaction among impulses. The slow potentials which occur in fine fibers such as the ramified branches, arborizations, of dendrites find therefore no obstacle for actual local interaction.

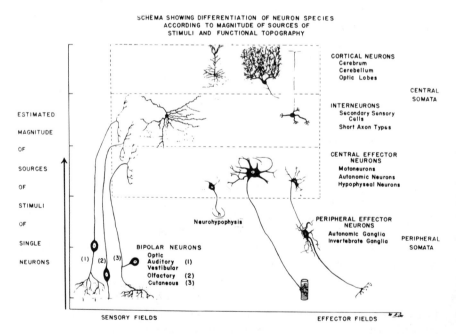

Fig. 1-9. Major neuron types in the mammalian central nervous system, arranged according to general role, hierarchical level, and probable extent of branching. From Bodian, 1967.

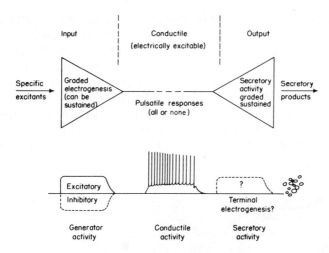

Fig. 1-10. Diagram showing the relationship between graded slow potentials, nerve impulses, and chemical secretions that act as boosters across structured junction between neurons (synapses). From Grundfest, 1967.

A somewhat simplified picture (Fig. 1-10) of the relationship between slow potential changes and nerve impulses based on these relationships looks like this: within a neuron the electrochemical events lead, on occasion, to membrane depolarization—graded changes increment until they become nerve impulses. Where neurons meet—either where fine, unmyelinated fibers form a feltwork and make contact in a relatively unstructured fashion called *ephaptic* (Fig. 1-11) or where the terminals of fibers actually make a structured contact through a *synapse* (Fig. 1-12) with other neurons— nerve impulses decrement into graded responses, i.e., they become small, slow potentials indistinguishable from the spontaneously generated local graded activity (see Chapter 3). In short, the effective *intra*neural mechanism is characterized by the incrementing of graded activity into a propagated nerve impulse; the effective *junctional* mechanism is characterized by the opposite: nerve impulses become decremented into local slow potentials. The junctional mechanism in turn influences the intraneural membrane depolarization but only after a period of time during which the opportunity for both spatial and temporal interactions among slow potential configurations has been realized. It is these interactions among configurations which give the slow potentials their special significance.

This view of junctional activity differs in emphasis from the commonly held approach to synaptic function. Most neurophysiological studies of the synapse have asked the question "how do nerve impulses—or the information carried by them—cross the synaptic cleft?" The present emphasis is on the slow potentials themselves—the suggestion is that the slow potentials produce patterns which serve a function in addition to a role in impulse transmission: the view taken here is that the slow potential pattern "computes" both the spatial neighborhood interactions among neural elements and, to some extent, the temporal interactions over a range of sites by a continuous (analogue) rather than a discrete, all-or-none (digital) mechanism.

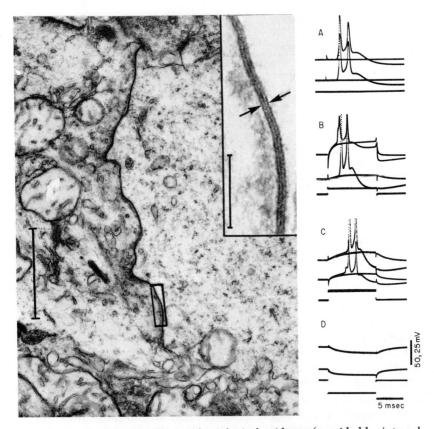

Fig. 1-11. Electrophysiological evidence (provided by intracellular recordings from two neurons for ephatic transmission across an unstructured contact between neurons depicted by electromicroscopy. Electrical pulses (B,C) and current (D) supplied to either cell, recording from the other. Remote stimulation (A) evokes spikes nearly simultaneously in both cells. From Grundfest, 1967.

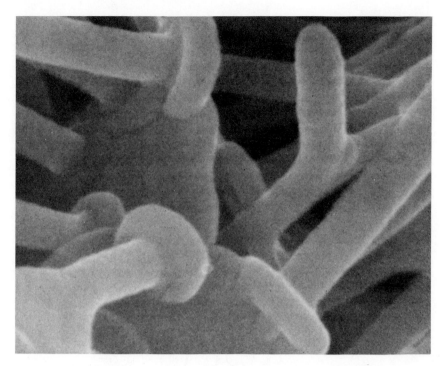

Fig. 1-12. Synaptic knobs at the intersection of two nerve fibers in the neuropil of the abdominal ganglion of *Aplesia Californica.* Magnification approximately 35,000. From Lewis, 1970.

The aggregate of slow potentials present over an extended location at any moment can be described as a state which has a microstructure. The arrival of impulses at ephaptic or synaptic junctions is never a solitary event. Axonal terminations are usually multiple—i.e., axons branch at their ends. As many as 1000 synapses may characterize the junctional possibilities between a pair of neurons. Dendrites are tree-like almost by definition, displaying many fine fibered branches which crisscross, making multiple contacts among neurons, contacts which for some cells (e.g., the amacrine of the retina) include structured synapses (Fig. 1-13). Thus ephaptic and synaptic events, those that are composed at the junctions between neurons, form a pattern. Inferences about the nature of such a pattern can be made from the known fine structure of the brain and the electrical activity recorded from it. Several such inferences suggest that these patterns make up wave fronts, a suggestion which becomes especially useful in dealing with the problems of equivalence in Part II. This

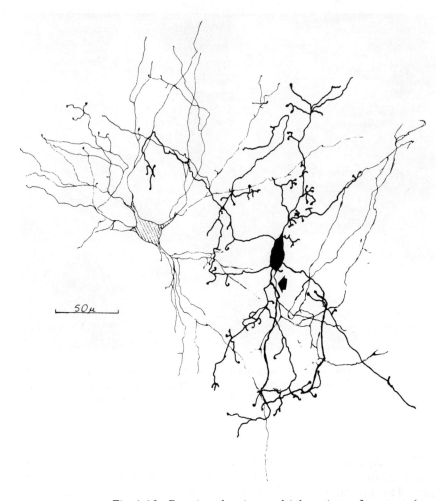

Fig. 1-13. Drawing showing multiple points of contact (synaptic and ephaptic) between two neurons in brain. From Ralston, 1968.

does not mean that the slow potential microstructure must be conceived of in wave mechanical terms, only that it may be useful on occasion to do so. If nothing else, interpreting slow potential patterns as constituting wave fronts helps to visualize what is occurring:

> The neuron is characteristically an 'all-or-nothing' relay. An impulse arriving across a synapse produces a very small and transient electrical effect, equivalent to .001 volt and lasting .01 to .02 second. It requires an excitation of about 10 times this voltage to cause the neuron to fire its discharge . . . .

Since convergence of many impulses on any one neuron is required to make it discharge, chains of single neurons cannot propagate a wave of activity through the cortex. Rather the propagation resembles an advancing front of multilane traffic, with many cells activated in parallel at each synaptic linkage in the chain . . . . (Fig. 1-14)

We can see immediately the explanation for one remarkable property of a neuronal network: how two completely different inputs (one to cells A_1 and A_2, the other to A_3 and A_4) can be transmitted through the same pattern of cell connnections, crossing each other and emerging as completely different outputs (D_3-D_4) . . . . (Fig. 1-15)

The transmission of a wavefront in the cortex is, of course, a much more complicated matter. With as many as 100 neurons involved at each relay

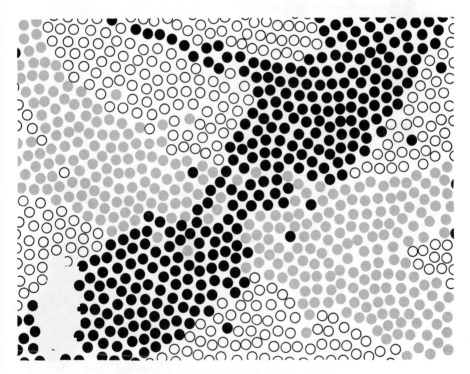

Fig. 1-14. In this schematic diagram the synaptic domains of the cortex are imagined as laid out as dots in one plane. The multilane traffic in one, evolving a specific neuronal pattern, is shown in black, and in another as dark gray. The unfilled domains are not activated by either pattern. Note that at the crossing of these two lanes the same domains should participate in both and so each should be represented as a very large gray dot, not just dark gray or black as shown. From Eccles, 1970.

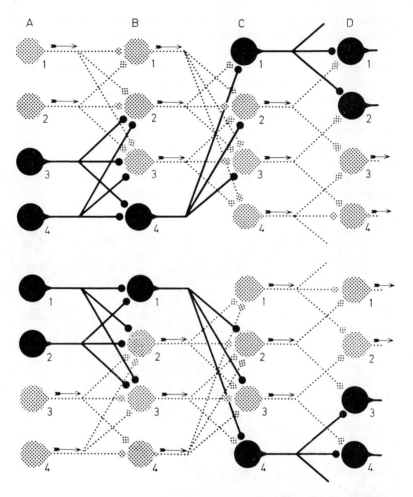

Fig. 1-15. Model of a highly schematic neuronal network to illustrate the simplest case of propagation along a multilane pathway. There is exactly the same anatomical network in the upper and lower diagrams. The synaptic connections of the twelve cells in columns A, B, and C are drawn, cells with impulses (note arrows) being shown in light grey, while the silent cells are black. The assumption is that a cell fires an impulse if it is excited by two or more synapses (also light grey). Thus an imput $A_1 A_2$ results in an output discharge of $D_3 D_4$ (upper diagram), whereas an input of $A_3 A_4$ gives an output of $D_1 D_2$ (lower diagram). Neurons B_2, B_3, C_2, C_3 are activated in the crossing zone for both these inputs. This diagram suffers from the serious defect that it ignores inhibition. From Eccles, 1958.

stage, an advancing wave may sweep over 100,000 neurons in a single second. Such a wave has . . . rich potentiality . . . . [Eccles, *Scientific American*, 1958, pp. 4–7]

Another inference suggests a nonpropagative standing or plane wave model derived from an idealized version of the anatomical distribution of connections between neurons (Sholl, 1956). The assumptions basic to this model are all reasonable ones: (1) neurons are randomly distributed; (2) the richness of connections between cells decreases with distance; (3) the spatial pattern of distribution of the processes of each cell is different in the way it scatters excitation to other cells; (4) there is a time decrement in excitation—i.e., the junctional potential change has a finite duration; and finally (5) the excitation is self-maintaining.

With this last assumption and no information about inhibitory interactions it can be shown that any equilibrium state would be unstable and that one would "soon find that the activity has died away in some places and flared up in others. It is for this reason that activity with some form of spatial and temporal organizations will always be favored . . ." (Beurle, 1956).

Detailed study of the electrical as well as the anatomical structure of some of the more regular appearing brain formations has in general supported the validity of these inferences:

It can be best envisaged by imagining that the cerebellar cortex is . . . continuously troubled by microwave production; each wave is a little ridge 3 mm long of Purkinje cell activation and has an inhibitory trough on either side. These waves do not propagate, but of course they competitively interfere, so greatly modifying the pattern of wave forms, and furthermore, even apart from such interference, a wave subsides in less than 100 msec. This competitive patterned operation must be a key feature of the action of the neuronal machinery . . . . [Eccles, Ito, and Szentagothai, 1967, p. 342]

Indeed, electrical recordings made from arrays of electrodes arranged so that their output can be displayed simultaneously over an area (a toposcope) demonstrate the occurrence of some sort of wave of activity (Walter and Shipton, 1951; Lilly, 1949; Livinov and Ananiev, 1955; Rémond, 1961). In what respect this form of wave corresponds to the nonpropagated standing wave inferred by Beurle remains to be investigated. The important consideration here is that, when appropriate, a wave-mechanical description of slow potential neural activity can be invoked—either as aid to picturing the nature of the slow potential microstructure or more formally as a model

LEVELS

$\bar{x}$ = 10

ρ = 30

M = 100

$\searrow$ = 300

$\triangle$ = 1000

$\triangledown$ = 3000

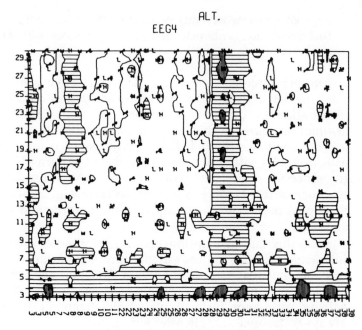

Fig. 1-16. Coherence plot of the EEG of Astronaut F. B. over a 70 minute period in an altitude chamber simulation of a Gemini flight. Forty records were made during this period; each was a recording of 20 seconds of the EEG. Note wave front characteristic of the plot and compare with Fig. 1-5. From Adey, 1967.

that adds precision to the interpretation of data. Thus the wave mechanical approach though not necessary to the description of the slow potential microstructure, promises to be useful on occasion (see Chapter 8 and Fig. 1-16).

In summary, most ordinary views of brain function are based on the generation and transmission of nerve impulses in neurons. Although sophisticated neurophysiologists have occasionally, albeit rarely, warned against oversimplification, these standard views curiously ignore junctional activities except as they pertain to further nerve impulse transmission. According to such views, the primary task of the synapse (or of the dendrite) is to transmit (or generate) impulses.

By contrast, George Bishop (1956), in a definitive review that discusses the "natural history of the nerve impulse," states that "the chief and most characteristic functions of neurons and other excitable tissues are performed by means of graded responses." He suggests that graded slow potentials are "more general as well as more primitive than the all-or-none response and that the latter probably developed when an early metazoan became too large . . . ." He reviews the evidence supporting the contention that the cerebral cortex "still operates largely by means of connections characteristic of primitive neuropil, the most appropriate mechanism for the maintenance of a continuous or steady state, as contrasted to the transmission of information about such states." The dendrites, rather than the "impulsive axon," are probably the essential elements of graded response tissue.

The approach taken in the present enterprise is in accord with Bishop. Junctional activities, because their effective mode is one in which continuous waxing and waning graded slow potential mechanisms predominate, provide the locus for a rich and neglected source for understanding the state part of the two process mechanism of brain function. This state is not some unformed overall condition of the brain. Quite the contrary—it is a microstructure composed of junctional slow potentials. There is therefore no longer the need to attempt to understand the neurophysiology of all psychological processes exclusively in terms of the operations of conducted nerve impulses. This added latitude given by a *two* process mechanism is most welcome.

synopsis

The unit of analysis for brain function has classically been the neuron. The present proposal for a two-process mechanism recognizes an additional unit: the neural junction, whose activity can become part of an organization (the slow potential microstructure) temporarily unrelated to the receptive field of any single neuron. Neural junctions are thus much more than just way stations in the transmission of nerve impulses.

neural modifiability
and
memory mechanisms

the search for the engram

One of the fundamental properties of states is that they can be modified. Modification of brain states accomplishes that most basic property of the nervous system, its time-binding function. This second chapter, therefore, takes a closer look at the tissue in which the slow potential microstructure develops in order to assess its modifiability.

Until the immediate past, evidence for the occurrence of neural modification by an organism's experience was not forthcoming despite considerable effort. As recently as 1950 Lashley concluded his famous paper on the search for the engram by stating: "I sometimes feel, in reviewing the evidence on the localization of the memory trace, that the necessary conclusion is that learning just is not possible at all. Nevertheless, in spite of such evidence against it, learning does sometimes occur"(Lashley, 1950, p. 501).

The picture has changed. An active field of investigation has opened several routes of inquiry into the problems of how the brain becomes modified by experience. The problems divide into three temporally distinct phases: the present chapter will deal with the development of permanent changes in the nervous system during learning; Chapter 3 describes a mechanism of intermediate duration which allows the tuning of neural circuits so that they can respond differentially to subsequent input; and Chapter 4 covers the temporary registrations which allow organizing operations to take place.

Why has the problem of the biology of memory, the search for evidence that experience produces permanent modification in neural tissue proved so difficult? Elsewhere in the body, when a structure changes in a healthy way over time we look to the growth and

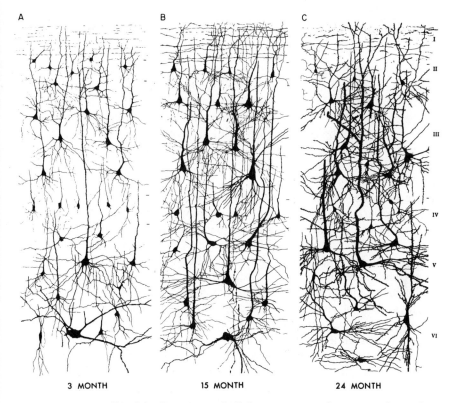

Fig. 2-1. Drawings of Golgi impregnated sections from the cerebral cortex of children 3, 15, and 24 months old. Note increased arborization and thickening of dendrites. Until recently attempts to correlate such growth with experience had failed. From the work of Conel. (A) 1947; (B) 1955; (C) 1959.

development of tissues. But in the brain the number of neurons fails to increase after an initial period subsequent to birth. Thus practically all behavioral development and learning must occur in the absence of obvious evidence of neural growth (Fig. 2-1).

The paradox has been met in three ways. The first denies the importance of the failure of neurons to reproduce and attempts to establish that some other form of *neural growth* does indeed occur as a function of experience. The second turns to a study of *neuroglia,* the nonneural elements of neural tissue that can increase in numbers over the lifetime of an individual. Finally, a powerful alternative has been the exploration of the possibility that the important modifications take place in terms of *chemical* storage processes.

neural growth

The possibilities for neural growth are not completely proscribed by the fact that neurons do not continue to replicate as do other cells in the body. Neurons are distinguished by their long fibers, branching extensions based on the cell body and these can be observed in tissue culture and even *in situ* to possess at their tips amoeboid structures called growth cones (Fig. 2-2). A growth cone pokes and shoves into the tissue in front of it and on occasion succeeds in opening a path into which the cone can then ooze, elongating the nerve fiber tip. Thus growth can occur provided there is space—when there is none, the amoeboid tip retracts only to push forward again and again. In the central nervous system growth is ordinarily precluded because tissue elements are extremely closely packed. In fact, considerable doubt has been cast, as a result of electron microscopy, that the extracellular spaces which are found everywhere else in the body, actually exist around neurons.

Brain scientists have therefore attempted to provide space in the brain and to observe nerve fiber growth after such injury. But until recently these efforts yielded little—the routine reaction of brain tissue to insult is to destroy the injured parts and to liquify them, leaving a hole or cyst whose capsule walls off any attempt at penetration. Now, however, modern technology has inadvertently provided a tool to circumvent this usual reaction. A cyclotron emits radiation that decelerates abruptly in soft tissue. At and only at the locus of deceleration destructive energy is emitted, thus circumscribed lesions can be made. With this instrument layers of adult rabbits' cortical cells have been killed without apparent damage to neighboring layers. With this method tissue damage is sufficiently local so that the usual reaction to grosser injury of neural tissue does

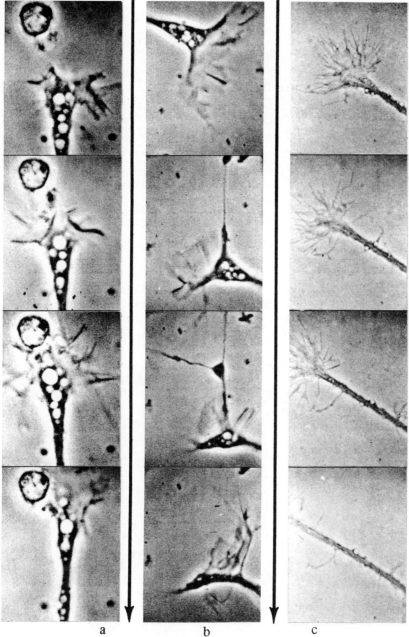

Fig. 2-2. Growth cones in action. Frames from a time-lapse photographic film. Note marked changes in form from frame to frame. From Pomerat, 1964.

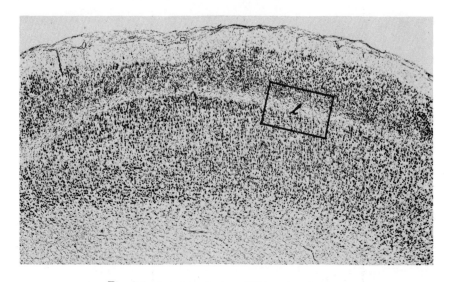

Fig. 2-3. Laminar lesion (*1*) in the fifth layer of the post-central region in rabbit cortex, 132 days after irradiation with a peak dose of 48,000 rads. Closer inspection reveals that numerous dendrites enter the laminar lesion. Thionin stain, 30X. From Rose et al., 1961.

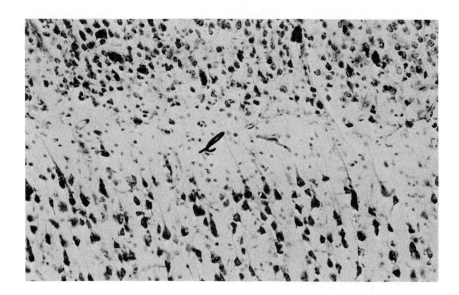

Fig. 2-4. The enclosed area in Fig. 2-3 shown under magnification of 200X. Notice the apical dendrites entering the laminar lesion. From Rose et al., 1961.

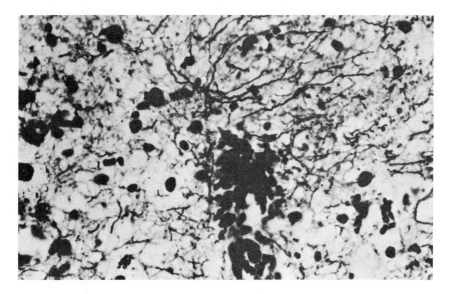

Fig. 2-5. Axonal sprouting in a laminar lesion in the rat striate cortex, 19 days after irradiation with 9000 rads alpha particles (surface dose). Bodian stain. X390. From Kruger, 1965.

not take place. Rather, space is made for active growth of nerve fibers (Figs. 2-3, 2-4, 2-5).

Sections made some weeks and months after injury show that fibers not destroyed become thicker (Kruger, 1965). This thickening appears to be a fairly normal increase in fiber size. Since fiber diameter is often an indicator of the length of the fiber, the thickening indirectly suggests that growth may have taken place. More direct evidence of growth is seen in the presence of large numbers of normal appearing, well-directed fibers which were invisible either before or immediately after the exposure to the cyclotron (Rose, Malis and Baker, 1961). Thus fiber growth *is* possible in the mature brain if the circumstances for growth are favorable.

These experiments cannot, of course, indicate whether growth actually occurs as a result of experience; another type of study has to be performed. Conditions of rearing rats were manipulated so that some of the animals received much stimulation (play, problem-solving experience) while others were relatively restricted. This restriction was sometimes limited to one or another sensory mode (e.g., rats reared in total darkness) to test whether the effect could be differential upon some areas of the brain. Comparison of the brains of animals reared under the different conditions showed that stimula-

	Percentage diff. EC > IC	P	Number EC > IC
Weight	6.4	<0.001	133/175
Total protein	7.8[a]	<0.001	25/32
Thickness	6.3	<0.001	45/52
Total AChE	2.2	<0.01	102/171
Total ChE	10.2	<0.001	118.5/132
Total hexokinase	6.9[b]	<0.01	17/21
DNA/mg	−6.1	<0.001	4/23
RNA/mg	−0.7	NS	10/23
RNA/DNA	5.9	<0.01	19/23
Number of Neurons	−3.1	NS	7/17
Number of Glia	14.0	<0.01	12/17
Perikaryon cross section	13.4	<0.001	11.5/13

[a]Weight difference 7.0% in these experiments.
[b]Weight difference 5.5% in these experiments.
(From: E.L. Bennett and M.R. Rosenzweig, Chemical alterations produced in brain by environment and training. In A. Lajtha (ed.), *Handbook of Neurochemistry.* New York: Plenum Press, 1970, p. 183.

Fig. 2-6. Effects of differential experience on occipital cortex of S_1 rats kept in enriched [EC] or impoverished [IC] conditions from 25 to 105 days of age. AChE, acetylcholine esterase; ChE, choline esterase; P, statistical probability level of significance. From Bennett and Rosenzweig, in A. Lajtha (ed.) *Handbook of Neurochemistry,* 1970, Plenum.

tion results in a measurable thickening of the cortex (of appropriate parts) in subjects given the richer experience (Bennett, Diamond, (Krech, and Rosenzweig, 1964).

Detailed histological analysis of the thickened cortex showed—as would be expected because neurons do not multiply after birth—that the number of nerve cells per unit volume actually decreased slightly. An increase in the number of branchings of basal dendrites, neurons that extend their fibers horizontally in the cortex, has, however, been reported as has an increase in the number and distention of dendritic spines, small hairlike protrusions on dendrites which are presumed active junctional sites. But a large part of the thickening resulted from an increase in *non*-neural cells—the glia (Figs. 2-6, 2-7. 2-8).

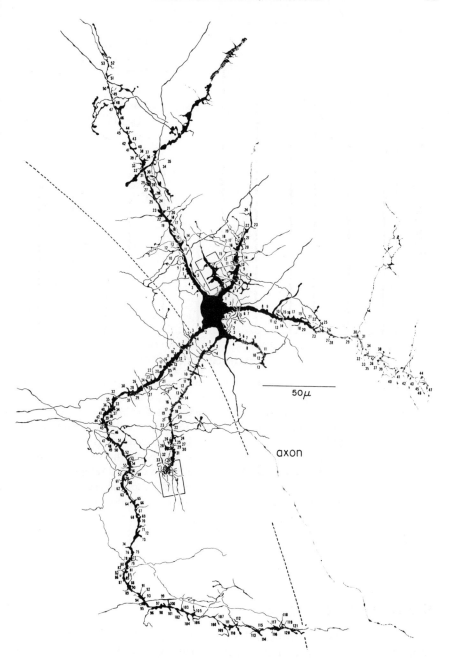

Fig. 2-7. Highly developed dendritic system of a neuron showing 121 spines each of which can act as a contact point with other dendrites. From Calvin after Valverde, 1967.

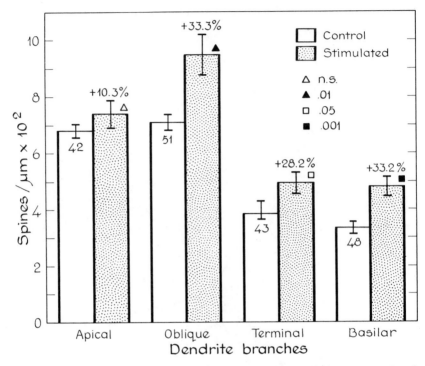

Fig. 2-8. Effects of environmental stimulation upon spine development of four different dendritic branches of the cortical pyramidal cells. Animals were treated in enriched (stimulated) or in impoverished (control) environments. The numbers in the bar graph are the numbers of neurons from which the indicated values for dendritic spines on the various branches were determined. Animals are 8 days old. All values shown for dendrite branches include standard errors and are derived from five control and five stimulated animals. Redrawn after Schapiro and Vukovich, 1970.

the role of neuroglia

The non-neural cells called neuroglia (or just glia) present in neural tissue have become the second focus for inquiry into the problems of memory storage. Glial cells originate from the same embryonic tissue as do nerve cells and glial function was for a long time thought of exclusively as nutrient support given to neurons. This nutritive function has been amply documented (e.g., Hydén, 1965). Glia are ideally situated to carry out this role—some of them (astrocytes) surround blood vessels and so can exchange metabolites with the circulation. Others, the oligodendroglia (which have a paucity of branches), are closely wrapped around nerve fibers especially at their tips, thus precluding the existence of extracellular space around neurons in these locations. In addition to exchanging metabolites with nerves, the oligodendroglia help manufacture the insulating material (myelin) which sheaths larger nerve fibers (Fig. 2-9).

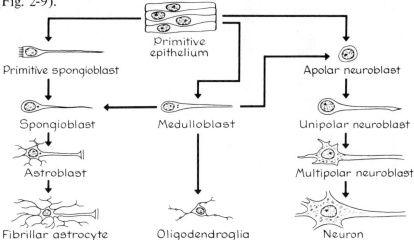

Fig. 2-9. Development of neurons and of neurologia. Redrawn from Bailey, 1933.

Another important function of oligodendroglia may be that they direct the growth cones of neurons. In the peripheral nervous system, a close relative of glia called Schwann cells, are known to guide the direction of growth of nerve fibers that regenerate after injury. The sequence of events is as follows: a cut or injured nerve fiber dies off, degenerates back to the cell body from which it originated. This cell body may be located in the spinal cord as far as several feet distant from the injury. Immediately, a special type of reparative cell present in the sheath of the nerve begins to multiply and take up the space left by the dying fiber. These make a column of tissue during the phase of degeneration. When regeneration begins at the cell body a pathway is ready for the growing tip of the nerve fiber to follow. When such a column is not present to guide growth, the nerve's growth cone pushes off into every which direction and forms a tangle which is, of course, nonfunctional and often painfully sensitive.

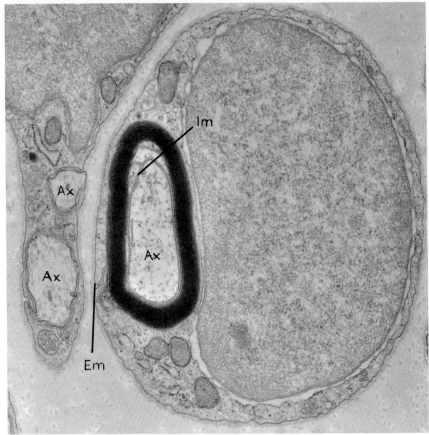

Fig. 2-10. Electron microscope photograph of cross section of peripheral nerve axon (Ax) showing Schwann cell wrapping (Em and Im). From Truex and Carpenter, *Human Neuroanatomy*, 6 ed.©1969 The Williams & Wilkins Co., Baltimore, Md.

These special reparative cells, the Schwann cells, are derived embryologically from the same source as is neural and glial tissue. Further, these Schwann cells are wrapped around nerve fibers (Fig. 2-10). And they aid in the formation of myelin sheaths much as do oligodendroglia in the central nervous system. Such considerations have led most investigators to classify oligodendroglia and Schwann cells together. The real possibility exists therefore that oligodendroglia perform as guides for neural growth in the central, much as Schwann cells do in the peripheral, nervous system.

The fact that glia are wrapped around the tips of nerve fibers poses an interesting problem. Except where nerve-to-nerve contacts are made by way of special structures called synapses the electrical potential changes produced in and by neurons occur in a medium of glial cells. How much influence do these cells exert, especially on the configurations that junctional potentials take?

Although questions such as these have not yet been answered, they have given rise to the speculation that glia, once they are modified, might permanently alter the activity of the neural aggregates with which the glia are so intimately bedded.

chemical modification

A series of experiments implicates glia directly in the memory mechanism. One of the substances involved in glia-neuron interactions turned out to be ribonucleic acid (RNA, a chemical that establishes the configuration of proteins) which itself is produced by desoxyribonucleic acid (DNA), the genetic memory molecule. In fact, these investigations showed that, when stimulated, neurons produce more RNA than any other tissue in the body (Hydén, 1961). And after stimulation stops and RNA production diminishes in the neuron, large concentrations of molecularly similar RNA begin to appear in the adjacent glia (Hydén, 1969).

Specifically, these experiments on the brains of rabbits and rats were accomplished by teasing apart under the microscope glia from neurons in the vestibular nucleus—an aggregate of neurons that

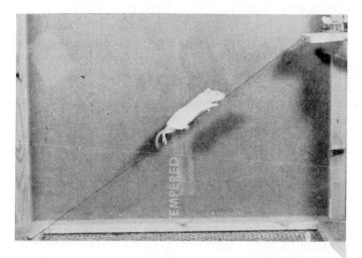

Fig. 2-11. Experimental situation showing rat climbing wire to reach food. From Hyden, 1965.

controls the postural balance of an animal. Stimulation of this "balancing" mechanism initially involved placing the subject in a centrifuge and whirling it about. In later experiments rats were required to climb an inclined wire; if successful they reached a platform supplied with food. Failure meant falling to a mildly electrified grid at the bottom of the cage. At various stages of the experiment the animals' vestibular neurons and glia were analyzed by microchemical methods for RNA concentration. During passive cen-trifugation the total amount of RNA in neurons was increased; for some hours after rotation the RNA was found to be augmented. Active wire-climbing not only increased the total amount of RNA, but also changed the relative amount of fractions of RNA which can be identified because of differences in the side chains which label the molecule (Fig. 2-11).

There appears to be no question that RNA production is somehow involved when nerves are stimulated physiologically or when the organism performs a task. However, the story is not simple. Within 24 to 48 hours after cessation of stimulation the effects on RNA concentration and type are no longer discernable—even in glia. The suggestion has been made, therefore, that RNA functions only as an intermediary between DNA and proteins which form the basis of a more permanent record. RNA determinations are nonetheless useful in indicating that the memory process has become active.

This view of RNA function proposes that storage takes place in other macromolecules such as polypeptides, proteins, lipoproteins and mucoids (see Bogoch, 1968; Glassman, 1967). All of these molecules are complex and must be synthesized by many metabolic steps. Experiments are therefore possible in which antimetabolites can be directed at one or another stage in synthesis. The antimetabo-lite can be injected before, during, or after the training of rats. Using this technique it was found, for instance, that an antimetabolite that interferes with protein synthesis can disrupt remembering if the injection is made within five or six hours after the rat experiences the task. This suggested that protein synthesis was blocked. However, it was later shown that if retention is tested some weeks after the injection, memory for the task shows little impairment. The anti-metabolite injection apparently interfered with retrieval rather than with the construction of a memory molecule (Agranoff, Davis, and Brink, 1965).

The possible role of proteins and other macromolecules (especially brain lipids) in memory ought not, however, to be restricted to the hypothesis tested by the antimetabolite experiments. Because of their complexity macromolecules have unique configurations, con-

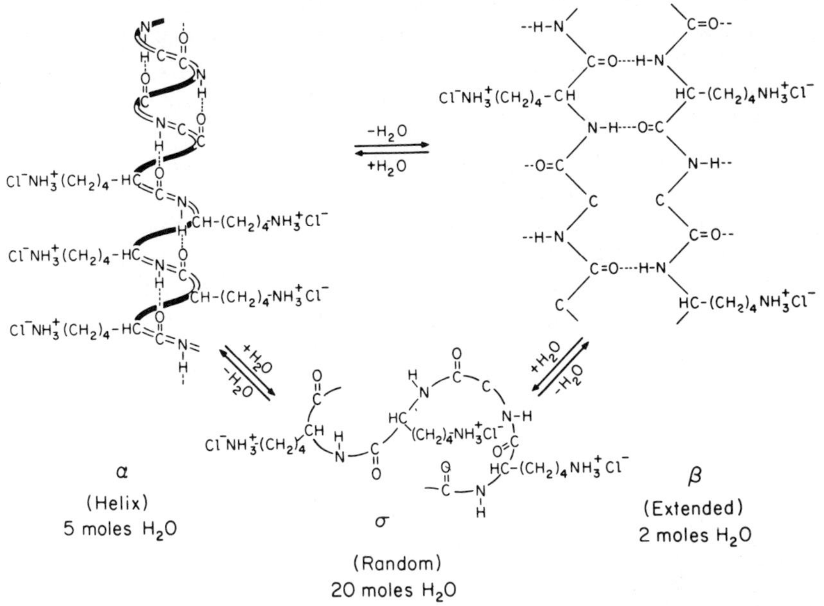

Fig. 2-12. Diagram of different conformations that can be taken by an amino acid (the polymer poly-L-lysine hydrochloride). From Blout, 1967.

formations that can be temporarily altered to produce a different state (Fig. 2-12). Conformational changes may well account for the temporary memory involved in imagery such as that found to an enhanced degree in persons with a "photographic" (technically known as "eidetic") memory. One such eidetically endowed student at Harvard has recently been shown by experimental test to retain every detail of a visual experience for as long as eight days. Part II will delve more into this topic of temporary twisting of molecules. As of now, investigations of conformational changes in brain tissue are barely possible—techniques are developing at such a pace, however that this field of inquiry promises much in the immediate future (Sjostrand, 1969).

Despite the considerable evidence against it, some continue to hold the hypothesis that RNA serves directly as the memory storage device. They base their view on a highly controversial series of "transfer" experiments made with flatworms, rats, and monkeys in which RNA is extracted from animals who have learned a task and from controls. These extracts are injected into naive subjects. Those injected with the "experienced" RNA sometimes, although by no means always, show superiority in the task over those injected with "control" RNA. Further, this differential effect has been reported to be countered by treating the extract with a substance which selectively destroys RNA (see review by McConnell, 1970).

A final alternative proposed by investigators holding the chemical storage hypothesis focuses on neural transmitters. Nerve impulses decrement in speed and amplitude as they reach the terminals of axons because of the marked decrease in terminal fiber size diameter. Presynaptic potentials are, therefore, for the most part insufficient in themselves to induce a postsynaptic potential. The presynaptic electrical charge is, however, sufficient to trigger the release of a chemical transmitter which is stored at the axonal ending in small vesicles

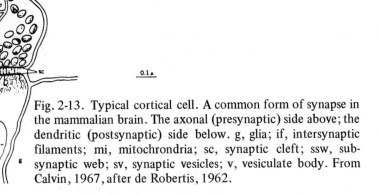

Fig. 2-13. Typical cortical cell. A common form of synapse in the mammalian brain. The axonal (presynaptic) side above; the dendritic (postsynaptic) side below. g, glia; if, intersynaptic filaments; mi, mitochrondria; sc, synaptic cleft; ssw, subsynaptic web; sv, synaptic vesicles; v, vesiculate body. From Calvin, 1967, after de Robertis, 1962.

(Fig. 2-13). Memory could be based on the ease with which the transmitter is released or with the amount released. Experiments are thus possible, and are being executed, in which the transmitter is either neutralized by pharmacological agents or its destruction (which ordinarily takes place so that the nervous system does not become one large pool of transmitter substance) blocked while an animal is being trained (Deutsch, Hamburg and Dahl, 1966). Results of such manipulations do show altered learning rates, but just as in the case of the antimetabolite studies, the question arises whether the administration of drugs causes side effects that alter brain function and consequently remembering—side effects, such as the production of local electrical seizures in parts of the brain, that are not directly related to memory storage per se but which interfere with retrieval at the time of testing.

induction—a model for memory storage

My response to the wealth of experimental results obtained in the search for the engram during the 1960s is twofold. First, there need not be only a single memory mechanism, a single memory molecule. Neural modifiability is multifaceted, and memory is not a unitary process. Imaging, recognition, recall partake in

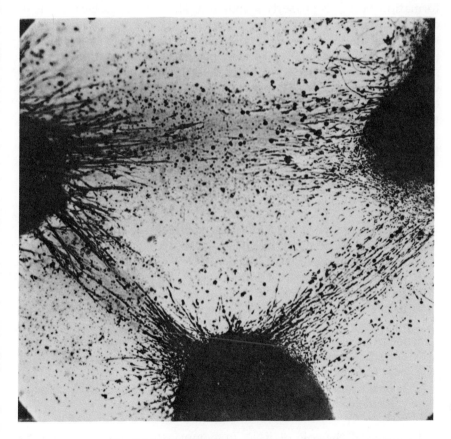

Fig. 2-14. A triangular connection formed among three embryonic spinal ganglia in vitro. This illustrates the tendency of neural tissue to form patterned pathways. From Weiss, 1967.

different ways of some or all of the basic modes of modifiability of neural tissue. Thus, the first conclusion to be reached is that memory in the brain is how you find it—no single mechanism serves all of the processes that allow an organism to bind experience.

Second, a simple model of the steps that involve *permanent* modification of brain tissue at the neural level can be formulated even now. Such a model must assure not only that storage can occur but that access to the stored change is readily retrievable. Further, the model must be based on already available data and make good biological common sense. At present the most likely source of such a model lies in an analogy with a process that occurs during the embryological development of the organism (See Fig. 2-14). Structures such as the eye will form only when the tissue out of which the formation occurs is properly stimulated. Most embryological tissue is equipotential—i.e., the DNA in all cells of the body is essentially the same. This implies that the potential to develop is ordinarily repressed. "Derepression," or release, occurs when the proper circumstances develop. Delineating what these circumstances are has kept embryologists busy for almost a century (see Hamburger in *Encyclopedia Britannica,* 1961). At present RNA and some endocrine secretions are the best known inductors of derepression. That these chemicals carry all the information necessary for induction is unlikely; a great deal of the specificity of the process must reside in the substrate. For instance, RNA extracted from a *calf's* liver can be used to induce the lens of a *rat's* eye. The relationship between inductor and substrate appears to be:

1. Inductors evoke and organize the genetic potential of the organism.
2. Inductors are relatively specific as to the character they evoke but are relatively nonspecific relative to individuals and tissues.
3. Inductors determine the broad outlines of the induced character; details are specified by the action of the substrate.
4. Inductors do not just trigger development; they are a special class of stimuli.
5. Inductors must be in contact with their substrate in order to be effective; however, mere contact is insufficient to produce the effect—the tissue must be ready, must be competent to react.
6. Induction usually proceeds by a two way interaction, by a chemical conversation between inductor and substrate.

Evidence of the rôle of RNA in memory storage can at present be suggestively explained by recourse to a model based on this embryogenetic process of induction. The model states that excitation of nerves is accompanied by RNA production. This neural RNA induces changes in the surrounding oligodendroglial cell commencing a chemical conversation indicated by the reciprocal nature of the variations in concentration of RNA (and a host of metabolites) between neuron and glia. A change is induced in the functional interaction of the glial-neural couplet. This change may in the first instance induce comparable RNA in the glial cell which then over a longer period of time produces alterations in the conformations of lipids, proteins, and lipoproteins, all large molecules which make up the membranes interfacing neuron with glia. Such macromolecular changes can alter the ease with which chemical neurotransmitters are released or destroyed. These configurational changes are reversible and can fade or be superseded. When maintained by repetition of the same pattern, however, the alterations in molecular conformation will endure long enough to produce an effective change in membrane permeability which, in turn, allows more RNA, metabolites, and neurotransmitters originating in the excited neuron to affect its glial surround to the point where glial cell division is actually induced. Once divested of its encapsulating glia, the growth cone of the neuron is free to plunge between the newly formed glial daughter cells and to make new contacts with the neurons beyond. Thus the induced cell division of oligodendroglia is assumed to guide the growth cones of central nervous system neurons much as those in the periphery are guided by the related Schwann cells (Fig. 2-15).

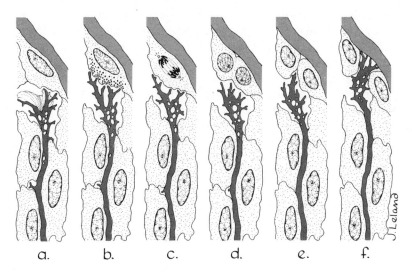

a. b. c. d. e. f.

Fig. 2-15. Six steps in the hypothesized induction process.

consolidation

Any change in glial-neural organization will be registered as a change in the microstructure of junctional slow potential activity. As noted, such changes can be temporary, or they may lead to more permanent organizations through neural growth. Much evidence is available to show that memory traces—engrams—require time to fix in the brain. This evidence is compatible with the induction model of memory storage because it shows that at least two and perhaps more processes can be distinguished on the basis of the time course of their occurrence.

Following a moderately severe head injury a person is unable to recall events that occurred during the period immediately prior to the injury. The duration of this period varies with the severity of the injury. This phenomenon is called retrograde amnesia and provides a lever for study of memory fixation, i.e., consolidation.

The most common method for producing retrograde amnesia in the laboratory is to administer electroconvulsive shock to rats, although other methods such as blows to the head, rapid anesthesia with ether, and the administration of certain amnesia-producing drugs have also been used. The evidence suggests that the sooner after an experience the convulsion occurs, the greater is the interference with later performance relative to that experience. For instance, in one investigation (Chorover and Schiller, 1965) a maximum effect was produced when convulsions followed within 15 seconds of an avoidance trial; the effect is practically gone when an hour intervenes between conditioning trial and convulsion. The effect depends to a large extent on the complexity of the experience that is to be remembered.

This is still not the whole story, however. A more complex two stage process of consolidation occurs under the appropriate conditions. A subject is taught to press a lever for a food-reward presented at slightly varying intervals. A signal is turned on at some point during the performance and is invariably followed after a given time by a foot-shock. As a rule, the subject's response radically diminishes or ceases entirely while the signal is on. The assumption is that an emotional state has been induced. A normal rate of response resumes once the shock has been experienced and the signal is off. When convulsions are administered 48 hours after the last trial and testing is resumed four days after the completion of the convulsive series, all convulsed subjects fail entirely to react "emotionally" to the signal. If, on the other hand, retests are delayed until 30, 60, or 90 days after completion of the convulsive series, the conditioned emotional response is again obtained in full force. These experimenters (Brady, 1951), exceeded the crucial hour during which the consolidation process can be maximally affected—however, their results can be interpreted as indicating that some mechanism necessary to the retrieval of the memory trace upon which the emotional reaction is based is still fragile for as long as a day or two after an experience.

The results of these experiments on memory consolidation can be interpreted according to the induction model in the following way: immediately after a trial, convulsive shock, anesthesia, etc., interfere with the metabolic exchange taking place between neuron and oligo-dendroglia, inhibiting induction by way of the RNA secretion in nerve and its reciprocal activation in glia. Engram formation is therefore eliminated and remembering precluded. When, on the other hand, the convulsion is produced later on, the RNA phase of the induction process has been completed. Now glial cell division is temporarily arrested, the ameboid explorations of the neuron's tip are temporarily halted, and the growth cone retracted. When these mechanisms recover, however, the process of establishing the engram continues where it left off and remembering can be demonstrated when the process is completed.

To firmly establish that consolidation really occurs, one ought to be able to find techniques to *improve* learning. This can, in fact, be done. When experimental subjects are injected with strychnine sulphate or similar excitatory drugs in a period from 10 minutes prior to or 30 seconds after receiving maze or discrimination trials, the strychnine-injected rats learn significantly more rapidly than do their controls: consolidation takes place faster. (McGaugh and Petrinovich, 1959).

These experiments form an impressive body of evidence that consolidation must occur in laying down a memory trace. The brain must be involved in consolidation—but just what is achieved during the process that makes remembering possible? An answer to this question may lie in the following observations.

In my laboratory different areas of the brain cortex of monkeys have been treated with aluminum hydroxide cream to produce local irritations which, when extreme, produce epilepsy. These irritations are manifested by altered electrical activity—abnormal slow waves and spike discharges. Such irritative lesions, while they do not interfere with a monkey's capacity to remember the solution to problems repeatedly solved prior to the irritation, do slow their original learning of these problems some fivefold (Pribram, 1966). Moreover, problem-solving in general is not affected; the defect is specific for those solutions to tasks which cannot be remembered when that particular part of the brain has been removed. Further-more, the impairment is restricted to the early part of the learning process, the part before there is actual demonstration that learning is occurring. Thus the irritative lesions do not permanently block the manifestation of consolidation. Could it be that a single engram restricted to one neural locus is insufficient to be manifest? A good deal of evidence from human learning experiments indicates that considerable rehearsal must take place for an experience to be remembered (Trabasso and Bower, 1968). What appears to occur during rehearsal is a distribution of the rehearsed material so that it becomes linked to a larger assortment of previously stored experi-ence. The results of the irritative lesion experiments can thus be interpreted as showing that the process of reduplication and distribu-tion of the engram has been retarded. A test of this interpretation would come from a comparison of learning by irritative-lesioned monkeys under spaced and massed trial conditions.

Histological analysis of the brain tissue treated with aluminum hydroxide shows tangles of nerve fibers much as those described in peripheral nerves when growth is not properly guided by an adequate Schwann cell column. Could it be that oligodendroglia are selectively killed off by the treatment, allowing the disordered growth to occur? Chemical analysis of the tissue implanted with aluminum hydroxide cream is of course impractical. But an ingenious experiment designed to answer this question has been achieved (Morrell, 1961b, Fig. 2-16). An irritative lesion made in one cerebral hemisphere produces, after some months, a "mirror focus" of altered electrical activity in the

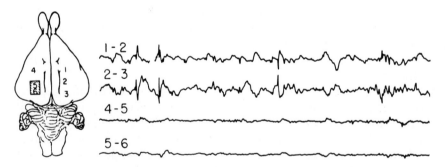

Fig. 2-16. Independent discharge in a secondary epileptogenic focus. The secondary focus (upper two channels) continues to fire despite cessation of discharge in the primary lesion (lower two channels). Calibration: 100 μV and 1 sec. From Morrell, 1961.

contralateral cortex by way of the interhemispheric connections through the corpus callosum. This "mirror focus" has not been directly damaged chemically, yet it possesses all of the irritative properties of the initial lesion. The RNA in this mirror focus is considerably altered when compared to that found in normal brain tissue. Could the altered RNA be responsible for the irritation and the consequent interference with reduplication of the memory trace?

Memory induction, just as embryological induction, appears to be a multistage process which takes time to run off. Each stage in such a process would be expected to show its own vulnerabilities that can be demonstrated by appropriate techniques applied at the critical moment. Much has been learned about the occurrence of "critical periods" in the development of embryos and of behavior in the early years after birth. A rich field of exploration and experimentation lies ahead in determining the nature of critical, i.e., sensitive periods in the development of the memory store.

Much more can and will be said about consolidation and the induction model, but first we need a more complete picture of the workings of the brain and the structure of the psychological process. Let us consider in the next chapter therefore some of the more reversible ways in which the brain can be modified by experience.

synopsis

It is in the junctional mechanism that long lasting modifications of brain tissues must take place. Although adult nerve *cells* do not divide, a mechanism of permanent modification of brain tissue does display many of the properties of the mechanism of differentiation of embryonic tissue. Experientially initiated guided growth of new nerve *fibers* does take place and alters the spatial pattern of junctional relationships among neurons. Long term memory therefore becomes more a function of junctional structure than of strictly neural (nerve impulse generating) processes.

the decrementing of neural activity and inhibitory interactions

the orienting reaction and its habituation

The first chapter examined the two basic classes of variables exhibited by the brain in the course of its functioning. As a model, the production of spoken language pointed out the power that can be achieved simply by modifying these two variables. The second chapter detailed evidence for modifiability, even permanent modifiability, but did not discuss the characteristics of the instrument that allows modifications to become actualized. The basic variables manipulated in playing a violin, flute, or organ are the same as those used in speaking, yet the instruments differ as do their products.

This chapter begins, therefore, the examination of organizations of the nervous system that allow it to be the instrument from which derives the richness of experience and of behavior. A good deal of this organization depends on semipermanent constructions that develop in the input and output systems by which the brain is in touch with its environment. Because of their accessibility. these

48

systems can, in addition, serve as models-in-miniature—and therefore guides to investigation—of more central processes whose complete specification is sometimes more difficult to attain. Since so much organization takes place during an initial contact between the organism and his environment, this is a good place to start inquiry.

Experimental evidence shows that, at any moment, current sensory excitation is screened by some representative record of prior experience; this comparison—the match or mismatch between current excitation and representative record—guides attention and action:

Eugene Sokolov (1960) performed the following simple demonstration that uncovered one of those discrepancies which form the fruitful paradoxes that guide experimentation in the neurobehavioral sciences. A person is exposed to the beep of a horn; he ordinarily orients toward it. The electrical activity of his brain displays a characteristic pattern—activation of the record obtained from the lateral surface of the cerebral hemispheres (as shown by an increase in the low amplitude high frequency components of the EEG) and hypersynchrony of the record obtained from medial and basal brain structures (and indicated by an increase in observable rhythmicity giving high amplitude to waves in the middle frequency range). Additional physiological characteristics of orientation occur: the flow of blood to the head increases at the expense of flow to the fingertips; changes take place in the electrical resistance of the skin and in heart and respiratory rate. But should the horn beep be frequently repeated, all these reactions markedly diminish. The subject is said to be habituated to the stimulus.

The resulting absence of reaction to the continuing beep turns out to be deceptive, however. Actually a great deal is still taking place. For if the stimulus changes slightly (the beep becomes softer) all the initial alerting reactions recur. This, of course, is the paradox. Until Sokolov's demonstration the assumption was always made that habituation simply raises the threshold of the nervous system to input. Sokolov's findings mean that the person who has habituated must be matching the current sound against a stored representation of prior tone beeps—why else would a diminution in intensity call forth again the full-blown orienting response? He tested his interpretation by habituating the person to a tone of a certain length. Then, suddenly he presented a shortened tone. Now orienting reactions occurred when the tone ceased, i.e., alerting responses were recorded at the onset of silence. The reactions continued for the "expected" length of the tone, then slowly disappeared. We have all experienced this surprising reaction to sudden silence (Fig. 3-1).

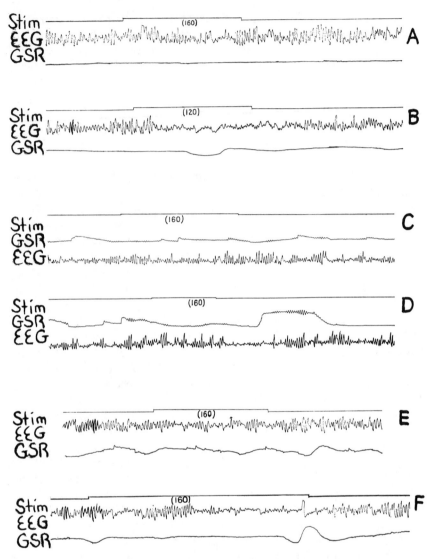

Fig. 3-1. (A) Habituated response (EEG and GSR) to stimulus intensity arbitrarily indicated as 160. (B) Dishabituation (orienting) when stimulus intensity is lowered to 120. (C) Same as A. (D) Orienting to the shortening of the stimulus duration. (E) Same as A. (F) Orienting to the unexpected lengthening of the stimulus duration. Note that GSR is also delayed. This is due to the sluggishness of the autonomic nervous system. From Sokolov, 1960.

I like to call this the "Bowery-el phenomenon." For many years there was an elevated railway line (the "el") on Third Avenue in New York that made a fearful racket; when it was torn down, people who had been living in apartments along the line awakened periodically out of a sound sleep to call the police about some strange occurrence they could not properly define. The calls were made at the times the trains had formerly rumbled past. The strange occurrences were, of course, the deafening silence that had replaced the expected noise.

A large body of evidence suggests that orienting reactions and their habituation are moderately long lasting and exquisitely specific. Each part of the brain shows a different electrical sign and a different time course of electrical events during orienting. Once habituation has taken place, dishabituation (the orienting reaction) recurs during a period as long as six months thereafter whenever any change in the situation takes place; a change in the sequence of occurrence, of the context in which the events happen, or of the intensity, duration, or configuration of the events themselves will result in dishabituation.

The neurophysiology of habituation has been studied extensively and has generated a good deal of controversy because of the various experimental approaches taken to the problem. Several factors must be untangled in order to enable interpretation. Most neurophysiologists have called habituation any progressive decrementing of response over the repeated presentation of the same stimulating event. Psychologists, on the other hand, have limited their definition to occasions when the decrement takes place within a few trials and when dishabituation can be clearly demonstrated. More recently some brain scientists, including myself, have emphasized Sokolov's even more stringent criterion: dishabituation must occur in the face of sudden diminution, shortening, or absence of the stimulus.

The locus from which the electrophysiological record is taken is also important. In my laboratory, for instance, we found that in way stations of the monkey's visual system between retina and cerebral cortex, habituation is indeed characterized by a decrementing response. In the cortex, however, some electrode placements show a decrement, others show an increment, and still others show no change at all. At the cortex, therefore, a patterned change is set up as a function of stimulus repetition; dishabituation effects a disruption of this pattern (Grandstaff and Pribram, in preparation). Had we lumped together the records from all the cortical sites or made our recordings from the scalp rather than through electrodes implanted directly into the cortex, we would have failed to find any effect, as indeed some investigators have reported.

At the cellular level a considerable amount of work has also been accomplished. Unit recordings have been made from the spinal cord and various brain sites. Nerve cells in many locations have been found to decrement their responses to the repetition of stimulation. This reaction occurs even in invertebrates such as the sea slug (Pinsker et al., 1970; Kupfermann, et al., 1970; Castellucci, et al., 1970). Once habituated, however, will most neurons dishabituate? Recent evidence gathered by Richard Thompson (Grove and Thompson, 1970) indicates that at least three populations of neurons can be distinguished—those that simply decrement, those that initially increment, and those that first increment and then decrement. Only the last of these populations are subject to dishabituation. Such experiments have thus far been performed only on the spinal cord; other reports of experiments on brain stem structures (superior colliculus) suggest that perhaps, though not certainly, decrementing single neurons can in these locations become dishabituated (Gerbrandt, Bures, and Buresova, 1970).

What has become clear from these data and from other work of Thompson's (Thompson and Spencer, 1966) is that habituation is dependent on the interactions among several neurons. Thompson used the sort of preparation which Sherrington made famous: an animal whose spinal cord is severed from its brain. Repetitive stimulation with electrical pulses administered to the cord's input fibers resulted in a progressive decrement of the strength of reflex flexion

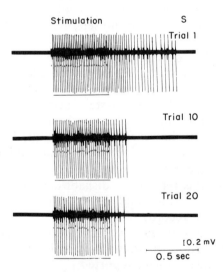

Fig. 3-2. Decrementing of response of efferent unit to repeated electrical stimulation of skin. From Thompson, 1967.

of the limb (produced much as is the knee-jerk of a patient undergoing a physical examination). This preparation proved ideal for exploring the spinal cord for the locus and physiological nature of the change involved in habituation (Fig. 3-2). Neither the input nor the output neurons involved in the reflex change are responsible for habituation—interneurons that connect input and output neurons are critical. Second, contrary to expectation, pharmacological manipulations ordinarily used by neurophysiologists to study pre and postsynaptic effects failed to have any effect: the response decrement indicative of habituation was not wiped out by the drugs. This suggests that habituation is not a function of changes occurring in junctional slow potentials. Similar evidence has been obtained by Sokolov (Sokolov, Pakula and Arakelov, 1970), using a different preparation (an invertebrate mollusc neuron). He finds that the slow potentials imposed on the membrane of the neuron body and the generator potentials recorded from its axon which give rise to nerve impulses can be manipulated *independently* of each other. In addition, his evidence shows that the generator mechanism responsible for nerve impulses becomes habituated.

Thus, in some instances the decremental processes involved in habituation appear to depend on mechanisms other than simple pre or postsynaptic changes. In other instances, however, contrary evidence is obtained. Depletion or augmentation of the supply of transmitter substance is sometimes, but not always, involved. Seth Sharpless (1967; 1969) has shown that in vertebrates neither sensitization nor desensitization of synaptic membranes occurs with use. On the other hand, Eric Kandel (Castelluci, et al., 1970; Kupfermann, et al., 1970; Pinsker, et al., 1970) has shown that in invertebrates the locus of habituation and dishabituation is presynaptic and involves the efficacy of the secretion of excitatory substances at synapses.

So the evidence is not yet coherent. A number of questions need answers. How can the generator mechanism be influenced at all if not by way of slow potentials? Is some biochemical buildup within the nerve cell body triggered and, if so, how (in a system that is ordinarily spontaneously active and therefore generating potentials anyway)? What is the nature of the biochemical change and what is its time course? Sokolov suspects the RNA mechanism. If he is correct, are the first steps of the induction process engaged during habituation or is the habituation mechanism completely independent of the process of permanent storage? Perhaps only under the conditions of prolonged and repeated habituation is the permanent storage mechanism engaged. If so, how? Finally, how does the change in nerve impulse configuration produced by habituation operate on the slow potential microstructure at the next synaptic level? For some possible initial answers to these questions let us explore the neural organization of the retina, a small "piece of brain" much more accessible to study than the central nervous system itself.

adaptation

What we sense of our environment is limited by the potentialities of receptor surfaces to engage one or another configuration of energy change. Thus the optics of the eye focus electromagnetic energy of a restricted band of wave lengths on the retina; wave form compressions of fluid are distributed across the cochlea of the ear; patterns of deformation of the skin excite free or specialized nerve endings in the somatic system and so forth. These configurations of energy changes interact with the ongoing activity of the receptors to produce modulations which are sufficiently reliable so that the organism can identify the energy changes.

Take again the simple model of speech production described in Chapter 1. Two basic variables are involved: steady state and discrete. The model was applied to brain function; now transpose it to the sensory mechanism. Replace the steady-state tensions of the vocal cord with steady-state distributions of energy configurations organized within extended receptor surfaces; for discrete plosions of air puffs, substitute discrete neural discharges in the form of nerve impulses. In short, assume that what goes on in the sense organ is not altogether different from what happens elsewhere in the nervous system, that sensory neurophysiology can provide a detailed model-in-miniature of the process of orienting and its habituation.

We are all familiar with the process of adaptation: the sensation of stepping into an almost too hot bath only to find a few minutes later that we must add warm water to be comfortable; the fading of the sensation of a pressure point applied to the skin; the walking into a pitch black movie theater and having to wait a few moments to be able to see an empty seat. These are all instances of sensory adaptation. The most striking example of adaptation is again paradoxical and is obtained in an experiment in which the image projected on the retina is stabilized by means of mirrors and lenses (Ditchburn and Ginsborg, 1952; Riggs, Ratliff, Cornsweet and Cornsweet, 1953). Surprisingly, our eyes are ordinarily in constant movement—even when we fix on a point, small tremorlike oscillations of the eyes can be recorded. These and other movements are in some people large enough to be conspicuous to others, but—and here is the paradox—the person with the exaggerated movements is unaware of them until

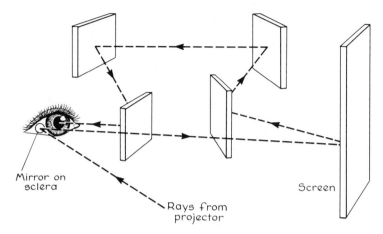

Fig. 3-3.   By first reflecting the stimulus image off a mirror mounted on the eye, the movements of the eye may be compensated for precisely, so that the image is stationary on the retina. Redrawn after Riggs, et al., 1953.

they are pointed out to him while he looks into a mirror (which usually sends him to his doctor who, if he knows of the abnormality, reassures his patient that there are no harmful concomitants). The eye movements prevent any single receptor element from being stimulated by the same pattern of bright and dark for any length of time—except, of course, in situations such as a dense fog, where light is not patterned at all and vision becomes limited to an appreciation of brightness. In order to study the effect of circumventing these eye movements, a mirror is pasted on the sclera, the white part of the eyeball which is insensitive. A pattern is projected to the mirror, reflected back through a compensating prism onto a flat surface which is viewed by the observer. The compensating prism corrects the excursions of the viewed display to correspond directly to the excursions made by the eyeball. In this way the image of the display falls always on the identical retinal locus—the image has been stabilized (Fig. 3-3).

A stabilized image quickly becomes an unobservable image. The visual mechanism adapts in a few seconds so that the pattern can no longer be visualized—it disappears, adaptation is complete. A similar experience can be obtained in the somatic mode: place an object in the hand and hold it very still. Soon the feel of the object disappears.

Were it not for some such mechanism, the organism would constantly be bombarded by an intensity and duration of input which would swamp any ability to make fine discriminations. In fact, the ability to make visual discriminations despite a change in background illumination over a range of about 10 billion to one constitutes another one of those discrepancies that opens the door to a flood of research. In this instance studies on retinal adaptation led to the discovery of the neural mechanisms responsible. The discrepancy involved the conception that retinal adaptation was thought to be due entirely to bleaching and regeneration of photosensitive pigments present in retinal receptors (Hecht, 1934). Recently, however, evidence began to accrue that nonphotochemical factors are needed in order to explain the time course of the adaptive mechanism and that these factors are basic to the operation of the photochemical effects (see Rushton, reviewed by Dowling, 1967).

The primary tool for these investigations has been a large electrode placed outside the eye. This electrode records changes in potentials generated by the entire retina as an electroretinogram. With the appropriate analytical methods answers as refined as those using the microelectrode technique are obtained.

Briefly, the mammalian retina is composed of several layers: a receptive one made up of rod and/or cone shaped cells in which photosensitive chemical pigments are found; an interactive layer made of cells whose processes extend horizontally to interconnect a host of neighboring retinal cells with each other; a bi-polar layer made up of cells which connect one or more receptors with ganglion cells which serve as the origin of the retinal output to the brain (Fig. 3-4).

The electroretinogram includes two components: a small "a-" and a larger "b-wave." The a-wave appears to be generated more peripherally in the retina than the b-wave. This is determined by placing a clamp on the optic nerve, a procedure which destroys the blood circulation of the retina except for vessels (from the choroid) which nourish the receptors. In such a preparation only the a-wave remains.

A similar procedure can be used to destroy the ganglion cells which make up the deepest layer of the retina; cutting the optic nerve close to its origin will result in the degeneration of most of the parent ganglion cell bodies. The electroretinogram appears undisturbed by this procedure; in fact, adaptation remains normal in such preparations. Thus this deepest layer of the retina cannot account for either the a- or the b-waves. This leaves the retina's middle layers as generators of the b-wave.

The course of adaptation of the a- and b-waves differs. The adaptation of the a-wave does not reflect the course of psychophysical adaptation and is therefore of less concern here. B-wave adaptation, on the other hand, parallels psychophysical adaptation and its mechanism is central to the argument. A series of ingenious

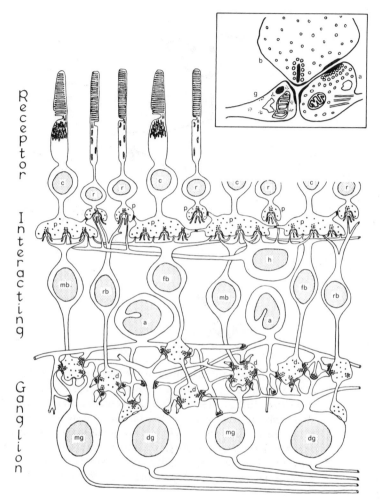

Fig. 3-4. A summary of the nature of the connectivity pattern of the primate retina, showing the synapses between the different types of cells as observed with the electron microscope in serial sections. Note the contacts between receptors, the widespread connexions of the horizontal cells and of the amacrine cells, and the vertical arrangement of the bipolars. The swollen central terminals of the bipolar cells form so-called dyad synapses (see box) with a ganglion cell and simultaneously with an amacrine cell. 5, rod; c, cone; mb, midget bipolar; rb, rod bipolar; fb, flat bipolar; h, horizontal cell; a, amacrine cell; mg, midget ganglion cell; d, dyad synapse; dg, diffuse ganglion cell; p, pedicel. The inset at top right shows details of a typical dyad synapse. From Horridge, 1968; Dowling and Boycott, 1966.

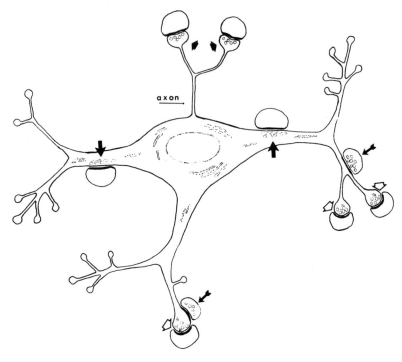

axon

Fig. 3-5. Drawing of a neuron in the visual system of the brain (lateral geniculate nucleus) showing synaptic connections. Note that, just as in the retina, the vesicles containing booster chemicals are sometimes on the far side and sometimes on the near side of the synaptic cleft, showing that the neuron both sends and receives signals (indicated by the direction of the arrows). This bidirectionality of connectivity (the dyad synapses) makes feedback possible. From Ralston, 1971.

experiments has provided evidence for the conception that adaptation is not a function of individual retinal cells but of pools of neurons in the retinal network. A typical experiment shows that sensitivity to light is the same whether the retina is exposed to a striped pattern of alternating dark and light bands or to an evenly spread light of an average intensity. This type of experiment reaches its logical climax when it shows that the threshold of a part of the visual receptive field of a single ganglion cell (as determined with a microelectrode) becomes adapted when another part of that receptive field has been illuminated.

The bulk of evidence indicates that the bi-polar and interactive cells in the middle layer of the retina are the generators of the *b*-wave and the locus of psychophysical adaptation. Several investigators (e.g., Fuortes and Hodgkin, 1964; Rushton, 1963; Dowling, 1967) have suggested that neuronal adaptation results from the operation of a feedback mechanism in which the signal at one stage feeds back onto a previous stage and thus reduces its sensitivity or gain. Recently John Dowling and Brian Boycott (1965) have shown with the electron microscope that the bi-polar, amacrine, and ganglion cell contacts can function in just this fashion. Reciprocal synapses were discovered which make possible the feeding back of excitation to a bi-polar cell from an amacrine cell which had initially received that excitation from the very same bi-polar. The inference is that this feedback is negative, constituting a servomechanism; but this remains to be established more directly. (See also Fig. 3-5.)

the enhancement of contrast

     The decrementing of neural responses would by itself fail to account for the construction of a "neuronal model" type of memory trace against which subsequent input becomes matched. As already noted, behavioral data show that dishabituation occurs with even the slightest change in a complex stimulus to which the organism has become habituated. Some transformational organization of neural events is required. How is this organization achieved?

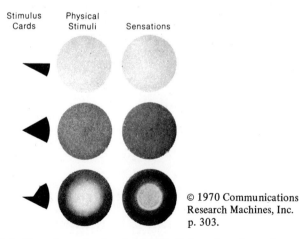

Fig. 3-6. Rotation of stimulus cards (left column) produces the physical stimuli and sensations shown (2nd and right columns). From *Psychology Today*, 1970.

An answer to this question begins with the observation of yet another of those discrepancies upon which brain research seems so to thrive. In this instance the observation was made by Ernst Mach, a Viennese physicist. Mach noted that when a person is confronted with an area over which there is a more or less abrupt change of luminance, the observed change in brightness is accentuated. Whereas the physical change as measured by instrument can be described by:

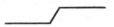

the perceived change looks more like:

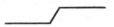

(See Fig. 3-6).

In other words, the area appears to have dark and light "bands", known as Mach Bands, at the points of change.

The psychophysical discrepancy could be resolved by the suggestion that the visual apparatus (probably the retina) functioned to

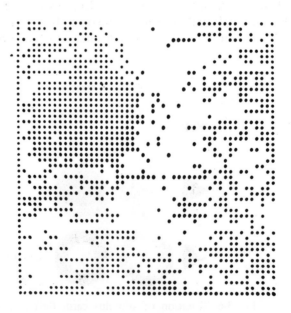

Fig. 3-7. Map of points on the retina at which a light spot produces responding in a particular lateral geniculate cell in the brain of a monkey. After Spinelli and Pribram, 1967.

differentiate, in the mathematical sense, light intensity with respect to area. According to this explanation the perception of visual contrast would be due to a neural mechanism which accomplishes differentiation. The mathematical model has been amended and updated as more refined analyses of the psychophysical discrepancy have been undertaken—yet Mach's fundamental approach and even the elements of his solution have been upheld by these studies which have also added the neurophysiological demonstration of the mechanism responsible for visual contrast (and, by extrapolation, contour).

By implanting a microelectrode in a nerve fiber originating in a ganglion cell, an experimenter can map the area of the visual field— i.e., the area in front of the eye—in which the transient appearance of a light will cause a change in the rate of impulse discharge (firing) of that ganglion cell. Such a map is known as the visual receptive field (see Fig. 3-7). A variety of maps is obtained when different cells are sampled: *most* maps are more or less round in shape, but some are star-shaped or linear, or display a long edge which divides the part of the receptive field where light produces an effect from the part where it does not. Generally, two classes of visual receptive field can be distinguished: those in which a light primarily inhibits the firing of the ganglion cell, and those in which the light primarily enhances the firing. Further, each of these primary reaction areas is surrounded, either in part or in entirety, by another region in which the response of the cell is opposite that shown in the primary zone. Thus, the majority of ganglion cells can be classified into on-center or off-center units; the on-center, as a rule, show an inhibitory penumbra; the off-center units often display a surround of enhanced activity.

These visual receptive field maps recorded from ganglion cells tell a good deal about the functional organization of the retina. Obviously such records are not simple manifestations of the activity of single receptors. Ganglion cells are third-order neurons and must be activated by the excitation of any of the large number of receptors with which they have anatomical connections. The receptive fields are generally large compared with the dimensions of photoreceptors and neighboring fields overlap considerably. Thus any one particular region of the receptor mosaic does not belong exclusively to any one particular ganglion cell (Ratliff, 1965, pp. 173–74).

The presence in the receptive field map of a surround which is opposite in sign to that of the central effect suggests that antagonistic excitatory and inhibitory influences are organized in such a way that stimulation of one receptor site reduces the effective excitation received by the ganglion cell from the neighbors of the stimulated

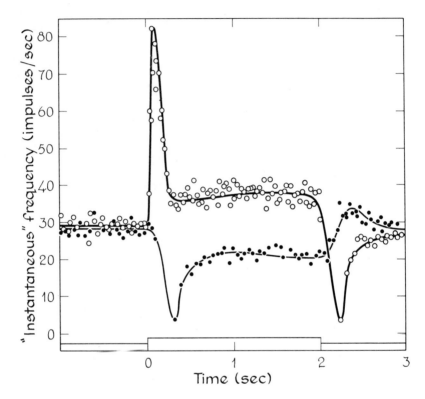

Fig. 3-8. Simultaneous excitatory and inhibitory transients in two adjacent receptor units in the lateral eye of limulus. One receptor unit (filled circles) was illuminated steadily through-out the period shown in the graph. The other unit (open circles) was illuminated steadily until time 0, when the illumination on it was increased abruptly to a new steady level where it remained for 2 sec and then was decreased abruptly to the original level. Accompanying the marked excitatory transients in one receptor unit are large transient inhibitory effects in the adjacent, steadily illuminated receptor unit. A large decrease in frequency is produced by the inhibitory effect resulting from the large excitatory transient; during the steady illumination the inhibitory effect is still present but less marked; and finally, accompanying the decrement in the frequency of response of the element on which the level of excitation was decreased, there is a marked release from inhibition. From Ratliff, 1965.

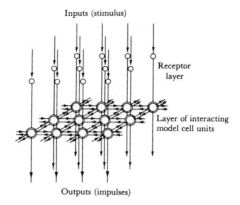

Inputs (stimulus)

Receptor
layer

Layer of interacting
model cell units

Outputs (impulses)

Fig. 3-9. Schema of the receptor and interacting (horizontal) layers of the retina. Vertical arrows indicate direction of signal transmission, horizontal arrows the inhibitory interactions. From Ratliff, *Mach Bands,* 1965, Holden-Day.

cell. In other words, stimulation of a retinal locus produces *inhibition* surrounding that locus. This process of "surround" or "lateral" inhibition has been directly observed in the eye of the horseshoe crab, *Limulus* (Fig. 3-8). In this creature retinal elements are spatially separate from one another—each element forms its own encapsulated unit, called an omatidium. Each omatidium can therefore be separately illuminated during microelectrode studies of the retinal output fibers. Shining a light on one such omatidium will produce excitation if the recording is made from a fiber whose receptive field includes that omatidium. When the light is moved to neighboring omatidia, the microelectrode records inhibition—and the resulting maps are similar to those obtained from mammalian ganglion cells when the receptors within their receptive fields are scanned by a transient light.

This process of "surround" or "lateral" inhibition is not restricted to the visual system. In hearing, the cochlear mechanism and in touch sensation the skin receptors show a similar functional organization (Bekesy, 1967). Within the central nervous system, the cells of cerebellar and cerebral cortex also respond in this fashion. In short, lateral inhibition is one characteristic of neural networks— especially those organized in flat sheets (as those in cortex, which in Latin means bark) whose neuronal depth includes several stages of processing.

What properties of these neural networks account for lateral inhibition? Several explanations have been given and they are not mutually exclusive; for precise (mathematical) description and evaluation of each separate explanation, the reader is referred to Ratliff (1965, Ch. 3). What must be accounted for by any explanation is the occurrence of lateral inhibition; its apparent dependency on the distance from the center of excitation; the observability of the interaction between excitation and inhibition. The most direct explanation holds either that branches from each receptor make inhibitory connections with their neighbors or, much more likely, that inhibitory neurons do the job—e.g., the amacrine and horizontal cells of the retina whose spreading arborizations of dendrites and absence of axons make them ideally suited to serve these functions (Fig. 3-9). Both in the retina (Svaetichin, 1967) and elsewhere in the nervous system (e.g., the cerebellum) these axonless dendritic networks have been shown to serve just such a function. In fact, recent experiments (Werblin and Dowling, 1969) using intracellular recording show that horizontal cells function exclusively by hyperpolarization, that is, by the generation of inhibitory slow potential changes. (In fact *only* slow potentials, no nerve impulses can be recorded from retinal elements peripheral to the ganglion cell layer.) And the imposition of inhibition by dendritic feltworks where slow potentials are generated by input fibers leads to an accentuation of the wave forms produced and, essentially, to the creation of interference effects which in their simplest form constitute surround inhibition.

In summary, the sensory mechanism semipermanently modifies its response to input by two processes: contrast enhancement and adaptation. The anatomical arrangements of the mechanism make it likely that these processes function reciprocally; the greater the decrementing of a unit's responses during adaptation, the less its inhibiting effect on neighbors to produce contrast enhancement (Fig. 3-10).

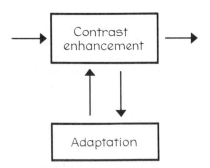

Fig. 3-10. Reciprocity of contrast enhancement and adaptation

Thus, the progressive damping, decrementing, of excitation prevents prolonged discharge and makes possible the successive comparisons of input patterns and in this manner enhances temporal contrast by simple subtraction. Further, the inhibitory interactions among adjacent neurons prevent spreading or irradiation of excitation through the receptive networks—the inhibitory interactions facilitate the sharpening of spatial patterns. Thus the processing of contrasting transformations on inputs is made more reliable than if the raw representations of changes in energy configurations per se were involved.

These properties of adaptation and contrast enhancement are not exclusive to receptors. Throughout the input systems and especially at the cerebral cortex, the decrementing and inhibitory interactions have been found to be operative (Brooks and Asanuma, 1965). This has led to the suggestion made earlier that the operations of adaptation and contrast enhancement as found in receptors might serve as models-in-miniature of the psychological processes of orienting and habituation.

The next chapter shows how these elementary processes, coupled with others still more temporary, come to have such an important and pervasive role in the functioning of the organism.

synopsis

Brain organizations of intermediate duration are largely the result of decremental and inhibitory neural processes. When monotonously stimulated, many neuronal aggregates show a decrementing of activity (adaptation and habituation) and thus become sensitive to novelty (the orienting reaction). In many parts of the nervous system, localized neural excitation inhibits surrounding neural activity and thus sharpens the contrast between excited and nonexcited tissue. Decrementing appears to be a function of the generator potential of neurons which initiate (by depolarization) nerve impulses; inhibitory interactions appear to depend on hyperpolarizations occurring in the junctional network.

codes and their transformations

what a code is

How can we characterize the forms which neuro-electric configurations temporarily take (and the relationships between forms) that make possible such very short term memory mechanisms as holding onto a sentence written in German until the verb finally appears? Research on the conditions that influence human memory has demonstrated the overriding importance of questions of configuration; whether something is remembered is in large part a function of the form and context in which it is experienced. We turn therefore to the problem of the substitution of one configuration for another by operations of the nervous system. In technical language this is the problem of the transformations or transfer functions that make coding and recoding possible.

Coding operations take place in the nervous system continuously. Physical energy is sensed by receptors and transformed into nerve impulses. These impulses, in turn, reach synaptic networks where the discrete signals become coded into the form of, i.e., encoded in, the slow potential microstructure. Before this encoded representation can be of influence elsewhere in the brain a decoding operation must take place, nerve impulses must again be constituted and in such a fashion that previously encoded information is not lost.

Two classes of transfer functions can be used to describe the coding operations used by the nervous system. Some transformations allow reasonably simple calculations of the correspondence between codes. Such calculations make it possible to decode the encoded form and vice versa. A sort of reversibility, a secondary functional isomorphism is maintained between codes by a one to one mapping between ciphers of the code.

The second class of transfer functions is entirely anisomorphic and arbitrary. Transformations in this class are irreversible unless one has the key to decipher the code produced in this fashion.

Reversible transformations occur in physical optical systems, in hi-fi transducers, and, as will become clear, in the encoding of neural configurations in the slow potential microstructure of the brain. Irreversible transformations occur in ordinary languages composed of arbitrary alphabetic combinations, in Morse code, in telephone and TV transmission signals, and the like. In the nervous system, as subsequent chapters will detail, irreversible transformations take place whenever an abstractive process such as feature detection occurs.

To what purpose would the brain engage in so many substitution schemes, so many coding and recoding operations? Any transformation risks a loss of fidelity. Why, then, the ubiquity of this property in the nervous system? What is to be gained by recoding? The answer must be in some improved efficiency or effective functioning.

That recoding is a far from trivial operation was brought home to me when I was confronted with the use of a general purpose computer. This instrument can be manipulated only in the language it understands, a spatial or temporal sequence of ons or offs, of yeses or nos, of ups or downs, of a set of switches which the instrument presents. If there are twelve such switches we must remember how to set each for each operation we want the computer to perform. Communication becomes therefore a series of

```
D  U  U     D  D  D     U  D  D     U  U  U
D  D  U     D  U  D     D  D  U     D  U  U
D  U  D     U  U  U     D  U  D     D  U  D
                                          Etc.
```

The task confronting the operator of the computer is therefore a

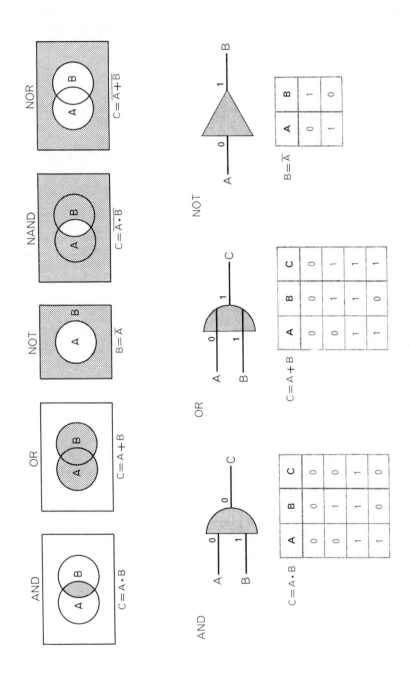

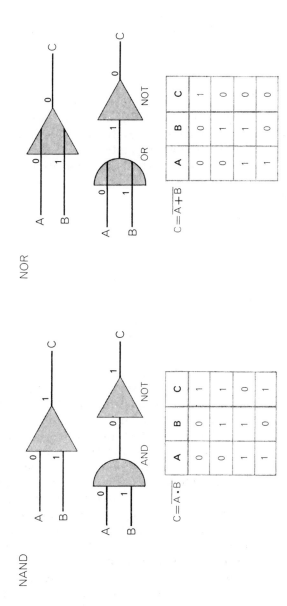

Fig. 4-1. Representation of "AND," "OR," "NOT," "NAND," and "NOR" binary logic elements. Input signals, either 0 or 1, enter the circuits at left and are logically combined to produce output at right. "Truth table" below each circuit lists all possible logical operations that can be performed. The "NAND" and "NOR" elements are formed by combining the "NOT" element with the "AND" and "OR" as shown. From Evans, "Computer Logic and Memory," D.C. Evans. Copyright ©1966 by Scientific American, Inc. All rights reserved.

formidable one of remembering long lists of ups and downs, strings of "binary" numbers:

$$011 \quad 000 \quad 100 \quad 111$$
$$001 \quad 010 \quad 001 \quad 011$$
$$010 \quad 111 \quad 010 \quad 010$$

Programmers were quick to get around this confusing way of managing their instrument: they divided the twelve switches into sets of three and labelled the up position with an integer increasing geometrically from right to left. Thus in each triad the up position indicates 4–2–1. When two or three switches are up simultaneously, the sum of the integers is represented. Thus

```
0 means D  D  D
1 means D  D  U
2 means D  U  D
3 means D  U  U
4 means U  D  D
5 means U  D  U
6 means U  U  D
7 means U  U  U
```

and any sequence of twelve ups and downs can be described and remembered by four numerals, e.g., the sequences presented earlier become 3047; 1213; 2722. This transformation called "octal" coding of a binary system is a tremendous economy—just how is it possible to achieve such a remarkable feat? (The superlative is not used lightly; by repetition of the process, classification into hierarchical schemes is provided for—and classification is a most fundamental logical procedure.) To obtain an answer, let us pose the problem more specifically: How can one transfer from a pattern where complexity resides in the *arrangement* of simple elements to a pattern where complexity resides in the unique meaning of each component element? A simple arrangement of convergent inputs (called by engineers "and" functions because inputs from two sources must add before an output is produced) crossed by parallel inhibitory arrays ("nor" functions, a combination of an "or" function in which output is determined by either of two inputs and a "not" function which negates, thus inhibiting output when either input is activated) will begin the job (see Figs. 4-1 and 4-2). This arrangement is so

DECIMAL		BINARY		
	A_3	A_2	A_1	A_0
0	0	0	0	0
1	0	0	0	1
○ 2	0	0	1	0
3	0	0	1	1
4	0	1	0	0
5	0	1	0	1
6	0	1	1	0
7	0	1	1	1
8	1	0	0	0
9	1	0	0	1

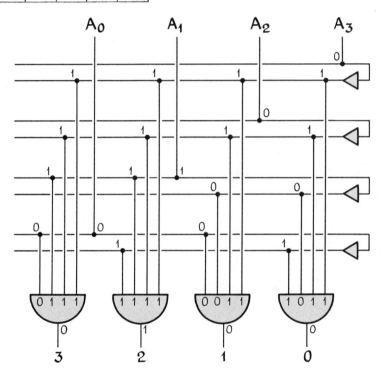

Fig. 4-2. Conversion of binary to decimal digits is accomplished by this circuit, made of four "NOT" circuits and four "AND" circuits. The "truth" table at left shows the binary equivalent for the decimal digits from 0 to 9. To show the principle involved in decoding binary digits, the circuit carries the decoding only as far as decimal digit 3. The signal at each of the numbered outputs is 0 unless all the inputs are 1. In the example this is true for the third "AND" circuit from the rt., labeled 2. Thus the binary digits 0010 are decoded to yield the decimal digit 2. Redrawn after Evans, 1966.

71

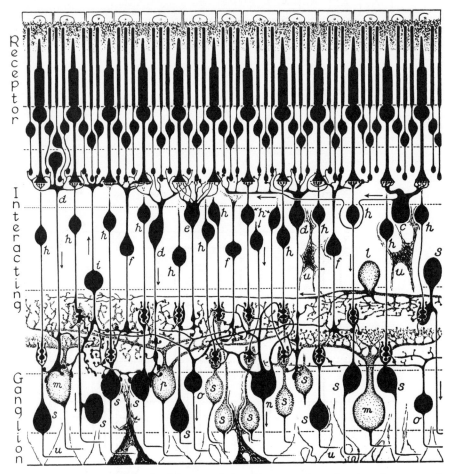

Fig. 4-3. Scheme of the primate retina, showing the types of the neurons and their synaptic relationships, so far revealed by means of the method of Golgi. From Polyak, 1941.

reminiscent of the configuration of the retina—our window to the brain—that one is tempted to label the "nor" function "horizontal layer hyperpolarization" and the "and" functions "ganglion cell discharge." Of course the retina is not nearly as neatly wired as this diagram—yet the organizations are amazingly comparable with respect to the process under consideration (compare Figs. 4-2 and 4-3).

Thus recoding turns out to be a powerfully effective part of the memory process, which the nervous system appears to be superbly constructed to perform. In fact, the forms of recoding, of representation, which are possible to the nervous system may be limitless. Nonetheless, certain classes of codes can be made out.

types of neural codes

We have already separated codes into two classes: those involving the discrete, impulse characteristics of nerve discharge, and those involving the steady-state microstructure produced at neural junctions.

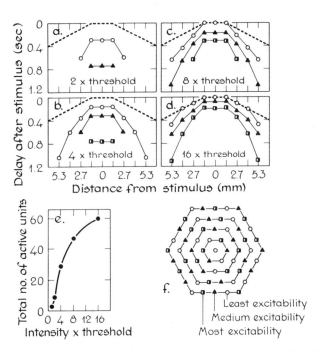

Fig. 4-4. Coding intensity and locus in parallel fibers. The spatial representation as found in tactile afferents from the cat's footpad when excited by mechanical pulses at one point; diagram based on quantitative experimental data. Assuming a number of equidistant receptors of three levels of excitability (f), a stimulus twice threshold will give the number of impulses at the distances from the stimulated point and at the time after stimulus shown in (a). The dotted line is the latency due to the traveling time of the mechanical wave in the pad. Stronger stimuli bring in responses shown in (b) to (d). The total number of impulses at each stimulus strength is given in (e). From Gray and Lal, 1965.

Impulse coding is not just a question of the presence or absence of a signal; an impulse code can utilize a diversity of variables which characterize trains of pulses. Don Perkel and Theodore Bullock (Perkel and Bullock, 1968) have identified the following types of coding in studying the signals emitted by the electric organs of certain fishes. Shifts in latency, the duration of bursts, the overall probability of firing and the variation in this probability, the incrementing or decrementing of firing or its rate of change are all altered in one or another set of conditions. For the most part these conditions are distortions of the electric field produced by these same signals sent by the electrical organs—distortions registered by the lateral line system of the fish, a radar-like process.

In addition to these purely temporal codes, spatial coding occurs when arrays of parallel lines—nerve fibers—produce what Perkel and Bullock call "ensemble" processing which depends on differences in the distributions of impulse trains among lines (See Fig. 4-4).

Spatial coding and especially the coding which involves differences in timing between neighboring ensembles of nerves becomes intimately related to the whole group of non-impulse coding processes— the steady-state slow potential microstructures which make up so much of the activity of the grey matter of the mammalian brain. For, as Perkel and Bullock point out, there must be a readout, some mechanism in the central nervous system which "reads" the impulse coded messages. These chapters argue that this readout takes place at neural junctions in the production of slow potential microstructures, momentary states resulting from the interactions among ensembles of neighboring and successive impulse coded signals.

spontaneity in neural activity

To be effective most codes need some sort of a stable base against which the coding operation can take place. The work of DeLisle Burns and others has established beyond reasonable doubt that neural activity furnishes such stability. Neural tissue spontaneously generates electrical potential changes. The brain, just as the heart, pulses continually. And, just as in the heart, slow potentials are responsible for initiating the pulsations and these slow potentials are dependent for their occurrence only on certain constancies in the chemical environment of the initiating tissues (Fig. 4-5).

A series of carefully controlled studies from Burns' laboratory (1958) definitively answers an age-old science fiction question: can the brain be kept active even when it is completely isolated (neurally) from other nervous tissue? The immediate answers were, as

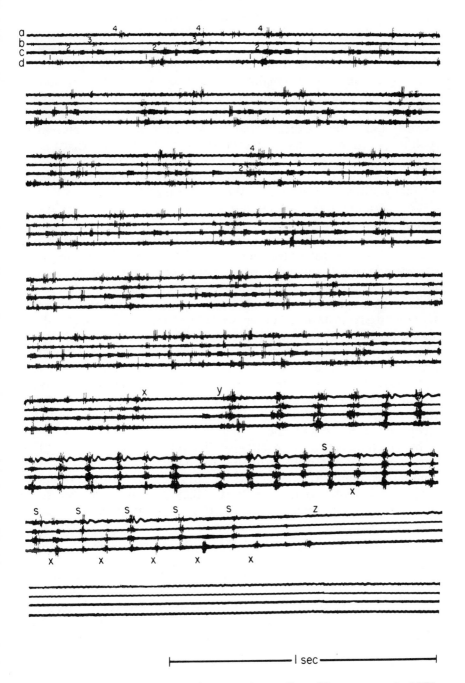

Fig. 4-5. A cerebral symphony. From Verzeano, et al., 1970.

they so often are, neither completely supportive of the notion that cerebral activity is "spontaneous" nor entirely supportive of the axiom of a quiescent *tabula rasa* upon which sensory experience becomes written. Burns found even in the unanesthetized animal, the isolated cortical slab remains inactive unless briefly stimulated, although there are some other reports (Echlin, et al., 1952; Gerard and Young, 1937; Henry and Scoville, 1952; Ingvar, 1955; Libet and Gerard, 1939) that indicate that spontaneous activity is present in such preparations. In any case, even taking Burns' conservative result, a few strong electrical stimuli applied to the cortical surface will produce a series of bursts of neural activity which usually continues for many minutes (or even hours) after stimulation has stopped.

The periodic waves of excitation that follow a few infrequent stimuli given to the unanesthetized cerebral cortex also occur whenever diffusely organized nervous tissue is stimulated. Effects lasting many hours have been observed after brief stimulation in the intact sea anemone (Batham and Pantin, 1950). Recently the luminescence response of sea pansies (a colorful soft coral) has been described: after a series of stimulations, these colonies begin to luminesce spontaneously instead of doing so only in response to stimulation. To explain this behavior, a slow change of state in the neural tissue (a primitive form of the slow potential memory process?) must be invoked. These changes of state are accessible to environmental influence and are, of course, influenced by the previous activity of the organism, but they also have intrinsic properties and their own time course of activity that determine recurrence apart from the environment of the moment.

In short, neuronal aggregates of the type found in the cerebral cortex are conservatively estimated to be quiescent in the absence of continuous input. However, these aggregates are easily aroused to prolonged activity. Hence, at "rest," they may be conceived to be just below the threshold for continuous self-excitation. In the intact mammal, a mechanism exists to insure central nervous system excitation beyond such a resting level. This mechanism is the spontaneous discharge of receptors.

Ragnar Granit (1955) has detailed how "the idea of spontaneous activity as an integral part of the performance of sensory instruments has grown upon us." He traces the history of this subject from the early observations of Lord Edgar Adrian and Yngvar Zotterman (1926) and Adrian and Brian Matthews (1927a, 1927b) on muscle and on optic nerve preparations to his own extensive experimental analyses. In addition, his evidence supports the suggestion that this "spontaneous" activity of sense organs makes them one of the brain's most important "energizers" or activators. To this we can now add the probability that this spontaneous activity forms the substrate, the stable base upon which and within which neural codes operate.

Again Burns has furnished the evidence (1968). Using micro-electrodes he found that approximately one-third of a large sample of brain cells showed a consistent overall rate of discharge over the time he recorded from them. Whenever such cells were stimulated to fire more rapidly or were inhibited, they compensated for the change by generating its reciprocal during the period after excitation or inhibition. These cells thus constitute the powerful stable base upon which the basic property of coding and recoding depends: spatial patterns can be generated by excitation in one location and simultaneous inhibition of spontaneous activity in another.

pacemakers and dominant foci

But the property of spontaneity has greater importance than just to provide a background for more active operations of the nervous system. There is good evidence that the spontaneous activity of neuronal aggregates can be recruited into the service of one or another coding mechanism. For instance, under certain conditions (the imposition of a direct current to polarize the tissue) neurons can be shown to "remember" by repeating the initial frequency to which they had been recruited when subsequently a pulse of different frequency is imposed (Chow, 1964; Chow and Dewson, 1964; Dewson, Chow, and Engel, 1964).

A study by Dominick Purpura (1962), however, illuminates the flexible nature of this modifiability. A population of brain cells was stimulated electrically and recordings were made from single units nearby. At the same time polarizing currents were imposed on the unit from which the recording was being made. The results of the experiment showed that in the presence of consistent stimulating conditions the unit response (6 per second discharge) remained consistent despite the imposition of polarizing currents. The technique thus allowed Purpura to demonstrate that the distribution of input to his unit was shifting from moment to moment (compensating for his artificially imposed polarizations) and that no fixed set of pathways was responsible for initiating the response of the unit (Fig. 4-6).

Whenever at any location the spontaneous activity of neuroelectric potential becomes sufficiently stable to organize the activity of other neural aggregates, it is known as a pacemaker. Some pacemakers, such as the one that governs the contractibility of the heart, are inborn and function throughout the life of the individual. They

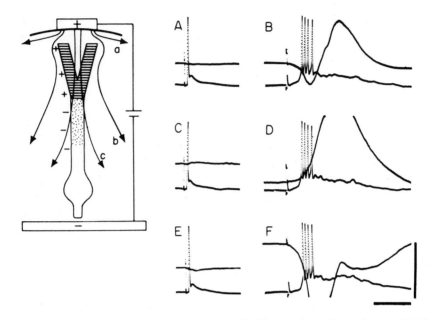

Fig. 4-6. Dissociation of effects of weak surface polarizing currents (50 μA/mm^2) on evoked cortical responses and intracellular activities of a pyramidal tract neuron. Upper channel records are surface responses to stimulation of ventrolateral thalamus. Patterns of intracellularly recorded activities are uninfluenced during dramatic changes in surface evoked responses. A, antidromic spike with a prominent delayed depolarization; B, patterns of synaptic drive during stabilization phase of augmenting response; C and D, during weak surface anodal polarization; E and F, during surface cathodal polarization. Calibrations: 50 mv; 20msec. Diagram, upper left, shows probable distribution of currents during weak anodal polarization: a, fraction of current flow; c, proportion of current inward at terminals of apical dendrites, outward across proximal dendritic regions. No effect of this current is observed at the soma level with weak intensities as indicated in D. From Purpura, 1967.

organize the organism's relationships with his environment and make him much more than a passive switchboard addressed by the exigencies of his experience.

Other pacemakers are somewhat less permanent, forming "temporary dominant foci" as a result of convergence of excitation upon them. A simple example of the experimental production of such a temporary dominant focus was performed many years ago (Zal'man-son in Ukhtomski, 1926). A dog was conditioned to raise his right hind leg to the sound of a tone. After this conditional response was well established, his right motor cortex (which controls the left side of the body) was exposed. Then during the performance of the conditioned reaction a patty of strychninized filter paper was placed on the area which controls the left forepaw in order to chemically excite it. Immediately the dog switched the responsive leg; he now raised his left forepaw to the conditional signal. This is usually interpreted to mean that the focus of neural activity which had been

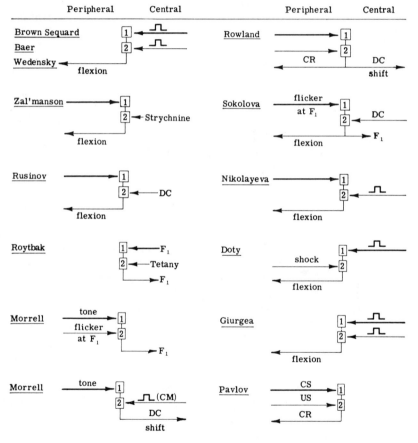

Fig. 4-7. Methods of conditioning that have been used by various investigators to establish and produce shifts in cerebral dominant foci. The example in the text refers to Zal'manson's experiment. From John, 1967.

established through conditioning and which dominated the functions of motor cortex was now overshadowed by a new "temporary dominant focus" established in this brain area by the chemical excitation caused by the strychnine. (See Fig. 4-7 for a summary of methods used to produce dominant foci.)

But most pacemakers are characteristically cyclic. In their simplest form they serve as biological clocks (Richter, 1955; Pittendrigh, 1960). In arrangements whose output interacts with current input, they perform the functions of neuronic shutters that periodically let some impulses pass (as in a movie camera; Lindsley, 1961) and scanners that spatially sample input systematically (as in a TV set; McCulloch, 1965). When their output is less recurrently regular but is programmed, the system is described as showing "voluntary" characteristics.

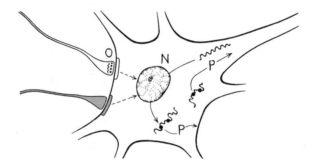

Fig. 4-8. One model of intracellular control of neuronal rhythms. N is the nucleus and P can be either polypeptide or protein. The wavy line represents messenger (informational) RNA with or without attached ribosomes (●). Coupling between the subsynaptic membrane and the nucleus and soma membrane or axoplasm is shown by dashed arrows. Synaptic vesicles (0) shown in nerve terminal on upper right. Redrawn after Strumwasser, 1967.

For many years it was impossible to distinguish between generator potentials and those pacemakers originating in the waxing and waning of the neuroelectric states occurring in the junctional microstructure. But as already noted, Sokolov (1970) indicates that the mechanism of generation of axonic nerve impulses may, under certain laboratory conditions, proceed relatively independently of manipulations of cell body membrane slow potentials. According to this evidence the generator potential originates within the structure of the nerve cell body and not at its surface, and is therefore not directly attributable to alterations in nerve cell membrane properties and the dendritic influences upon these properties (See also Fig. 4-8).

Another interesting dissociation between impulse generation and electrical state fluctuations has been observed during one of the phases of sleep. This phase is characterized by rapid movements of the eyes, often by jerky body movements (observe your dog sleeping sometime) and by electrical rhythms recordable from the brain which paradoxically look like those obtained in the waking state. When awakened during this phase of sleep, human subjects almost invariably report that they have been dreaming whereas when awakened during other phases such reports are rare.

When microelectrode recordings are made from most neurons in the brains of monkeys during waking (Evarts, 1967) no recurrent regularities in discharge are discernible. During ordinary sleep, these same cells will discharge in spaced bursts with intervening periods of relative inactivity. These intervals of bursting roughly correspond to the fluctuations recorded simultaneously with gross electrodes. During the paradoxical phase of sleep, however, single units display intense bursting at intervals recurring about four times a second—but the gross electrical recording (EEG) does not reflect this dominant rhythm. This is interpreted to mean that although single units display a strong temporal pattern, these units are discharging out of phase with each other, their activity is decoupled from that of their neighbors. Some sort of coupling mechanism must therefore exist independently of nerve impulse generation. Such couplings are most likely effected through the junctional slow potential microstructure. Thus it is unlikely that the steady state and the discrete neuronal processes are simply reflections of one another. The rules of transformation which allow recoding of one process into the other must be empirically determined for each condition of interest to investigators. At this time any general statements about the types of transformations involved are likely to be premature.

the organization of neural codes

This need for empirical information about specific instances does not preclude the possibility of forming hypotheses about the types of transformations most likely to characterize nontrivial recoding operations; such hypotheses are needed to guide research. By definition they will fit only the category of reversible transformations, since irreversible operations are arbitrary and must therefore simply be discovered. Practically any psychological process that can be described in words could be coded neurally by an irreversible operation. The question remains whether in fact this is the mechanism in any specific instance.

Reversible transformations, and especially some classes of linear transforms, have especially useful properties in explaining psychological phenomena as will become evident in subsequent chapters. Some of the possible rules of reversible transformation are readily stated and tested now that computers are available to help analyze the matrices of data involved. Here are examples:

1. Successive nerve impulses are accumulated (or subtracted) into amplitude fluctuations of state in the postsynaptic microstructure.
2. Successive slow potential states in the junctional microstructure are correlated into potentials sufficient to modulate a neuron's generator potential.
3. Nerve impulses arriving simultaneously at neighboring locations are spatially superposed, i.e., neighborhood interactions of an additive (or subtractive) nature take place.
4. When two sources simultaneously evoke a state in the slow potential microstructure, correlation between them takes place and the correlation becomes decoded into nerve impulses.

Evidence suggests that some active neural mechanisms, many of them built in at birth, can make these rules operative. The next chapter, therefore, details the form taken by some of the most basic modules of which the nervous system is composed.

synopsis

Evanescent neural organizations take place as each neural aggregate recodes its input. Recoding is a surprisingly powerful adaptive and constructive instrument which the organism uses to act in and on his world. Some coding operations maintain a functional isomorphism and are reversible, provided the appropriate transformations have occurred. Junctional inhibitory interactions result in such transformations.

the logic of the
nervous system

the organization of reflexes—the classical view

Chapter 3 showed the benefits of using receptor structure and function as models-in-miniature of some aspects of central nervous system organization. Continuing this pattern, this chapter turns to output mechanisms in the belief that here also is a rich source of data on the construction of the brain mechanisms that make coding possible. The models derived from the two sources are markedly similar, a fact that gives added weight to the validity of the approach. When considering output mechanisms the accessibility of observable behavior makes it possible to spell out even more clearly the formal characteristics, the logic of the neurophysiological process. This logic, classically conceptualized as a reflex arc, is now viewed as a process which accomplishes analytic and control functions. The resolution of a discrepancy between new data and then current theory highlights the story of this change in views.

Sherrington's *Integrative Action of the Nervous System* stated the classical theoretical conception of the organization of reflexes.

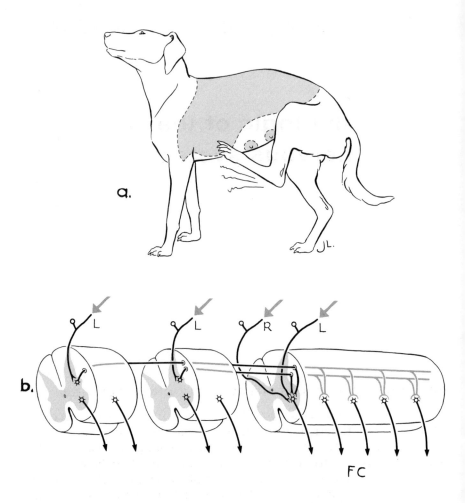

Fig. 5-1. (A) The 'receptive field,' as revealed after low cervical transection, a saddle-shaped area of dorsal skin, whence the scratch-reflex of the left hind-limb can be evoked. (B) Diagram of the spinal arcs involved. *L,* receptive or afferent nerve-path from the left foot; *R,* receptive nerve-path from the opposite foot; receptive nerve-paths from the opposite foot and from hairs in the dorsal skin of the left side; *FC,* the final common path, in this case the motor neurone to a flexor muscle of the hip. Redrawn after Sherrington, 1947.

Though this conception has guided much neurophysiological research (e.g., D. P. C. Lloyd, 1959), it has had an even more profound influence on psychological thought. Sherrington viewed the organization of the reflex (attempting to define a unit of analysis for the behavior of the "spinal" preparation he was studying) as follows:

> A simple reflex is probably a purely abstract conception, because all parts of the nervous system are connected together and no part of it is probably ever capable of reaction without affecting and being affected by various other parts, and it is a system certainly never absolutely at rest. But the simple reflex is a convenient, if not a probable, fiction [Sherrington, 1947, p. 7].

Sherrington's view relied on earlier experiments by Bell (1811) and by Magendie (1822). These investigators used to advantage the anatomical circumstance that every somatic peripheral nerve splits into two major divisions at its junction with the spinal cord: a ventral (towards the stomach) and a dorsal (towards the back) root. Selective cutting of the dorsal roots of the nerves of a limb of a dog produced anesthesia (complete loss of feeling) of that limb without any marked change in patterns of movement (motor function). Selective cutting of the ventral roots of the limb nerves produced paralysis without any alteration in sensitivity. The results of these experiments were so dramatic that they became generalized into a "law" (the Law of Bell and Magendie) which states that input and output from the central nervous system are carried by noninteracting pathways. Hence, input nerves are called afferents (*ad* + *fero* = to carry in) and output nerves are called efferents (*ex* + *fero* = to carry out; See Fig. 5-1).

A long- and often implicitly held generalization of the Law of Bell and Magendie holds that all afferents are sensory (i.e., connected to sensory receptors) and all efferents are motor (i.e., connected to contractile muscles) a generalization Sherrington made explicit in his famous fiction, the reflex arc. And the reflex arc is the neurological counterpart of the behaviorists' approach to the analysis of psychological processes in terms of simple correlations between input to the organism (stimuli) and output (responses).

efferent control of input—the feedback loop

A revision of the reflex arc concept becomes necessary because of data not available to Sherrington. These data show that all of the organism's input mechanisms are directly controlled by the central nervous system. Thus, output fibers, efferents, regulate the organism's receptor and therefore sensory functions, as well as his movements.

This revision began in experiments which further analyzed the functions of the nerve fibers which make up the ventral root. (See Fig. 5-2.) Anatomical observation showed that one-third of these fibers, a group characterized by their small diameter and called γ fibers (as opposed to the larger α and β groups), ended not in contractile muscle tissue per se but in specialized receptors called muscle spindles. These spindles sense the amount of tension in the muscle fibers among which they are located. That such a large bulk of the ventral root innervated these spindles posed a puzzle to reflex-arc oriented physiology, and experiments were begun to solve the problem. The most dramatic data resulted from electrical stimulation of the distal end (the end towards the muscle) of a cut ventral root from which the larger fibers had been removed by dissection. Such stimulation had no direct effect on muscle contraction—the γ fibers are, therefore, efferents whose function is not motor. More

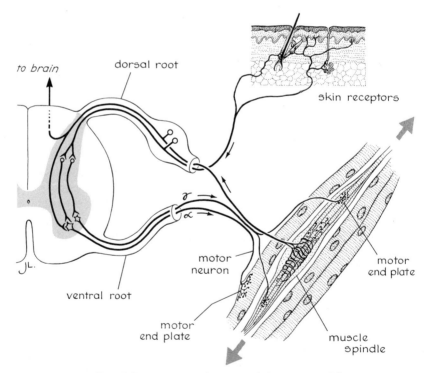

Fig. 5-2. Summary diagram of the gamma (γ) motor neuron system. Redrawn after Thompson, 1967.

interestingly, the electrical activity of the dorsal root was monitored during stimulation of the γ efferent fibers, and indeed the spontaneous rate of activity of the dorsal root afferent activity was markedly decremented by this ventral root stimulation (Granit, 1967). Thus the γ system effects a negative feedback on input derived from the muscle spindles, much as do the mechanisms of adaptation and habituation discussed in Chapter 3. Further, the rate of activity of muscle spindle afferents could be influenced, via the γ efferent after connections by stimulations made within the spinal cord (small ventral horn cells), the brain stem, cerebellum, and even the (motor) cortex (Kuffler and Hunt, 1952; Leskell, 1945). As Chapters 12 and 13 will cover in detail, these experimental results make it necessary to view the regulation of motor functions of the organism, his behavior, as being effected through those receptors intimately concerned in movement, rather than as a direct manipulation of muscle contractions. We will therefore defer further considerations of the neural control of behavior until we have discussed in detail the mechanism by which receptor events become organized.

At first it was thought that the motor system was unique and that central control over receptors pertained only to movement. Very quickly, however, evidence accrued that skin receptors (Hagbarth and Kerr, 1954), the auditory afferent mechanism (Galambos, 1956; Rasmussen, 1946; Desmedt, 1960; Dewson, 1968) and the olfactory sense (Kerr and Hagbarth, 1955) were also subject to direct regulation by the central nervous system. Success was not as immediate in demonstrating efferent control over visual input: pioneering studies (Granit, 1955; Hernandez-Peon and Scherer, 1955) were criticized because efferent fibers to the retina could not be identified anatomically. Studies were therefore undertaken in my laboratory in the hope that efferent control over visual input would become a more plausible reality. These studies utilized recently available computer and microelectrode techniques. Nonvisual inputs (clicks and taps to the paw) evoked responses in the optic nerve of cats (whose muscles, including those of the after pupil had been immobilized). Further, the electrical activity of the retina (measured by the electroretinogram) and of afferents originating in the retina was altered by such nonvisual stimulation (Spinelli, Pribram, and Weingarten, 1967; Fig. 5-3). Finally, as in the case of other sensory modalities, stimulation of the appropriate part of the cerebral cortex resulted in changes in the receptivity (e.g., size of the receptive field) of the retinal ganglion cells (Spinelli and Pribram, 1967). The results of these experiments strengthen the belief that the organization of the visual mechanism resembles the other sensory systems in that central control of input does exist.

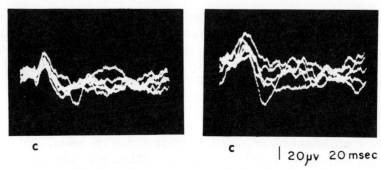

Fig. 5-3. Recording made with bipolar electrode implanted in the *optic* nerve, of electrical responses to *auditory* click stimulation (c). This record was made directly from he oscilloscope face by superimposition on photographic film. The left record was made when the animal appeared to be "attending" while the right record was made with the animal "distracted." From Spinelli, Pribram, and Weingarten, 1965.

the feedforward bias

One process involved in neural control over input is different from the feedbacks so far considered. Interest in this process stems from a paradox in the perceptual realm discovered by Hermann von Helmholtz, the great German physician, physiologist, and psychologist. Helmholtz noted that the visual world jumps when we push our eyeballs about with a finger. By contrast, when we move our eyes voluntarily or in response to an external cue the visual world remains stationary. In both the manipulative and the ordinary movement of the eyes the patterns of light projected on the retina are identical. Helmholtz reasoned that the ordinary perceptual process must therefore include some mechanism which counters and corrects the retinal signals to just the extent necessary for the final image to remain still.

Merton (Brindley and Merton, 1960) took Helmholtz's observation into the laboratory. He paralyzed his own eye muscles, then tried to move his eyes. The visual world jumped in the direction of the intended movement.

It would have been logical to assume that feedback from the eye muscles is involved in producing the correction necessary to perceive the ordinary stationary world. However, the results of the experiment on eye muscle paralysis cannot easily be accounted for in this fashion, since the movement of the visual world was perceived independent of any change in muscular contraction. Further, proprioceptive impulses from the eye muscles have not been traced very

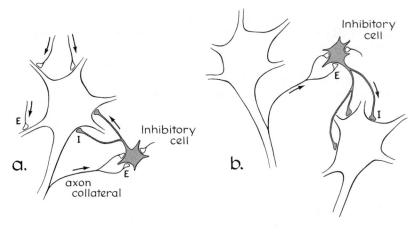

Fig. 5-4. (a) The decrementing of neural activity through inhibitory feedback via Renshaw cells. (b) Contrast enhancement via Renshaw cells, where axon collaterals of a nerve cell effect inhibition of its neighbor. This narrows the central field of discharging cells and creates alternating bands of enhancement and inhibition in the neural network.

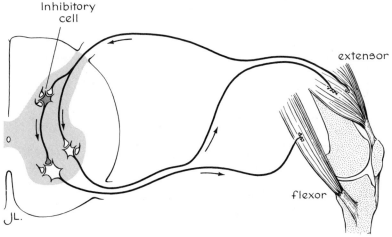

Fig. 5-5. This illustrates the operation of forward inhibition. Impulses flowing along a pathway are partly diverted along collaterals that excite inhibitory interneurons. These interneurons inhibit cells that sometimes have a function opposite to that of cells directly excited by the main operation channel of the input. This feedforward inhibition, just as lateral inhibition, is a parallel kind of inhibitory action in distinction to feedback inhibition which is the basis of serial processing.

far into the brain in spite of many unsuccessful attempts to do so. These facts all suggest that some sort of "feedforward" process biases perception (Mackay, 1966; Mittelstaedt, 1968).

Neurological evidence in support of a feedforward, or "corollary" discharge as Teuber (1960) has called it, has been obtained recently but is as yet indirect and incomplete. Neurons within the central stations of the input systems discharge whenever eye movements occur (Bizzi, 1966a, 1966b; see also Figs. 5-4 and 5-5). Furthermore, identifiable neurological patterns occur in the visual cortex *prior* to the onset of a response; these patterns appear to be specific to a particular response and are present only after the organism (a monkey) has learned the solution to the task in which the responses are made (Pribram, Spinelli, and Kamback, 1967). These "intention patterns" will be discussed in detail in Chapters 7 and 17.

a test–operate–test–exit process (TOTE)

The reflex arc has to cope with all this evidence. Obviously the simplest, most direct modification of Sherrington's fiction is to add an output from the central nervous system to the receptor. The consequences of this apparently minor addition are far from trivial. Imagine for a moment that, isolated from other stimu-

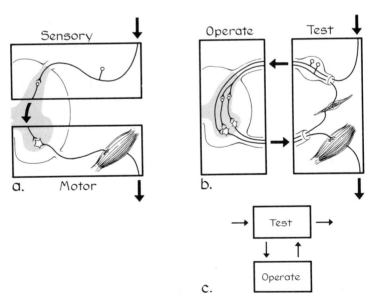

Fig. 5-6. Development of the TOTE from the reflex arc concept. Note that the γ-connectivity of the muscle spindle demands that a "test" be performed.

lation, you are monitoring receptor activity from its afferent. When a change occurs how would you know whether that change was the result of an event outside the organism or whether something within the central nervous system was modifying receptor activity? Some computation, some test must be applied to discern "reality"—i.e., a stimulus originating outside the organism (Fig. 5-6).

Much behavioral evidence supports the concept that some sort of active test is performed on input. Many of the pertinent observations result from experiments in which the visual image is distorted or inverted by prism glasses worn by the subject for a prolonged time. Given an opportunity to move about and manipulate his environment, an organism can right his perceptual world in a matter of hours or days (depending on the extent of the distortion). Should such manipulation or movement be proscribed, however, there is considerable delay in the correction of the distortion if it can be accomplished at all. The manipulative experience appears integral to some phase of the construction of the corrective mechanism (Held, 1968; Howard, Craske, and Templeton, 1965; Figs. 5-7, 5-8).

To gain some insight into the power of this testing mechanism, try the following. Next time you encounter a nonmoving "up" escalator step onto it and note that the stairs appear to be moving upward for a few seconds. You may indeed need to grab hold of the arm rail to keep from falling when the discrepant somatic sensation of nonmovement is felt. As you stand the moving sensation quickly stops. Now begin to ascend the steps; again you'll have a sensation of a moving staircase. The "movement" appears as a specific bias attached by experience to escalators (ordinary stairs are not sensed as moving), a bias enhanced by one's own movements with respect to the escalator.

The fact that the testing process depends so heavily on the opportunity for manipulation of the environment has led to the suggestion that perception is in essence a "motor" phenomenon (Sperry, 1952; Festinger et al., 1967). Such views maintain that perception per se is more a reflection of the response patterns instigated in the brain by an input than it is a resultant of the input patterns. This appears an extreme view—taken to its logical and absurd conclusion it would mean that we would perceive every woman on the street as Aphrodite (and in whatever state of dress or undress we are set to see her at the moment) and every man as Adonis. There is, of course, some truth to this—"beauty" is to a large extent in the eye of the beholder. Yet the distortions of perception that are ordinarily possible are limited. When they go beyond these limits we speak of them as illusions and hallucinations. And though any account of the perceptual process must take into consideration

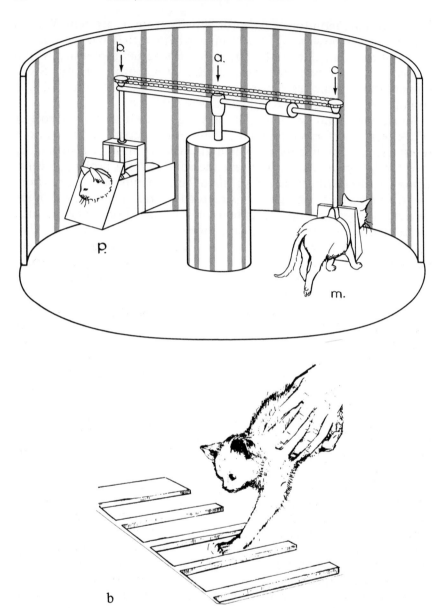

Fig. 5-7. (A) Apparatus for passively transporting one kitten (p) via mechanical linkage to an actively moving kitten (m). Movements are about the axes labeled a, b, c. (B) Apparatus for testing visually guided reach. From Hein, *Human Neuroanatomy,* 6 ed. © 1967 The Williams & Wilkins Co., Baltimore, Md.

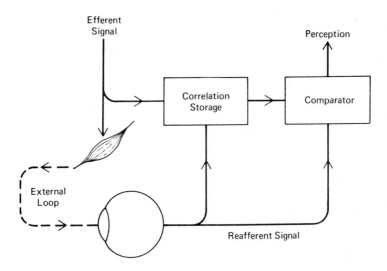

Fig. 5-8. Held's proposed model for the correlation and recor-relation of efferent signals with visual (reafferent) signals from the eye. Note similarity to connectivity shown in Fig. 5-5. The comparator represents the test phase of the feed-forward pro-cess. Held's conception differs from the TOTE (see Fig. 5-9) in that there is no feedback between comparator and correlation storage. From Dodwell, 1970. After Held, 1961 as reprinted in 1962.

the possibility of the production of illusions and hallucinations, the account need not make illusion and hallucination the perceptual way of life.

A generalized diagram of the reflex, the unit of neurobehavioral analysis, can therefore be attempted (see TOTE Fig. 5-9). To be effective, input must be compared to and tested against spontaneous or corollary central neural activity; the results of this comparison initiate some operation which then influences either other parts of the nervous system or the external world. The consequences of this operation are then fed back to the comparator and the loop con-tinues until the test has been satisfied—until some previous setting, indicative of a state-to-be-achieved, has been attained (exit).

This modification of the reflex arc results in a diagram familiar to engineers. Tracking devices of various sorts are built to just such specifications. The apparatus, known as a servomechanism, is essen-tially a mechanism whereby the effects of an input are matched against the effects of the outcome of an activity aimed to deal with that input. The thermostat is probably the most familiar available servomechanism.

The reflex arc was a conception used by Sherrington to explain data he had before him. The success of his explanations made the reflex arc an extremely useful fiction. The TOTE diagram is also a fiction when applied to neurobehavioral analysis. It is a somewhat higher-order fiction than the reflex arc—the reflex arc is the limiting case of a servo in which feedback can be accomplished only via the organism's environment and in which the operation performed is insensitive even to this feedback, i.e., the effect, once initiated, runs itself off to a predetermined state. The usefulness of a higher order fiction must lie in its ability to handle a larger range of facts. The TOTE concept was brought to bear for just this reason: the reflex arc cannot encompass the data that demonstrate the central control of receptor mechanisms. Further, the TOTE concept can handle a variety of other neurobehavioral observations, such as the treatment of adaptation and habituation in Chapter 3. Yet, it is important to bear in mind that the neurobehavioral TOTE just as the reflex arc, is but a fiction and should be supplanted or supplemented whenever it is found restrictive rather than useful. The expanded though still oversimplified TOTE shown in Fig. 5-9, for instance, more clearly diagrams the relationship between feedback and feedforward and the

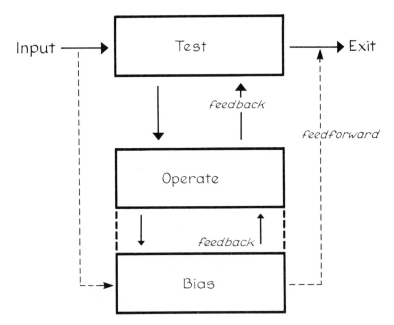

Fig. 5-9. The TOTE servomechanism modified to include feedforward. Note the parallel processing feature of the revised TOTE.

role of coding, memory, and bias in the neurobehavioral process than did our earlier version. As an overall improvement on the reflex arc, however, the TOTE conception is central to any development of a reasonably coherent view of neurobehavioral organization. (See Miller, Galanter, and Pribram, 1960, for one such coherent view.)

summary of the two process mechanism

Part I has has been concerned with bringing together a wealth of disparate facts about the brain and its control of behavior to form some simplified scheme that can serve as an anchor for further thought and exploration. The scheme adopted is the TOTE, a logic "element" made up of two reciprocally related processes: (1) the "test," a state composed of junctional (synaptic and dendritic) potentials, and (2) an "operation" on that state by nerve impulses generated by receptors or by the central nervous system. This two process logic element is, of course, an oversimplified abstraction from the data. But I want to emphasize the usefulness of this TOTE concept for our time and research purposes just as Sherrington emphasized the usefulness of the reflex arc for his.

The state or bias part of the mechanism has built into it contrast enhancement achieved through surround inhibition. Testing (comparing input against existing state) involves among other factors, a process of spatial superposition of the excitatory and inhibitory interactions among neighboring neural elements. The operator part of the mechanism involves, among other mechanisms, a decrementing process, a damping of the changes initiated by input in each neuron or neuronal pool. Spatial superposition enhances contrast and thus facilitates coding; decrementing serves as one of a number of forms of memory storage (Fig. 5-10).

Because of the spontaneous activity of neuronal aggregates, whether cyclic or programmed, changes in state are initiated not only from the environment but by the brain as well. This fact, in addition to the ubiquitous presence of central control over receptor function, makes almost useless the reflex-arc, stimulus-response conception of neurobehavioral organization, let alone of psychological function. The next parts will document this need to view behaving, sentient organisms—especially man—as other than passive responders to the exigencies of environment:

Western thought has alternated between two views of man's relations to his universe. One view holds that he is an essentially passive organism shaped by the exigencies of his environment. The other emphasizes his active role, manipulative and selective not only of artifacts but of sense data as well. The

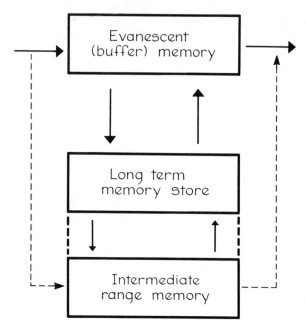

Fig. 5-10. Memory in a TOTE context.

neuropsychological contributions to behavioral science strongly support the active view and thus point to a resurgence of the dignity of man as a scientific as well as a political and humanistic tenet. [Pribram, Neuropsychology in America (Voice of America Lecture, 1959). In B. Berelson (ed.), *The Behavioral Sciences Today*. New York: Basic Books, pp. 110–11.]

synopsis

The two-process proposal of brain function derives from yet another set of data. Classically, the function of the nervous system has been conceived as a direct input-output, stimulus-response device expressed neurologically as a reflex-arc. The ubiquitous presence of feedback and feedforward mechanisms (e.g., central nervous system control of receptor function) necessitates a modification of this view. Feedback and Feedforward are best conceptualized as a Test-Operate-Test-Exit (TOTE) servomechanism, an elementary neural logic structure of which more complex neural organizations are composed. The Test phase of the logic expresses the junctional, the Operate phase the nerve-impulse portion of the two-process mechanism of brain function.

part 2

the organization of
psychological processes

"The brain is a machine for making analogical models."

Craik (quoted by McCulloch, 1965)

images

A major problem of neurobehavioral research is to determine in what respect and to what extent brain processes and psychological functions are coordinate. Part I sought to develop a coherent language, a coherent set of terms derived from observation and experiment on the brain's simplest organizing mechanisms. Part II addresses psychological functions by an experimental analysis of the verbal reports of subjective experiences. Over the past half century subjective experience has rarely been admitted as a legitimate field for scientific inquiry. Instead, the focus of study has been instrumental or verbal behavior per se. This approach has been generally successful in quantitatively delineating environmental variables that influence behavior, but somewhat less than successful when variables within the organism codetermine what happens. In such circumstances the data make considerably more sense when physiological as well as environmental variables are monitored. It is important to emphasize that the behavioral approach cannot, however, be dispensed with: many clinical neurologists and brain physiologists have neglected specification of relevant environmental circumstance, uncritically asserting an identity between what they observe physiologically and some psychological function. Thus the study of psychological processes had become polarized, with behaviorists at one extreme and physiologists at the other. On the one hand, most early behaviorists declared that operations defining subjective statements were impossible and that scientific psychological language should, therefore, entirely exclude mental terms; meanwhile, medically trained scientists would loosely refer to psychological functions such as voluntary action, affective feeling, or imagination on the basis of uncontrolled subjective reports without specifying the defining operations of their language, thus making it difficult for other scientists to know just what was being talked about.

During the 1960s behavioral psychology came to appreciate the dictum of Gestalt psychology that subjective awareness is an integral part of the biological and social universe and is too central to the operations of behavior to be ignored. Thus "respectable" psychologists began to work on problems such as cognition, thought, and attention. By the end of the decade even Imaging, our present subject, could be discussed openly at psychological meetings without undue risk.

This broadening of the base of psychological inquiry came about, of course, by a rigorous attempt to detail the defining operations that make possible scientific communication about subjective processes. My own procedure (Fig. 6-1) is to start with nonbehavioral means to describe categories of organismic and environmental circumstances. I then use behavior as a dependent variable to study interactions between the categories (which constitute the independent variables of the experiment). From data obtained in such experiments I *infer* psychological functions and examine their similarities and dissimilarities to verbal reports of subjective experience. When the fit appears right, I use mental language (Pribram, 1962; 1970).

This recourse to mental terms is not capricious. For one thing, much of clinical neurological analysis is based on the verbal reports of subjective experience when the brain is damaged or electrically stimulated. Further, I found the behaviorist jargon (with which I had been doing my thinking) replete with inconsistencies that couldn't be clarified until I admitted the relevance of the subjective mode. In other words, I had to come to terms with Gilbert Ryle's (1949) famous "Ghosts in the Machine." Images and feelings are ghosts—but they are ghosts that inhabit my own and my patients' subjective worlds. They are our constant companions and I want to explain them. They reside "in" that machine called the brain, yet they

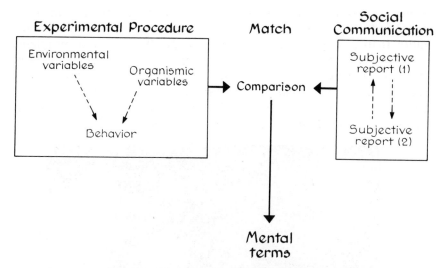

Fig. 6-1. Diagram of brain-behavior relationships

cannot be pointed at. If we ignore them, all we have is a behaving machine. I am interested in the ghosts, the psychological functions— not just the machine/brain nor just its regulation of overt behavior.

As this book developed it became clear that some progress could be made by considering the relation between brain, behavior, and psychological functions in the light of the two-process mechanism of brain function. Could it be that ghosts such as Images and feelings occur as a function of the organization of states in the brain? This part of the book pursues some answers to this question while Part III is based on its complement: could behavioral action be realized when neural operations based on these states take place?

awareness - an hypothesis

Much of the neurological and behavioral evidence regarding Imaging focuses on the techniques used to determine how pattern perception occurs. How do patterns come to be perceived? Not only psychologists and neurologists but also engineers are concerned with this question. Pattern "perception" by machine is obviously useful in such pursuits as language translation and the development of recognition devices. Currently, pattern sensing devices have become important to the construction of robots and automata which can function in lieu of man in a variety of limited situations. Even in these circumscribed endeavors, creation of a stored and available representation of the environment in which the robot is to function is essential. Such a machine (Fig. 6-3) can solve more than a very limited and circumstance-bound set of problems once it has some "map" of the terrain in which it is to operate. Pattern "perceiving" devices build up in one manner or another a spatially coded representation, a map, of their experience. Thus they can "learn" to respond differentially to a particular pattern: they can "recognize" the familiar, and distinguish the novel.

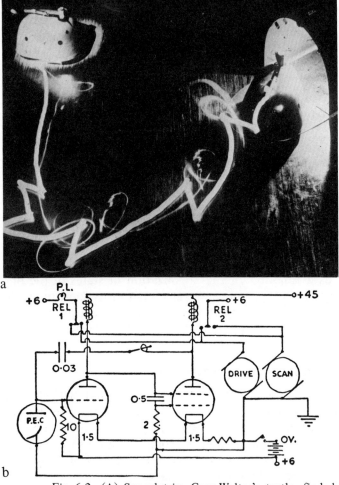

Fig. 6-2. (A) Speculatrix, Grey-Walter's turtle, finds her way home. (B) Circuit diagram of Speculatrix. From Walter, 1953. Reprinted from *The Living Brain* by W. Grey Walter. By permission of W.W. Norton & Company, Inc. Copyright © 1963, 1953 by W.W. Norton & Company, Inc.

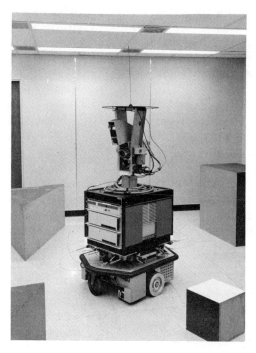
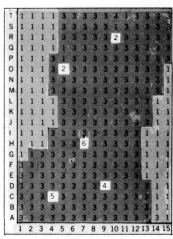

a   b

Fig. 6-3. (A) The Wanderer, a robot developed at Stanford Research Institute. (B) The Wanderer is a self-navigating robot that explores a strange room by dividing it into imaginary regions and registering in each region what it has perceived. This image then becomes the robot's cognitive "world map." From Block and Ginsburg, 1970.

Automata can, of course, be constructed without recourse to a map: Grey Walter's turtle (1953; Fig. 6-2) and Ross Ashby's homeostat (1960) are two early examples of a host of artifacts constructed to move, avoid objects, select paths. Unless fitted with another device—one that can react to patterns—these early artifacts were, however, limited in their behavioral repertoire.

Psychologists during the early period of the ascendency of behaviorism also attempted to explain the behavior of organisms and especially the learning process without using the concept "Image." Very quickly it became apparent that without some intervening construct such as a "map" (Tolman, 1932) the explanatory power of the behavioral observations were, though certainly possible, considerably limited in scope. Recently the importance of the Image concept has started to be recognized: cognitive psychologists analyzing the process of verbal learning have been faced with a variety of Imaging processes which demand neurological underpinnings.

Why, then, should there be any hesitancy in accepting Imaging as a worthwhile and powerful explanatory principle? Two very good reasons: (1) until recently there was little, if any, rigorous experimental evidence about how Imaging might occur, and (2) there was great difficulty in conceiving of a neurological mechanism that would make and store, in available form, a spatially encoded representation of experience.

The reasons for hesitancy no longer hold. Recent behavioral research has put a foundation under Imaging, and neurological research as well as insights derived from the information-processing sciences, have helped make understandable the machinery which gives rise to this elusive ghost-making process. This evidence forms the current and the next few chapters.

Any model we make of perceptual processes must thus take into account both the importance of Imaging, a process that contributes a portion of man's subjective experience, and the fact that there are influences on behavior of which we are not aware. Instrumental behavior and awareness are often opposed—the more efficient a performance, the less aware we become. Sherrington noted this antagonism in a succinct statement: "Between reflex action and mind there seems to be actual opposition. Reflex action and mind seem almost mutually exclusive—the more reflex the reflex, the less does mind accompany it." Thus the danger that a range of problems is ignored if the focus of inquiry is purely behavioristic. Here I want to dwell just on these often ignored problems. (Discrimination behavior, pattern recognition, and similar categorizations encompass more than what this and the next two chapters are about. However, what is said here is relevant to the larger problems which are discussed in Chapters 14 and 17.)

The reciprocal relationship between awareness and behavior is perhaps best illuminated by the psychological processes of habit and habituation. If an organism is repeatedly exposed to the same situation, is placed in an invariant environment, two things happen. If he consistently has to perform a similar task in that environment, the task becomes fairly automatic, i.e., he becomes more efficient. The organism has learned to perform the task; he has formed *habits* regarding it. At the same time the subject habituates: he no longer produces an orienting reaction; he no longer notices the events constant to this particular task in this environment. His verbal reports of introspection, his failure to move his head and eyes in the direction of the stimulus, and electrophysiological measures such as galvanic skin response, plethysmography and EEG, all attest to the disappearance of orienting when unvarying input in an unvarying situation is repeated. As noted, however, habituation is not an indication of some loss of sensitivity on the part of the nervous system but rather the development of a neural model of the environment, a representation, an expectancy, a type of memory mechanism against which inputs are constantly matched. The nervous system is thus continually tuned *by* inputs to process further inputs.

The habitual performance of the organism also results from neural activity. In the case of expectancy, input processing appears to diminish with repetition; in the case of performance, enhanced efficiency of output processing apparently occurs. So the question is: What is the difference between the two kinds of neural activity that make awareness inversely related to habit and habituation?

Nerve impulses and slow potentials are two kinds of processes that could function reciprocally. A simple hypothesis would state that the more efficient the processing of arrival patterns into departure patterns, the shorter the duration of the design formed by the slow potential junctional microstructure. Once habit and habituation have occurred behavior becomes "reflex"—meanwhile the more or less persistent designs of slow potential patterns are coordinate with awareness. This view carries a corollary, *viz.* that nerve impulse patterns per se and the behavior they generate are unavailable to immediate awareness. Thus, even the production of speech is "unconscious" at the moment the words are spoken. My hypothesis, therefore, is an old-fashioned one: we experience in awareness some of the events going on in the brain, but not all of them.

In short, nerve impulses arriving at junctions generate a slow potential microstructure. The design of this microstructure interacts with that already present by virtue of the spontaneous activity of the nervous system and its previous "experience." The interaction is enhanced by inhibitory processes and the whole procedure produces effects akin to the interference patterns resulting from the interaction of simultaneously occurring wave fronts. The slow potential microstructures act thus as analogue cross-correlation devices to produce new figures from which the patterns of departure of nerve impulses are initiated. The rapidly paced changes in awareness could well reflect the duration of the correlation process.

What evidence suggests that the junctional electrical activities of the central nervous system are involved in awareness? Joseph Kamiya (1968) and others (Galbraith, et al., 1970; Engstrom, London, and Hart, 1971) have shown, using instrumental-conditioning techniques,

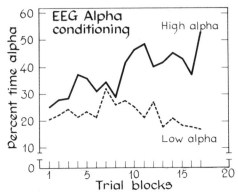

Fig. 6-4. Graph of results of one-minute trials in which subjects were asked to maintain the emission of alpha waves (unbroken line), then to suppress them (broken line). From Kamiya, 1970.

that people can readily be taught to discriminate whether or not their brains are producing certain wave forms which repeat approximately 10 times per second, the so-called alpha rhythms, even though they have difficulty in labeling the difference in the states of awareness they perceive. Subjects who have been able to label the "alpha rhythm state" claim that it is one of pleasantly relaxed awareness. More experiments of this kind are now being carried out in order to find ways to shorten the long educational process currently entailed in Zen, Yogi, and western psychotherapeutic procedures aimed at identifying and achieving pleasant states (Fig. 6-4).

More specific are some of Ben Libet's recent experiments (1966) that have explored a well-known phenomenon. Since the demonstrations in the 1880s by Gustav Fritsch and Eduard Hitzig (1969) that electrical stimulation of certain parts of man's brain results in movement, neurosurgeons have explored its entire surface to determine what reactions such stimulations produce. For instance, Ottfried Foerster (1936) mapped regions in the post-central gyrus which give rise to awareness of one or another part of the body (Fig. 6-5). Thus sensations of tingling or of positioning can be produced in the absence of any observable changes in the body part experienced by the patient. Libet has shown that the awareness produced by stimulation is not immediate: a minimum of a half second and maximum of five seconds elapses before the patient experiences anything. It appears that the electrical stimulation must set up some state in the brain tissue, and only when that state has been attained does the patient become aware (Fig. 6-6).

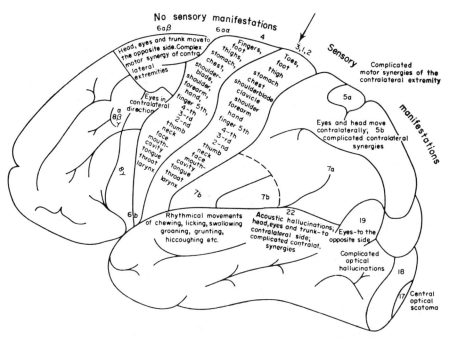

Fig. 6-5. Summary of data given by Ottfried Foerster on results of stimulation of various points of the human cortical hemisphere (1926). From Bernstein, © 1967. Reprinted with permission from Pergamon Press Ltd.

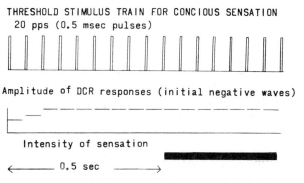

THRESHOLD STIMULUS TRAIN FOR CONCIOUS SENSATION
20 pps (0.5 msec pulses)

Amplitude of DCR responses (initial negative waves)

Intensity of sensation

⟵――――― 0.5 sec ――――⟶

Fig. 6-6. Diagram of relationships between the train of 0.5 msec pulses at liminal intensity applied to postcentral gyrus, and the amplitudes of the direct cortical responses (DCR) recorded nearby. The third line indicates that no conscious sensory experience is elicited until approximately the initial 0.5 sec. of events has elapsed, and that the just detectable sensation appearing after that period remains at the same subjective intensity while the stimulus train continues. From Libet, 1966.

perceiving

In many ways the hypothesis presented so far in this chapter is crucial to the consistent view of the functions of the nervous system being developed. It is also controversial. Part I of the book reviewed the logical operations performed by the nervous system. Here I want to show how these operations make it possible for the organism to be aware of the here and now, to perceive the existential present.

The problem is this: look at a friend, then look at his neighbor, and you are immediately aware that they are different. Further, there is little, if any, interference between what you see at one moment and what you see at the next. In the auditory mode such transient rapidly paced recognitions—of musical phrases, of phonemic combinations of speech, etc—are the commonplace of communication. Ordinary views of the functions of the nervous system have considerable difficulty explaining the immediacy, precision, and apparent multidimensionality of evanescent awareness. Here a unique process must be in operation. How might it work?

Donald Hebb reviewed the problem incisively in the first three chapters of his classic volume on *The Organization of Behavior* (1949). He states: "One must decide whether perception is to depend (1) on the excitation of *specific cells* or (2) on a *pattern of excitation* whose locus is unimportant." Hebb makes his choice: "a particular perception depends on the excitation of *particular cells at some point* in the central nervous system."

As neurophysiological evidence has accumulated (especially through the microelectrode experiments of Jung (1961); Mountcastle (1957); Maturana, Lettvin, McCulloch, and Pitts (1960); Hubel and Wiesel (1962)); this choice appears vindicated: the microelectrode studies have identified neural units responsive only to one or another attribute of a stimulating event such as directionality of movement, tilt of line, etc. Today, the body of neurophysiological opinion would, I believe, agree with Hebb that one percept corresponds to one neural unit (see, for example, Fig. 6-7).

The hypothesis brought forward in the first section of this chapter argues that Hebb's choice is a Hobson's choice, that patterns of excitation must, of course, depend for their origin upon the excitation of specific cells but that the patterns become to some extent independent of cells as units and become instead the designs imposed by the *junctional* anatomy, the synaptic and dendritic microstructure of the brain. These designs serve, in the proper circumstances, as the neurological equivalents of percepts. I will agree with Hebb's assumption that what one recognizes depends a good deal on the previous

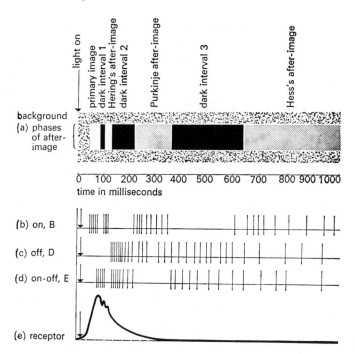

Fig. 6-7. Correlations of subjective visual after-image of man and neuronal discharges in retina and visual cortex of the cat, following a brief light flash of 300 lux (modified from Grusser and Grutzner, 1958). (a) Scheme of successive phases of after-images (according to Frohlich, 1929). Time in milliseconds. (b to d) Schematic responses of retinal on, off, and on-off neurons and different response classes (B, D, E) of cortical neurons. (e) Receptor response of the outer plexiform layer of the retina obtained with intracellular recording.

The light flash is marked by a descending arrow. In (b-e) the arrows are shifted to the right because in Frohlich's experiment latency of conscious experience is 20 to 40 msec. longer than the latency of cat cortical neurons. The shaded area surrounding the after-images signifies the background of observation and the Eigengrau of the eye.

The scheme combines retinal and cortical responses, although cortical neurons show lower frequency and stronger periodicity. A pause in the primary activation of cortical B neurons is concurrent with the initial E discharge. During longer illumination both correspond to the bande noire of Charpentier (Jung, 1961) and after short flashes probably to dark interval 1. The scheme of Grusser and Grutzner has been corrected appropriately as they also described a pause in on-off neurons between 200 and 450 msec. From Jung, 1969.

experience one has had, but I will differentiate from this the direct immediacy of an Imaged psychological present, its existential complexity upon which the holistic Gestalt argument on perception depends. In his approach Hebb has confused the historical development of the recognition process and what is Imaged. It takes many hours of labor to construct a program which allows a computer to make calculations—the calculations are performed by the built-in machinery of the computer in microseconds. It takes many hours to learn to recognize unfamiliar patterns, but infants a few weeks old (see Chapter 8) have been shown to correctly estimate the relative size of figures placed at various distances (size constancy) and to distinguish a figure presented in various rotations (shape constancy). Learning is only part of the problem of what is recognized. The Gestaltists were in large measure correct in their nativism. There are inherited built-in neural mechanisms that give rise to Imaging, but the Gestaltists were wrong in suggesting that this is the entire story of perception. Now, however, the pendulum has swung far in the other direction and there is danger that a whole bevy of interesting phenomena will be neglected because of an exclusive interest in the problem of how we *learn* to recognize.

When Hebb wrote his book there were two general views of the operation of the nervous system. One was well substantiated, the other was not. The well substantiated view dealt with the generation of nerve impulses and their transmission across connnections between nerves. The other view dealt with fields of electrical potentials. Wolfgang Köhler based his Gestalt arguments on these neuroelectrical fields and went out to prove their ubiquitous existence in the decade after the publication of Hebb's statement.

I was fortunate to be able to partake in these explorations. The experimental attack proved successful (Köhler, 1958), and others in my laboratory and elsewhere have recorded and imposed direct current fields and shown correlations with neural function and behavior (Gumnit, 1961; Stamm, 1961; Morrell, 1961). D.C. fields restricted to the appropriate region are generated when an organism is stimulated through one or another sensory portal (Fig. 6-8). The imposition of D.C. fields directly on the brain can retard or speed learning depending on the polarity of the imposed potential. But Köhler and I disagreed when he insisted on the connection between the D.C. fields and perception. Later, when I had finished the experiments in which I implanted aluminum hydroxide cream over the cortical surface, we were again able to come to terms. The experiments showed that pattern discrimination performance remains intact despite marked disruption of D.C. and E.E.G. activity

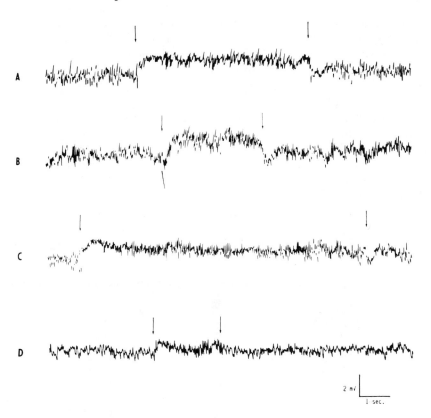

Fig. 6-8. Direct Current Field responses from auditory area in response to auditory stimulation. "Active electrode" on dura overlying middle ectosylvian gyrus; other electrode on frontal periosteum. Upward deflection indicates dura negative with respect to bone. (A) Shift in response to white noise. (B) Shift in response to tone of 4000 Hertz. (C) Shift in response to white noise returning to baseline before end of auditory stimulation. (D) Response to 50 clicks/sec. returning to baseline before end of stimulation. From Gumnit, 1960.

(Figs. 6-9, 6-10). Köhler had never accepted experiments performed by Lashley (Lashley, Chow, and Semmes, 1951) in which gold foil was used to distort neuroelectric fields as evidence against his theory, nor did he yield to Sperry's crosshatches (Sperry, Miner, and Meyers, 1955) into which insulating mica strips had been placed. But when faced with the evidence from the aluminum hydroxide cream implantations he exclaimed: "that ruins not only my D.C. field but every other current neurological theory of perception."

Let me briefly review the evidence which has accrued since that conversation to dispel for me this dismal view of the neurology of perception. As detailed in Part I, nerve impulse is but one of the important electrical characteristics of neural tissue. Another characteristic is the slow potential microstructure. Though slow potentials are akin to Köhler's D.C. fields, they differ importantly in that they are not diffuse but sharply localized at the junctions between neurons or in dendrites where they may even be miniature spikes that more often than not attenuate when they begin to propagate. Nerve impulse conduction leads everywhere in the central nervous system to the organization of a junctional slow potential microstructure. When nerve impulses arrive at synapses, post-synaptic potentials are generated. These are never solitary but constitute an arrival pattern. When post-synaptic potentials occur in dendritic fields of the brain they are often insufficiently large to immediately incite nerve im-

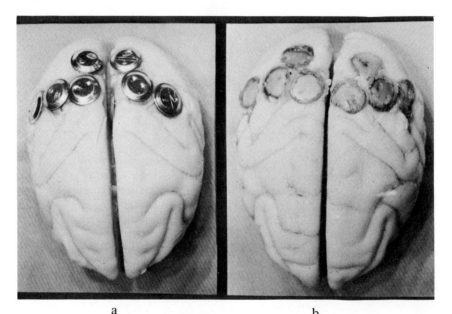

a   b

Fig. 6-9. (A) Photograph of monkey brain with implanted silver discs containing aluminum hydroxide cream. (B) Photograph of same brain after removal of discs. In this instance the implantations were performed on the parietal cortex. Other experiments on the occipital, temporal; and frontal cortex were performed in a similar fashion or else multiple minute punctate injections of aluminum hydroxide cream were made into the cortex. From Stamm and Warren, 1961.

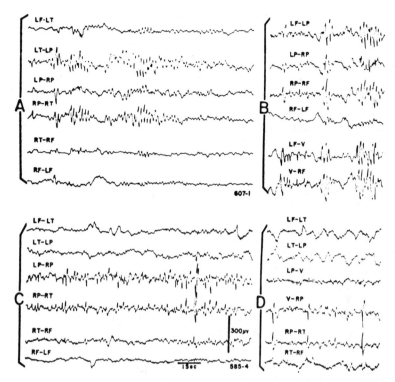

Fig. 6-10. Samples of EEG from two monkeys implanted as shown in Fig. 6-9. A and B are traces from one recording taken preoperatively. C and D show traces from a recording taken five months after implantation of alumina cream. Bipolar scalp recordings between locations indicated: L: left, R: right hemisphere; F: frontal; T: temporal; P: posterior parietal and V: vertex. Calibrations as indicated. From Stamm and Warren, 1961.

pulse discharge. So these patterns of post-synaptic potentials develop a design which resembles a wave front. But this design of slow potentials is not some esoteric field, a mirage superimposed on known neural function—it is a microstructure made up of classical neural slow potentials, the resultant of arrivals of nerve impulses awaiting axonic departure.

Arrival and departure patterns conceived as microstructures thus become a third force in the cell versus "floating" field argument about the possible neurological mechanism of the holistic properties of perception. The need for this third force has been recognized before. Lashley was profoundly troubled by the problem:

Here is the dilemma. Nerve impulses are transmitted over definite, restricted paths in the sensory and motor nerves and in the central nervous system from cell to cell through definite intercellular connections. Yet all behavior seems to be determined by masses of excitation, by the form or relations or proportions of excitation within general fields of activity, without regard to particular nerve cells. It is the pattern and not the element that counts. What sort of nervous organization might be capable of responding to a pattern of excitation without limited, specialized paths of conduction? The problem is almost universal in the activities of the nervous system and some hypothesis is needed to direct further research. [Lashley, 1942, p. 306]

Subsequently, he suggested that an interference pattern model would account for the phenomena more adequately than either of the more extreme views. He did not, however, have available to him a clear model of how the mechanism might work. He never specified the fact that the "waves" generated by arrivals of nerve impulses are constituted of well known and classical neurophysiological processes: synaptic and dendritic potentials. He thus never arrived at the argument for the existence of a junctional microstructure partially independent of nerve impulse conduction developed in these pages. This left his wave forms both too much tied to the neuronal circuitry he found unsatisfactory, and at the same time disembodied when flexibility needed to be accounted for. He was thus discouraged from pursuing his insight. Nonetheless, a most incisive insight it has proved to be as will become evident. Let me pause for a moment for a quotation that gives the essence of his thinking:

The anatomic studies of Lorente de No have revealed a system of cross connections in the cortex which will permit the spread of excitation in any direction along the surface. Many adjacent neurons are capable of mutual excitation and the whole system is organized as a network, with loops of various lengths and complexity, capable of transmitting impulses from cell to cell across the cortex, or of reexciting initial points of stimulation by the action of return circuits having diverse characteristics.

From such a structural organization functional properties may be inferred with some confidence. Excitation started at any point must spread from that point throughout the system, since extinction (through buildup of activity in reverberatory circuits) will occur only after the passage of the initial impulse. If the system is uniform throughout, a series of radiating waves should be produced, since the first wave of excitation will be followed by a wave of extinction, with excitation following again, either from successive volleys arriving over sensory pathways or by reexcitation at the retreating margin of the zone of extinction. The timing of the waves should be uniform, since it is dependent upon the speed of conduction and the refractory periods of the elements of the system. With several or many points of excitation, interference patterns will be formed.

Disregarding for the moment the effects of return circuits in order to get a simplified picture, the action should be somewhat analogous to the transmission of waves on the surface of a fluid medium. Interference of waves in such a system produces a pattern of crests and troughs which is characteristic for each spatial distribution of the sources of wave motion and which is reduplicated roughly over the entire surface. A somewhat similar patterning of excitations in the plane of the cortex is to be expected. Spatially distributed impulses reaching the cortex from the retina will not reproduce the retinal pattern of excitation in the cortex but will give rise to a different and characteristic pattern of standing waves, reduplicated throughout the extent of the functional area. An immediate objection is that the excitation of one part of the field may render that part refractory to impulses coming from other parts, and so block the formation of a uniform pattern. However, if the transcortical paths of reverberatory circuits are of random length, as they apparently are, not all in any region will be simultaneously in a refractory state and blocking will not occur. [Lashley, 1942, pp. 312–14]

The next chapters will develop what is perhaps a more currently tenable view of the "third force" in the neurology of perception, a view based on the existence both of neurons and of the junctional microstructure.

synopsis

Early behaviorists vehemently rejected the study of subjective experience. The resulting neglect severely restricted the scope of psychology. The two-process mechanism of brain function remedies this limitation by providing objective techniques and a conceptual tool, the junctional mechanism, with which to study perceptual Images and also emotional and motivational feelings.

features

some neuroanatomical problems in perception

Among the major deterrents to understanding the neurology of the perceptual process has been one of those discrepancies, one of the paradoxes which we have in these chapters recurrently encountered in the attempts to link functions of the nervous system with psychological processes. In the present instance the paradox concerns the neuroanatomical organization of the input system and the effects on behavior of disruptions of that organization (see Fig. 7-1).

In essence, the anatomical arrangement of input systems is one which preserves a topological correspondence between receptor surface and the cerebral cortex. This means, e.g., that an arrangement of points on the retina will be projected onto the cortex as a similar arrangement of points. Thus maps of retinal-cortical correspondence can be drawn—deriving the data for such maps from the effect of small lesions within the input systems on tracts made by the resulting degeneration of nerve fibers (Browuer, 1934; Browuer and Zeeman, 1926), or by electrically or photically stimulating points on the

116

retina and recording the cortical locus in which electrical responses can be evoked (Talbot and Marshall, 1941). Similar maps have been made in the somesthetic system; and the cochlear-cortical auditory mechanism is also arranged in this fashion (Rose and Woolsey, 1949).

This receptor-cortical organization is not accomplished via a point-to-point direct connection by a single nerve strand. Rather, a complex organization much as that we have already examined at the

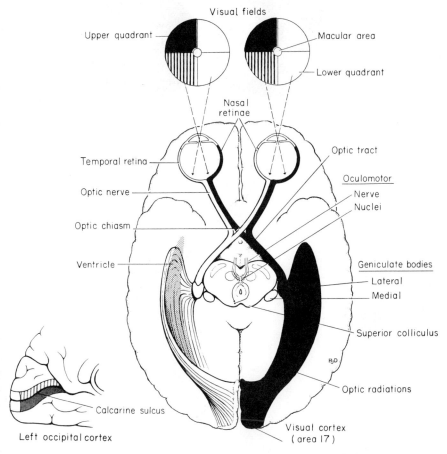

Fig. 7-1. Diagram of the visual pathways viewed from the ventral surface of the brain. Light from the upper half of the visual field falls on the inferior half of the retina. Light from the temporal half of the visual field falls on the nasal half of the retina, while light from the nasal half of the visual field falls on the temporal half of the retina. From Truex and Carpenter, *Human Neuroanatomy*, 6 ed. ©1969 The Williams & Wilkins Co., Baltimore, Md.

retina is replicated at every station of the input mechanism and also at the cortex. In effect, an overall reduction in the number of cells occurs between the receptor and ganglion cell layer of the retina (the reduction is approximately one hundred and fifty to one in man). From the ganglion cell layer to the lateral geniculate nucleus in the thalamus the number of optic elements remains essentially constant.

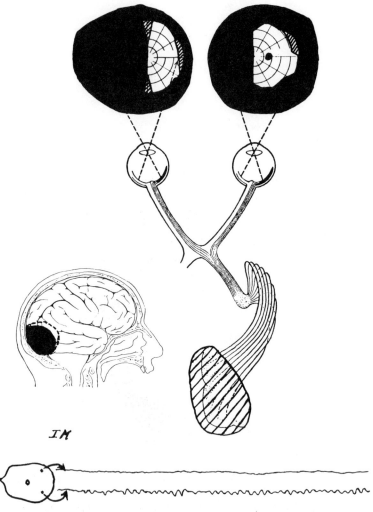

Fig. 7-2. Map of the visual field, diagram of the anatomy of the visual system showing lesion, and tracings of the EEG of a 20 year old girl with a lesion of the right occipital lobe. From Case, 1942.

From thalamus to cortex the reverse of the retinal situation holds: a single geniculate cell may contact 5000 cortical neurons, each of which is in contact with some 4000 others through its dendritic fields. This arrangement, aided by inhibitory interactions, insures that, despite some overlap, when two points in the retinal fovea of monkey are stimulated clear separation is maintained so that two minutes of retinal arc are separated at the cortical surface by 1 mm (Marshall and Talbot, 1941, p. 134). One would think such an arrangement to be compatible with projecting some sort of "image" from the receptor surface onto the cortical surface much as a photographic image is projected onto the film plane surface in a camera.

The paradox appears when the input systems become damaged, either through disease or surgery. True, as expected, a hole (scotoma) can, under the appropriate circumstances, be demonstrated in the visual field in the location predicted from the anatomical arrangement (Fig. 7-2). Yet with even the smallest part of the input mechanism intact, this hole is often unperceived even with the eyes held stationary, and pattern recognition, in many respects indistinguishable from the normal, remains possible. People with huge scotomata either are wholly unaware of them or can soon learn to get about easily by ignoring them. An animal in whom 80 to 98 percent of the input mechanism has been removed or interrupted is able to solve problems requiring discriminations of patterns differing only in detail. Lashley (1929) removed 80–90 percent of the striate cortex of rats without impairing their ability to discriminate patterns. Robert Galambos cut up to 98 percent of the optic tracts of cats and the animals could still perform skillfully on tests necessitating the differentiation of highly similar figures (Galambos, Norton, and Frommer, 1967). In a recent experiment, KaoLiang Chow (1970), also working with cats, severed more than three-fourths of the optic tract and removed more than three-fourths of the visual cortex; hardly any of the point-to-point projection system remained intact. Although visual discrimination of patterns became disturbed initially by such drastic interference, the animals relearned the task in about the same number of trials required to learn prior to surgery.

In my experience both in clinical neurosurgery and in the laboratory (e.g., Wilson and Mishkin, 1959), *limited* removals restricted to cortex that do not massively invade white matter leave the patient or experimental subject's perceptual abilities remarkably intact over the long range. After a temporary scotoma lasting a few weeks, very little in the way of deficit can be picked up.

As already noted, a variety of other methods for disturbing the

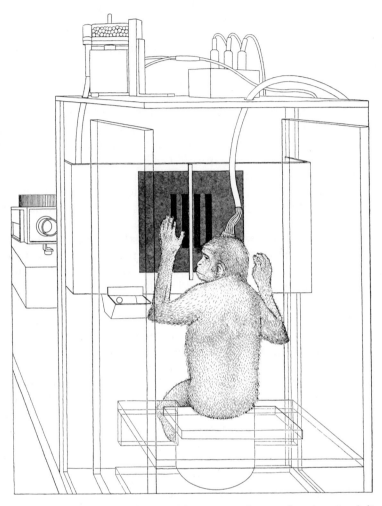

Fig. 7-3. Drawing showing monkey performing visual discrimination task. On the translucent panel in front of him the monkey sees, flashed for a microsecond, either a circle or a set of vertical stripes. He is rewarded with a peanut, which drops into the receptacle at his left elbow, if he presses the right half of the panel when he sees the circle or the left half when he sees the stripes. Electrodes record the waveforms generated by the flashed pattern that appear in the monkey's visual cortex as he develops skill at this task. Early in the experiments the waveforms show whether the monkey sees the circle or stripes. Eventually they reveal in advance which half of the panel the monkey will press and whether he was correct or incorrect. From Pribram, 1969d. "The Neurophysiology of Remembering." Copyright © 1969 by Scientific American, Inc. All rights reserved.

120

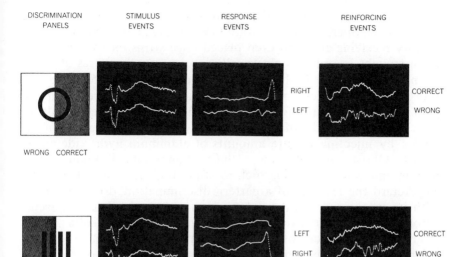

DISCRIMINATION PANELS   STIMULUS EVENTS   RESPONSE EVENTS   REINFORCING EVENTS

Fig. 7-4. Results of visual discrimination experiment illustrated in Fig. 7-3. The records under "Stimulus Events" are averages of three days' recordings of waveforms that appear immediately after circle or stripes have been flashed. The records under "Response Events" were those generated just prior to the moment when the monkey actually responded by pressing either the left or the right half of the panel. The records under "Reinforcing Events" were produced when the monkey was rewarded with a peanut if he was correct or not rewarded if he was wrong.

A difference in the second trough of the W-shaped part of the "stimulus" waveforms indicates whether the monkey has seen stripes or a circle. Only after he has learned his task do the response waveforms show differences in pattern and these appear just *prior* to the moment the monkey presses the right or the left half of the panel. These differences appear regardless of whether he has seen a circle or stripes. Thus the waveforms reflect his intention to press a particular half of the panel and do not indicate whether his response is going to be right or wrong. However, a third difference in waveforms does indicate whether a reward has been obtained: a slow shift in baseline following the movement of response indicates anticipation of reward and a 25-30 Hertz waveform indicates disappointment. From Pribram, 1969d. "The Neurophysiology of Remembering," Copyright © 1969 by Scientific American, Inc. All rights reserved.

presumed organization of the input systems has been tried to no avail: Roger Sperry and his group (1955) surgically cross-hatched a sensory receiving area and even placed mica strips into the resulting brain troughs in order to electrically insulate small squares of tissue from one another. Lashley, Chow, and Semmes (1951) tried to short-circuit the electrical activity of the brain by placing strips of gold foil over the receiving areas. And I have produced multiple punctate foci of epileptiform discharge within a receiving area of the cortex by injecting minute amounts of aluminum hydroxide cream (Kraft, Obrist, and Pribram, 1960; Stamm and Pribram, 1961; Stamm and Warren, 1961). Such multiple foci, although they markedly retard the learning of a pattern discrimination, do not interfere with its execution once it has been learned (whether learning occurs before or after the multiple lesions are made). These results make it clear that the effects of sensory input on brain tissue, the input information, must become distributed over the extent of the input system.

Electrical recording has also contributed substantially to the evidence that information becomes distributed in the brain. E. Roy John (John, Herrington, and Sutton, 1967) for instance, uses the technique of "labeling" an input to the visual system by presenting to cats stimuli which are differentiated not only by their geometric pattern but by the frequency of the flickering light which illuminates them. This differential frequency of illumination becomes reflected in the neuroelectric activity of the brain which follows the imposed frequency (or if this is fairly rapid, a subharmonic of that frequency). Thus the frequency encoded difference can be "traced" within the brain. This technique has yielded a number of interesting results, but of importance here is that careful analysis of the labeled wave shapes (computing possible differences between those occurring in one location in the brain and those occurring in others), shows that identical labeled wave forms occur in many brain structures simultaneously.

Another set of experiments performed in my laboratory (Pribram, Spinelli, and Kamback, 1967; Figs. 7-3, 7-4) shows, however, that once learning has occurred this distribution of information does not involve every locus within a system. Very small electrodes were used. Monkeys were trained to respond differentially to different geometric stimuli. In contrast to John's experiments, a very brief single flash illuminated the stimuli. Several distinct types of wave forms of electrical activity were evoked in the visual cortex. One type, obtained when the wave form was computed from the moment of stimulus onset, showed clear distinctions that were related to the stimuli. The other two types were obtained when the wave form was computed from the moment of response. One of these reflected whether the monkey received a pellet for responding correctly or whether he did not because he responded erroneously. The other type of wave form occurred immediately prior to the overt response. This wave form correlated with the particular response (pressing a right or left panel of a pair) which followed and was independent of the stimulus shown and the reward obtained. Important here is the fact that all of these characteristic wave forms did not appear everywhere in the visual cortex. One characteristic wave form was recorded from some electrodes, another wave form from other electrodes. Their distribution followed no discernible pattern. However, there was complete consistency from day-to-day—and week-to-week—of the recordings obtained from any particular electrode. Whatever encoding process had occurred, it had stabilized by the time of our recordings.

These experimental results are incompatible with a view that a photographic-like image becomes projected onto the cortical surface. The results do indicate that each sensory system functions with a good deal of reserve. Since it seems to make little difference to overall performance which part of the system is destroyed and which part remains, this reserve must be distributed in the system—the stored information necessary to making a discrimination is paralleled, reduplicated over many locations. It thus becomes likely that the retardation in learning resulting from the epileptic foci produced by aluminum hydroxide cream implantations indicates interference with this reduplication of information storage (Fig. 7-5).

The questions raised by these observations must be juxtaposed against another: how do objects appear sufficiently consistent so that we can recognize them as the same, independent of our angle of view or their distance from us? How do we recognize an object regardless of the part of the retina, and therefore of the brain, which is directly excited by the light coming from that object? The capacity for such size and object constancy is already developed in the human infant a few weeks of age. Thus any easy explanation of the constancy phenomenon in terms of learning is brought into question. Just what sort of mechanism would simultaneously allow for the existential flexibility of perception and the constancy of recognition once distribution has taken place?

Both the facts of pattern perception in the presence of scotomata and of perceptual constancy demand that there must be an effective neurological mechanism to spatially distribute the information contained in the input to the brain. If the facts of perception are to be

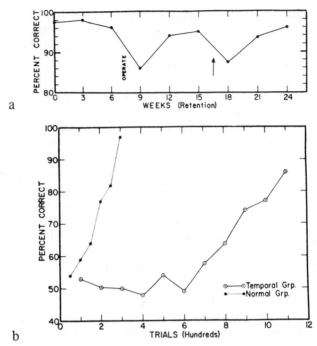

a

b

Fig. 7-5. (A) Retention scores on pattern discrimination tested at 3-week intervals in experiments similar to those illustrated in Figs. 6-9 and 6-10. Implantation of alumina cream is
indicated by "operate"; epileptoid discharges were first seen
during week indicated by arrow. (B) Learning curves obtained
on visual pattern discrimination task. (Scores are group med-
ians for successive blocks of trials.) Open circles indicate
performance of monkeys with epileptiform lesions of cortex
of the temporal lobe; filled circles indicate performance of
control group. From Stamm and Pribram, 1961.

accounted for, the simple correspondence of a point-to-point ikonic
isomorphism suggested by the anatomy of the system cannot be
sufficient. When 80 percent of the visual field is blinded by cortical
removal, recognition is mediated by the remainder of the visual field;
when the visual cortex is peppered with lesions, the part between the
lesions functions so well that little difficulty is experienced in
making discriminations; whether we view an object with one part of
our retina or another, or whether we view it from one angle or
another, we can still recognize the object. These are not the properties of ordinary photographic images—tear off 98 percent or even
80 percent of most photographs and try to identify them!

a feature detection process

One way out of the dilemma is to deny that the neural input mechanism is in any respect an Image maker, that the detection of patterns results from the extraction by single neurons or small groups of them of distinctive features of the input, and that pattern perception is accomplished by a hierarchy of such feature detectors. The convergence that takes place within parts of the input channels supports this view.

The mapping of visual receptive fields can be accomplished for units in the various stations of the input systems. In the brain cortex

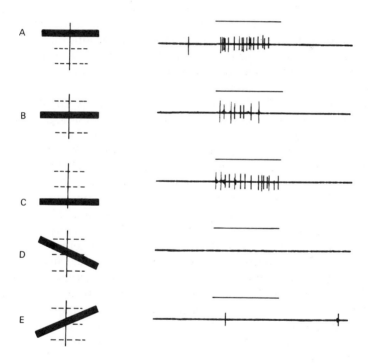

Fig. 7-6. Receptive sensitivity of cortical cell activated only by left (contralateral) eye over a field approximately 5 x 5°, situated 10° above and to the left of the area centralis. The cell responded best to a black horizontal rectangle, 1/3 x 6°, placed anywhere in the receptive field (A-C). Tilting the stimulus rendered it ineffective (D-E). The black bar was introduced against a light background during periods of 1 sec, indicated by the upper line in each record. From Hubel and Wiesel, 1962.

two types of units have been identified. Approximately half of these map as more or less circular fields, such as those of retinal ganglion cells but without as strong a surround (Jung, 1961; Spinelli, Pribram, and Bridgeman, 1971). The other half of the two major types of cortical units are much more likely to be activated by elongated than by circular spot types of inputs. These elongations must be presented to the eye in certain orientations to be maximally effective; different units respond to different lengths and orientations of lines, edges, and even corners (Hubel and Wiesel, 1962; Fig. 7-6).

The ready explanation of these observations is that the line and edge sensitive units are activated only when there is excitation of most or all of a linear array of spot sensitive units (recall Fig. 3-7, p. 60) whose connections converge on the line and edge receptors. The assumption is made that by virtue of further convergences, line and edge detector activity can be combined to produce cells sensitive to more complex patterns. This assumption has been supported by the finding of units especially sensitive to such complex patterns as corners and short segments of lines.

An explanation of perception in terms of a feature analysis mechanism thus becomes extremely tempting. Electrophysiological analysis of the receptive fields of units within the input channels indicates that, to some extent at least, feature selection takes place within these channels. Further, the evidence suggests that basic features such as those which determine color (DeValois, 1960; DeValois and Jacobs, 1968), contour, and direction are built into the organism. This type of basic feature detection is supplemented by feature selection which is sensitive to experience. There is some question as to whether experience modifies the builtin feature detectors per se or whether additional units are recruited by experience, causing a modification of the unit population sampled by the experimenter. It is clear, however, that in the mature organism feature analysis is not limited to builtin detectors. Feature analysis by memory units must also occur. Let us look therefore at the architecture of a neural logic composed of feature analyzers to see what it can and cannot account for in perception.

structures of feature analyzers

A sophisticated statement by Gerhard Werner (1970), based in part on his own extensive research and that of Vernon Mountcastle (1957) and of David Hubel and Torsten Wiesel, and in part on the TOTE formulation, describes a process for somesthetic feature analysis which applies with only minor modifications to the other input systems. He discerns a basic columnar structure in the brain cortex in which each neuron of the column displays a receptive field which makes up a unit of representation of the input. Columns of neurons tend to display identical or at least similar receptive fields and thus make up one level of representation. These columns are, in turn, combined into more complex structures by directionally sensitive units which serve as pointers connecting the activities of the columns (Fig. 7-7). These pointers, depending on the preferred direction of response, structure the electrical activities of the columns into various relationships to one another; if pointers with more than one direction are available, blocks of columns become connected to form "ring structures." Werner compares his cortical columnar structures to the list structures out of which computer programs are constructed. Each list contains items that point to other lists. Thus complex interactions, list structures, can be programmed by this simple device. In TOTE terms the static receptive field properties of the cortical columns form the basis of the test phase of the servo; their directional sensitive properties, the basis of its operate and exit phases. Spinelli (1970) has, in fact, designed a program (called Occam) to simulate a feature analyzer based on this cortical structure. By the presentation of patterns of nerve impulses or wave forms this program can be tuned to respond subsequently when certain features of the wave form are repeated (Fig. 7-8).

A somewhat simplified version of Werner's and Spinelli's feature analyzer is composed as follows: a cortical column is conceived to consist of input and operator neurons, and of interneurons and test cells. An input to a neural unit of the column that displays a receptive field is distributed to interneurons which in turn connect to an operator neuron. The interneurons are tunable—i.e., they adapt and habituate, they have memory. Each interneuron thus acts as does a bin in a computer that averages the patterns of input to which it is exposed. Only when a pattern is repeated does structured summation occur—nonrepetitive patterns simply raise the baseline and average out. Thus the operator neuron, sensitive solely to *patterns* of excitation is activated only when input patterns are repeated. The entire process is sharpened by feeding the output from the operator neuron back onto the input cell via a test neuron that compares the pattern of neural activity in the input and operator neurons. When match is adequate, the test cell produces an exit signal, otherwise the tuning process continues. Thus each cortical column comes to constitute an engram by virtue of its specific sensitivity to one pattern of neural activity, a "list" of interresponse times of a firing neuron or the wave form that describes the envelope of the firing pattern.

Each cortical column is conceived as being connected with others by horizontal cells and their basal dendrites, which are responsible

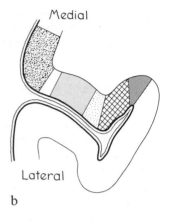

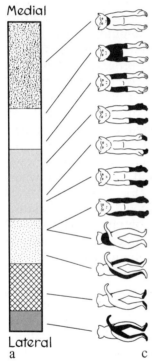

Fig. 7-7. Diagram showing experimental and analytical steps taken to reconstruct the organization of somatosensory cortex in terms of the receptive fields recorded from individual cells. *a* represents the experimental results; *b* represents the grouping of results according to cortical columns from several penetrations in one or more monkeys; *c* represents the cortical organization of the grouped results in TOTE terms and shows the relationship of this organization to the body surface. Such reconstructions lead to a conception of cortical structure comparable to the coding of information into "lists" (made up of TOTE units) from which computer programs are constituted. Compare with Fig. 7-8. Redrawn after Werner, 1970.

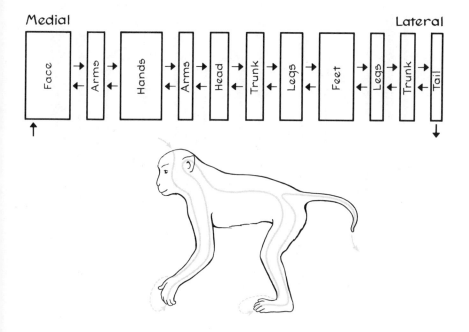

Medial   Lateral

Face → Arms → Hands → Arms → Head → Trunk → Legs → Feet → Legs → Trunk → Tail

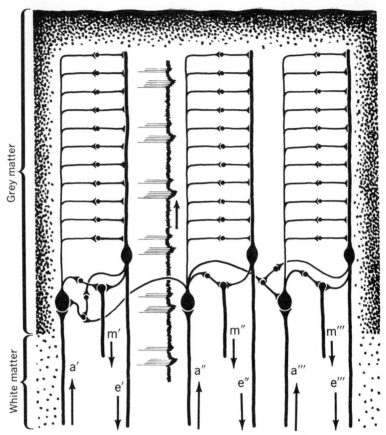

Fig. 7-8. Spinelli's OCCAM. See page 127 for explanation. Input neurons: a; output neurons: e; test neurons: m. Compare with Fig. 7-9. From Pribram, 1969b. *On the Biology of Learning,* © 1969 by Harcourt Brace Jovanovich, Inc. and reprinted with their permission.

for inhibitory interactions (Fig. 7-9). Whenever these horizontal cells are activated unsymmetrically, as they are by directional sensitive inputs, a temporary structure constructed of several columns is put together. These extended structures, dependent on hyperpolarization rather than on nerve impulse transmission, are composed therefore by the action of the junctional microstructure and constitute temporary neural states. But more of this in the next chapter.

We now have good evidence that the so-called association areas of the cerebral cortex exert a type of control over the input systems which is in many respects similar to that exercised when a zoom lens is extended and retracted. This function would have the effect of changing the number (and perhaps the complexity) of cortical columns that can be contained in such a temporary structure (Chap. 17).

The logic of the input systems can thus be conceived to constitute a filter on input, a screen that is being continually tuned by that input. One of the characteristics of the filter is that it constitutes a self-adapting system whose parameters of adaptation are controlled by its own past history and by the operations performed on it by

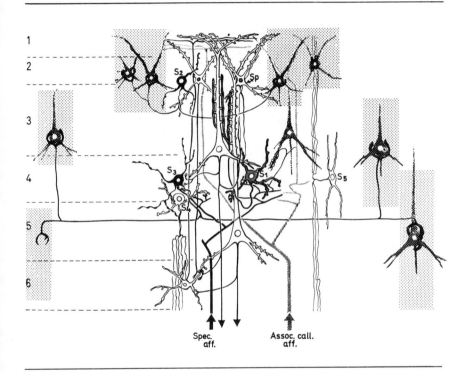

Fig. 7-9. Semidiagrammatic drawing of most important cell types of neocortex and their interconnections. Note especially the pyramidal cells' (output neurons) connections to stellate (test) interneurons (S_1, S_3) which receive input from specific afferents (spec. aff.). From Szentogothai, 1969.

other neural mechanisms. Another systems characteristic of the filter, because of the properties provided by the interconnections among logic elements, is Image construction. But this is getting ahead of the story. Let us first return to the problem of why an Imaging process is necessary at all and what limitations the feature analysis approach to perception encounters.

the limitations of feature analysis

What then is wrong with an imageless, feature analysis view of perceptual processes? Three things. First, the features analyzed are not the distinct features they appear to be. Second, the richness of the phenomena of perception is unaccounted for by the feature detectors so far discovered. And third, manipulations of sensory input during development have decoupled the effect produced on feature detectors as studied with microelectrodes from that produced on feature analysis as studied by behavioral discrimination.

Let us examine the problem of feature distinctiveness first. Irvin Rock (1970) incisively states the problem:

> ... Those who would claim that the response of neural detectors can account for why things look as they do may be unaware of precisely those facts about perception that the Gestaltists were at pains to point out. For example we know that phenomenal size is not simply a function of the size of the retinal image; phenomenal shape is not directly a function of the shape of the corresponding image; phenomenal speed is not directly a function of the rate of displacement of the retinal image and so forth. Instead, despite great variation of the proximal stimulus with changes of the observer's position, the world of objects maintains a surprising degree of constancy. These facts cannot be denied and they cannot be set aside as intellectual achievements if by that is meant that things do not *look* constant under these changing conditions, only that we *know* they are constant. The evidence is quite strong against such a formulation.
>
> Let us consider in detail some of the facts concerning the perception of movement. To begin with, there is position constancy, namely, the fact that when we move or move our eyes the retinal image of the entire scene moves but the scene does not appear to move. The converse also holds, namely, a *non*-moving image does lead to movement perception when we move our eyes or head, as in the case of following a moving object with the eyes or viewing an after-image while moving the eyes. Then there is stroboscopic movement, intermittent *stationary* images yielding a sense of movement. There is the further fact of movement *induced* in objects whose images are stationary by virtue of the displacement of surrounding objects, such as in the case of the moon appearing to move when the clouds displace in front of it . . . .
>
> One might entertain the hypothesis that the true sensory basis of movement perception was the stimulation of movement detectors but that the meaning of such stimulation is determined by other information. For example, one might say that no movement at all is perceived if the registration of retinal displacement is cancelled out by information to the effect that the organism's own voluntary movement has produced it, as von Holst, and before him, Helmholtz suggested. Or one might argue that in induced move-

ment, the detectors supply the crucial information that *something* has moved but for reasons as yet unknown, the movement is assigned to the nonmoving object.

Frankly I don't see how this is really tenable. It does not explain why I see my after-image moving when I move my eyes even in a completely dark room where there are no visible stationary objects whose images would displace over the retina. In the case of stroboscopic movement, if the eyes are held stationary, the only basis for stimulation of movement detectors would arise from the nystagmic tremor of the eye, but this would not do justice to the spatial extent of the movement perceived, namely *between* the two quite separate flashing stimulus objects. Nor can this hypothesis deal with induced movement in the manner suggested because the inducing object can be moved so slowly that it is below threshold when it alone is visible. Clearly then the basis of movement perception here is the change in location of the induced object relative to the inducing one, not stimulation of detectors of image displacement.

Consider next, the problem of the perception of an object's orientation. Is the basis of the perceived orientation of a line the orientation of its image on the retina? Obviously not, because when the head is tilted the vertical and horizontal lines on the wall continue to appear vertical and horizontal. We have here yet another constancy, in this case, of phenomenal orientation, despite variation in the orientation of the retinal image. To a considerable extent it holds even where a single luminous line is viewed with head tilted in an otherwise dark field. Therefore the conclusion is warranted that information about the observer's own position must be taken into account before the perceptual significance of a given retinal orientation is "deduced."

What then should we make of the discovery by Hubel and Wiesel of orientation detectors in the visual cortex? Clearly they cannot be signs of the orientation of objects in the environment. One might maintain that they are signs of the orientation of objects with respect to the organism, in other words detectors of egocentric orientation, and that they provide the necessary basis for the assessment of how objects are oriented in the environment when other information is available concerning how the observer himself is oriented. For example, one might say that when an image of a line is retinally vertical it will always appear egocentrically vertical, i.e., parallel to the long axis of the head; the line will then appear vertical in the world if the observer is upright and horizontal in the world if the observer is tilted $90°$.

While I think this is a plausible idea, it runs into serious difficulties because of certain additional facts. If the observer remains upright, a vertical line seen within a room which is tilted will look quite tilted in a direction opposite to that of the room. So here a vertical image will no longer signify a vertical object despite the fact that the observer is upright. Furthermore, the line will no longer appear egocentrically "vertical" either. To these facts should be added the finding that observers will adapt to a prismatically tilted image, so

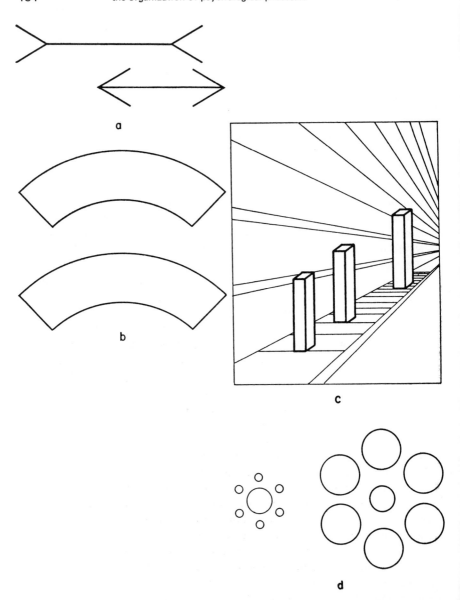

Fig. 7-10. Some size inconstancies (illusions) produced despite identical retinal images. In *a*, the classical Müller-Lyer illusion, two equal lines appear unequal because of the surrounding arrowheads; in *b*, the lower figure appears larger than the upper figure although both are the same size; in *c*, the three posts are all the same height; in *d*, the two center circles are equal. From Kretch and Crutchfield, 1962.

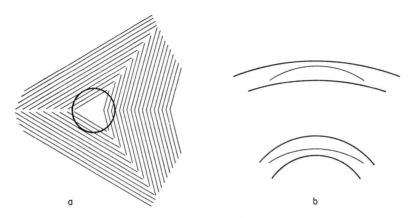

Fig. 7-11. Two examples of the influence of surroundings on perceived shape: in *a*, the figure lying on the striped background is an exact circle; in *b* the two inside arcs are identical. Illusions are hard to account for by a feature detection mechanism. From Kretch and Crutchfield, 1962.

that a vertical retinal image is no longer the sign of a vertical object when the observer is upright nor, in fact, is it any longer the sign that an object is oriented in a vertical direction with respect to the observer.

Are orientation detectors in the cortex relevant to form perception? One might suppose that perception of form reduces to the perceived orientation of the lines making it up. Thus, a square is perceived when two horizontal and two vertical line-detectors are stimulated. It is well known that figures look very different when their orientations are changed. Superficially this very fact might appear to be proof of the role of orientation-detectors in form perception because entirely different fibers would come into play. That could be said to be the basis of the altered appearance. But the fact is, that, by and large, it is *not* the change in the orientation of the image on the retina that accounts for the altered appearance. In experiments I and my associates have performed, it has repeatedly been shown that if the figure remains in an unchanged position in the environment but is viewed from a tilted posture, it does *not* look any different, or expressed more objectively, there is no decline in recognition. Why should this be true if entirely different detectors are responding? Conversely, if the figure is also tilted, by the same amount as the observer, so that the orientation on the retina is now *not* changed at all, it nevertheless looks entirely different and, therefore, is often not recognized. A simple demonstration is to form an after-image of a square with head upright and then to view it with eyes closed and head tilted 45°. It now looks like a diamond. Why should this be true if the *same* detectors are responding?

These findings make sense, however, if we say that the crucial fact about orientation is the perception of a certain region of a figure as the top, another as the bottom, etc. If we continue to correctly identify the same region as the top, as we do when we are tilted and the form is not, we see it unchanged. If however we take a different region of the figure as the top, as we do when the figure is tilted in the environment, we see it as a very different shape. This process would seem to have nothing to do with orientation-specific detectors.

The probable role of these detectors then is in providing the basis for our discriminating one image orientation from another. In the past we may have incorrectly thought that this discrimination was governed by the spatially different orientations of the projected cortical "images." In other words, neural detectors may be the mechanisms whereby certain stimulus information is received, in this case information that one orientation is the same as or different from another. Such information is, of course, necessary for perception as a starting point, but by no means is the response of these fibers to be thought of as the neural correlates of percepts. [1970, pp. 2–5]

The remainder of Rock's paper reviews additional interesting experiments difficult to account for on a feature detector basis (see also Figs. 7-10, 7-11).

The second deficiency of the imageless feature detection view of perception is that the tapestry of awareness is rich, but the pattern recognition process, dependent on classification, is relatively impoverished in the detail with which it operates. A pattern recognition mechanism that selects features can be wrong. All of us have waited for someone who is late in arriving at a crowded meeting place and misidentified strangers who share features with that person. We recognize A, *A* and a as the letter *A,* yet are keenly aware of the differences in the style with which the letter is written. Perception appears at the same time to allow not only a richness of experience and "a powerful preference to maintain a constant organization," but also a tendency toward "maximum simplicity," as the experiments of the Gestalt psychologists have shown. The evidence suggests that the richness of perception is related to the complexities that can be demonstrated independently in the environmental energy configurations exciting the receptor surfaces (see Gibson, 1966) which must engage some brain mechanism of equal capacity for richness. Evidence provided by Rock and others indicates that only the tendency toward simplicities, the frames of reference, are due to the feature analytic mechanism and even here another mechanism, a more "cognitive" process, plays a role.

The third limitation of relying on feature detection to account for the facts of perception comes from experiments in which newborn infants have been deprived of sensory input for varied periods of time. As noted in Chapters 6 and 8, human infants show the ability

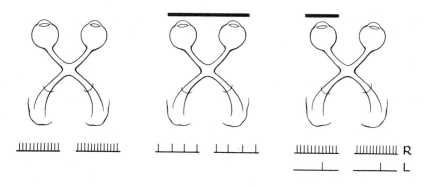

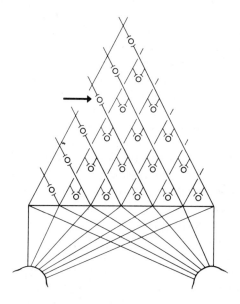

Fig. 7-12. Diagram of results of experiments in which both eyes or one eye are deprived of visual input during infancy. Note that unilateral deprivation leads to much greater suppression of activity recorded from cells in the visual cortex. This poses certain difficulties (see text) for a simple feature detection mechanism since cells are connected to both eyes (lower diagram) and continue to be normally responsive to stimulation via the undeprived eye.

to maintain size and shape constancy within a few weeks of birth. In animals the ability to make discriminations develops equally early; when the brains of these infants are studied a full blown set of feature detectors is found. When sensory input is restricted, however, this simple correlation between behavior and brain function breaks down. To be specific, when cats or rats are raised in complete darkness their ability to make simple brightness or contour orientations remains intact, but the ability to discriminate among more complex visual patterns is severely impaired. In such animals the receptive field orientation of cortical neurons though still discernible is less sharply tuned and the cells fatigue more rapidly than in normally reared animals. But when sensory deprivation is restricted for a comparable length of time to just one eye, all visual orientations and discriminations are severely impaired when that eye alone is used. This evidence correlates with the fact that few cortical units can be driven by stimulations of the deprived eye and, of those that can, scarcely any respond selectively to line orientation or movement. This reaction occurs even though a usual complement of such cells is present in the cortex as is shown by their normal responsiveness to stimulation via the experienced eye (see Fig. 7-12). Thus some sort of suppression of responsiveness must occur when an imbalance in the ordinary mode of excitation is produced, and this suppression exceeds the malfunction produced solely by disuse (as in the completely deprived animals). Unless some actual change in connectivity accounts for the monocular suppression of responsiveness at the cortex, some process other than simple feature analysis must be responsible for the suppressive effect.

Leo Ganz, in a recent review (1971) of these and other similar findings, makes an additional point. On the basis of the experimental results obtained with completely deprived animals, he distinguishes two types of tasks. Brightness and contour orientation demand only that the organism respond in terms of the reaction of the majority of his feature detectors. Discriminations of more complex patterns—e.g., between an upright and inverted triangle—cannot be accomplished on this basis. We need some sort of additional, more flexible brain mechanism which he calls "selective attention" that actively suppresses the dominant reaction of feature detectors, a reaction which is largely irrelevant to adequate solution of the discrimination.

We have therefore returned once more to the necessity for a mechanism additional and complementary to feature analysis. And so we come back to the possibility that the input systems are organized so that neural signals become coordinate with some sort of psychological "Imaging" process. The problem is to determine the neurological nature of the organization involved. Obviously on the basis of the data reviewed at the beginning of this chapter, this organization cannot be simply a mosaic of points generated at the receptor and propagated unchanged to the cortex to form a photographic picture-like image. And obviously it must take into account the line sensitive units and other feature detectors that make up the neural structure of feature analysis in the brain.

synopsis

Subtotal removals of brain tissue regardless of location within the input systems interfere remarkably little with perceptual recognition processes. The neural logic involved in any particular perception therefore appears to be distributed within the system. Direct evidence for distributed memory has also been obtained. This memory logic is composed of built-in detectors for elementary features (such as lines and corners) and of analyzers for more complex transformations of distinctive features (such as wave forms) which are tunable by experience.

holograms

an hypothesis

Let's return for a moment to our generalized model. The model specifies two basic processes: spatially organized states and operations on those states performed by pulsed neural transmissions. Part I described how these basic properties of neuronal aggregates could be combined into logical operations which enhance the analytical and the control (servo) functions of the nervous system. Because of their importance and because they are today so neglected by the neurobehavioral and neurophysiological community, I emphasized the point that constructions of configurational, topological, i.e., spatial representations in the nervous system constituted one form that brain states can take. I proposed that interactions among the patterns of excitation which fall on receptor surfaces become, after transmission over pathways organized in a parallel fashion, encoded by virtue of horizontally interacting processes in the slow potential activities of neuronal aggregates to form temporary microstructures whose design depends more on the functional organization of neural junctions than on neurons per se as units.

Chapter 7 detailed evidence that specified the existence of a feature detection and analyzer mechanism but also presented the argument for a need of a neural organization beyond that furnished by feature analyzers; Chapter 8 formulates the hypothesis that the mechanism of the junctional microstructure of slow potentials provides this organization. The hypothesis is based on the premise that neural representations of input are not photographic but are composed not only by an initial set of feature filters but by a special class of transformations which have considerable formal resemblance to an optical image reconstruction process devised by mathematicians and engineers. This optical process, called holography, uses interference patterns. It has many fascinating properties, among which the facility for distributing and storing large amounts of information is paramount. These properties are just those needed to resolve the paradox posed by the demand for functional lability, the rapidly paced transients, in the context of demonstrated anatomical constraints in neural input organization.

Before proceeding with the precise formulation, a few paragraphs explaining the general approach taken here may be helpful. Optical information processing by holography is described mathematically in wave mechanical terms. In physical optics, the equations used to describe the behavior of light in experimental situations can be couched either in quantal or in wave form. The physicist is not unduly concerned whether light *is* quantal or a wave, whether it comes in packets or as electromagnetic waves, or both. He is concerned in describing the results of his observations as quantitatively and fully as can be done and chooses his descriptive tools accordingly. Some observations can be crisply described as statistical probabilities of occurrences of quantal events; others yield more readily to the mathematics of wave formulations.

One observation in particular has been difficult to conceptualize by the quantum approach. When light of very low luminance is passed through a grating so that at most a few quanta would be expected to pass through a single slit, the equations describing the light on the far side of the grating must, in order to fit observation, take into account some interactions that appear to take place between the light passing through one slit and that passing through neighboring slits (Fig. 8-1). It is difficult, though not impossible, to account for this interaction by the quantal view: how can a quantum of light influence a neighbor separated from it by a grid? It seems as though each quantum exerted a (one is tempted to say "magnetic")

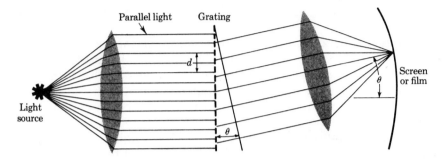

Fig. 8-1. Diffraction grating. From Murray and Cobb, 1970.

force on its neighbor. This phenomenon of neighborhood interaction has been studied extensively and given the name *superposition.* The mathematical equations that satisfactorily account for superposition are sets of linear equations called *convolutional integrals* that are ordinarily used to describe interactions among wave forms. The description of one wave form is convoluted with that of another. There is less of a conceptual problem in accounting for superposition when the smooth passage of a wave front of light is considered to be interfered with by the grating which causes small "eddies" of interaction to form. These eddies can be conceived to constitute the interference effect and to account for superposition—the neighborhood interaction.

The holographic hypothesis on brain function in perception takes the form of superposition. Whether in fact one chooses to account for the behavior of the brain's electrical potentials in statistical or in wave mechanical terms depends on the observations that need to be described. That formulation should be chosen which can most quantitatively and most fully do the job and at the same time be conceptually plausible. Chapter 3 described the occurrence of lateral or surround inhibition in receptors and in central stations of the brain. Lateral inhibition effects a neighborhood interaction among neural events. If this spatial interaction is adequately described by the convolutional integrals that define superposition in the physical sense, we can conceptualize the interaction in terms of interference effects. The plausibility of this choice is reinforced by evidence that in the retina, at least, neighborhood interactions in the horizontal cells are due exclusively to inhibitory interactions, by slow potential hyperpolarizations and not to depolarizations which lead to nerve impulses. This point deserves further exploration.

As in Chapter 3, receptor events serve as our model-in-miniature—

this time of the "neural holographic" process. We have already noted that excitation of one unit in the optic nerve affects the discharge rate of neighboring units. We have also noted that the receptive field of a particular unit is composed of this spatial interaction among neighbors. In the optic nerve these receptive fields usually consist of a more or less round central spot which reacts by either increasing (on-center) or decreasing (off-center) its spontaneous discharge rate, and a surround which shows activity of a sign opposite that of the center. Chapter 7 was directed toward the problem of what type of code, what type of organization (logic) would be composed by the operation of many such units. This chapter addresses a different set of problems: what is encoded in one receptive field, i.e., what features of the optical image does the shape of the receptive field represent?

This answer comes from a detailed mathematical analysis by

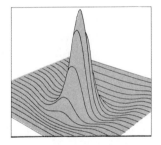

Fig. 8-2. Map of visual receptive field represents recordings made from the axon of a single ganglion cell in the retina of the eye when a point source of light is presented in various parts of the visual field. The map contains smooth contour lines because the ganglion cell integrates the response of its neighbors, with which it is interconnected; recall Fig. 3-4. The height of the contour at any point represents the number of times the individual nerve cell fires when the location of the point light source corresponds to that position on the map. Maximum firing occurs when the position of the light corresponds to that of the central peak. In mathematical terms, each contour line represents the "convolutional integral" of the first derivative of the shape of the stimulus figure. The interaction of many such convolutional integrals may produce hologram-like interference patterns within the visual system and elsewhere in the brain. Storage of such patterns could provide the basis of a distributed memory system. From Rodieck, in Pribram, 1969d. "The Neurophysiology of Remembering," Copyright © 1969 by Scientific American, Inc. All rights reserved.

Rodieck (1965) of the quantitative relationships which exist between specifiable moving and flashing visual stimuli and the shape of the receptive field generated by them. The resulting response curves (which represent a vertical section through the three dimensional display of the receptive field, Fig. 8-2) have a particular shape. When two or more stimuli are presented simultaneously, the response curve corresponds rather well to that which would have been produced by superposition of the response curves of separate presentations. Rodieck thus concludes that "it is possible to obtain from the response patterns to a small light spot flashed in various parts of a cell's receptive field, the response pattern of the cell to any shaped figure at any orientation moving at any velocity through any part of the receptive field." This finding allowed the reconstruction of the receptive field from moving spots and also enabled the recording by computer shown in Fig. 3-7. The shape of the receptive field thus turns out to be a convolution of the first derivative of the shape of the optical stimulus.

As already noted, convolution integrals that spell out the response relationships among neighboring events (spatial superposition) describe the basic process involved in holography, in optical informa-

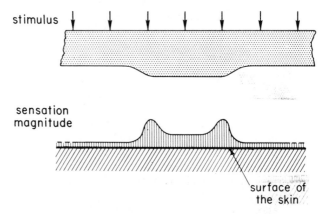

Fig. 8-3. Diagram of experiment showing the existence of Mach bands for skin sensation. The experiment uses a vibratory pattern with a point-to-point intensity as shown by the diagram labelled "stimulus." The sensation obtained when the vibratory pattern is placed on the forearm is indicated by the diagram labelled "sensation." A similar but somewhat attenuated effect can be obtained by direct pressure (of different intensities) with a nonvibrating stimulus. From Békésy, 1967.

tion processing systems (Gabor, 1949, 1951). More specific equations based on Fourier, Fresnel, and Laplace transformations also describe interference effects. It is an empirical problem to determine which transformation usefully describes a system's operation under any given set of circumstances.

In the visual system—and there is good reason to suspect from the work of Georg von Bekesy (1960, 1967, Fig. 8-3) in the auditory, somatic, and gustatory systems as well—these sorts of transformations describe to a remarkable degree of precision the interaction between the patterns of energy change which excite the receptor surfaces and the spontaneously occurring neuronal potential changes of receptor units. In optical information processing systems such transformations ordinarily refer to wave form analyses (e.g., interference effects) and there is no special need to ignore completely a wave mechanical approach to the superposition effect which occurs in neuronal aggregates. The advantages of this approach are that a physical process based on interference effects displays many of the attributes of the neural process in perception and thus makes the brain's Imaging mechanism a little easier to comprehend. Let us therefore look for a moment at the physical hologram.

the physical hologram

Most of us are familiar with the image generating aspects of optical systems. A camera records on photographic film placed *at* the image plane a copy of the light intensities reflected from the objects within the camera's visual field. Each point on the film stores information which arrives from a corresponding point in the visual field, and thus the film's record "looks like" the visual field. Recently studies have been made of the properties of records made on film which is placed somewhere *in front of* the image plane (e.g., in the focal plane) of an optical system. When properly exposed by a coherent light source, such a film record constitutes an *optical filter* in which information from each point of the visual field is stored throughout the filter itself (Fig. 8-4).

These filters display a number of remarkable characteristics. As we have all experienced, when a film does not lie exactly in the image plane of a camera, the image becomes blurred, boundaries become less sharp, contrast is less marked. In an optical filter the information is distributed so that the stored image does not resemble the visual image at all. The optical filter is a record of the wave patterns emitted or reflected from an object. "Such a record can be thought of as 'freezing' of the wave pattern; the pattern remains frozen until

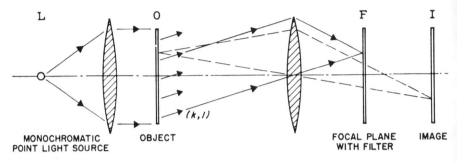

Fig. 8-4. Diagram of the method for producing an optical filter hologram. From van Heerden, 1968.

such time as one chooses to reactivate the process, whereupon the waves are 'read out' of the recording medium" (Leith and Upatnicks, 1965). Thus when transilluminated by a coherent light source, an optical filter reconstructs the wavefronts of light which were present

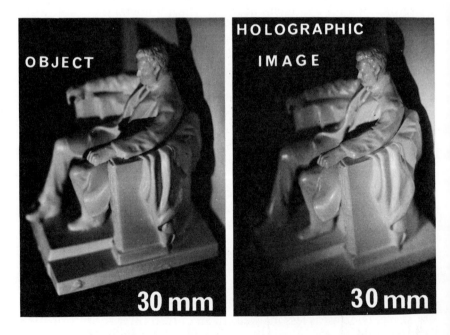

Fig. 8-5. Direct photograph (left) and photograph of virtual image of same object through hologram, both in laser light. Note high degree of perfection in holographic imaging attainable with contemporary techniques. From Stroke, 1969.

when the exposure was made. As a result, a virtual image of the visual field can be seen by looking towards the filter. This virtual image appears exactly as did the visual scene during the exposure, complete and in three dimensions (Fig. 8-5). In essence, all the information describing the visual field and from which an image of the visual field can be reconstructed, is contained in the filter.

As the observer changes his viewing position the perspective of the picture changes, just as if the observer were viewing the original scene. Parallax effects are evident between near and far objects in the scene: if an object in the foreground lies in front of something else, the observer can move his head and look around the obstructing object, thereby seeing the previously hidden object .... In short, the reconstruction has all the visual properties of the original scene and we know of no visual test one can make to distinguish the two. (Leith and Upatnicks, 1965, p. 30)

Even before the use of optical filters in the reconstruction of images had been practically demonstrated, Dennis Gabor (1949, 1951) had mathematically described another way of producing images from photographic records. Gabor intended to increase the resolution of electron microphotographs. He proposed that a coherent background wave be forced to interfere with the waves refracted by the tissue. (Reflection from an opaque object would serve as well.) The resulting interference pattern would store both amplitude and phase (neighborhood interaction) information which could then, in a second step, be used to reconstruct, when transilluminated with a coherent light source, an image of the original tissue. Gabor christened his technique "holography" and the photographic record a "hologram" because it contained all of the information to reconstruct the whole image.

Gabor holograms can be composed in two ways. A wave form is divided by a beam splitter (e.g., a half-silvered mirror) so that one part serves as a reference, the other is reflected off the object to be photographed (Figs. 8-6, 8-7). The reference alone can then be used to reconstruct an image. Or each part of the divided beam can be reflected off a different object. When one of the objects is used as a reference at the time of image reconstruction, the other appears as a "ghost" image. In this instance, the hologram can be used as a mechanism for associative storage of information.

The formal similarity between Gabor's refraction and reflection holograms and the various types of optical filters gradually became apparent. They are basically similar in that the resultant coding of information in each is a linear transformation of the pattern of light

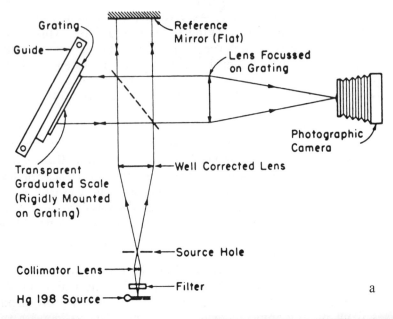

Grating
Guide
Reference Mirror (Flat)
Lens Focussed on Grating
Photographic Camera
Transparent Graduated Scale (Rigidly Mounted on Grating)
Well Corrected Lens
Source Hole
Collimator Lens
Filter
Hg 198 Source

a

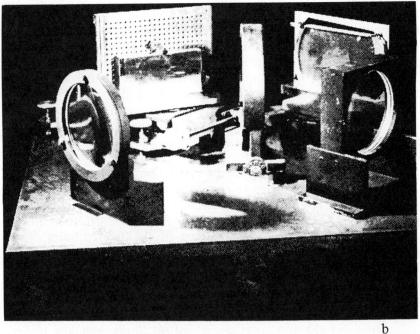

b

Fig. 8-6. (A) Diagram of method for producing Gabor-type holograms. (B) Photograph of apparatus. From Stroke, 1969.

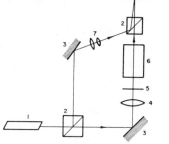

Fig. 8-7. A holographic microscope which allows one to observe the image at various depths. (1) Laser, (2) beam-splitting prism, (3) mirror, (4) condenser, (5) object, (6) microscope, (7) microscopic lenses, (8) hologram. From Stroke, 1969.

not only in terms of its intensity as in an ordinary photographic process, but also in terms of neighborhood interactions (spatial phase). The most intensively studied holograms have been those in which these phase relationships can be expressed mathematically as Fourier transforms. These are special forms of convolutional integral which have the property that the identical equation convolves and deconvolves. *Thus any process represented by the spatial Fourier transform can encode and subsequently decode simply by recurring at some second stage!*

All holograms (Fig. 8-8) have some interesting properties in com-

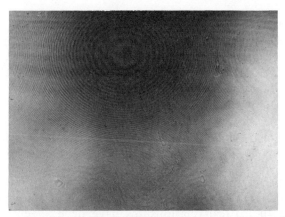

Fig. 8-8. A direct print of an actual holographic film. No image can be seen, yet despite the differences in appearance of different parts, essentially the same image is reconstructed from any part.

mon which make them potentially important in understanding brain function. First (and from the standpoint of this chapter most important), the information about a point in the original image is distributed throughout the hologram, making the record resistant to damage. Each small part of the hologram contains information from the entire original image and therefore can reproduce it. As the pieces become smaller, some resolution is lost. As successively larger parts of the hologram are used for reconstruction, the depth of field of the image decreases, i.e., focus becomes narrowed, so that an optimum size for a particular use can be ascertained (Leith and Upatnicks, 1965).

The hologram has a fantastic capacity to usefully (i.e., retrievably) store information. Information incorporated in a suitable retrieval system can be immediately located and accurately reconstructed. The density of information storage is limited only by the wave length of the coherent light (the shorter, the greater the capacity) and the grain size of the film used. Furthermore, many different patterns can be simultaneously stored especially when holograms are produced in solids. Each image is stored throughout the solid, yet each image is individually retrievable. As Leith and Upatnicks (1965) describe it:

> . . . several images can be superimposed on a single plate on successive exposures, and each image can be recovered without being affected by other images. This is done by using a different spatial-frequency carrier for each picture . . . . The gating carriers can be different frequencies . . . and there is still another degree of freedom, that of angle. [p. 31]

Some ten billion *bits* (a measure on the amount) of information have been usefully stored holographically in a cubic centimeter! As Pieter van Heerden points out, if we store during a lifetime as little as one bit per second, our brain requires approximately 3×10^{10} elementary binary (nerve impulse) operations *per second* to accomplish this. "If that sort of thing was going on it was [at first] incomprehensible . . . . However, once confronted with this paradox, it gradually became clear . . . that optical storage and processing of information can provide a way of accomplishing this 'impossible' operation . . ." (1968, pp. 28–29).

A final point about physical holograms. Optical systems are not the only ones that can be subjected to the holographic process. Now that the mathematical relationships have been specified, computer programs have been constructed that "simulate" optical information processes. One such program represents the intensity of an input by the size of a disc; spatial phase relationships are represented by the angular direction of a slit within that disc (Fig. 8-9).

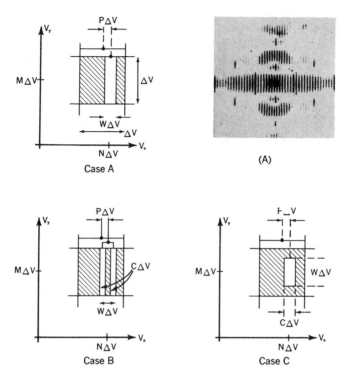

Case A

(A)

Case B

Case C

Fig. 8-9. One example of a non-optical hologram. The diagram shows three ways of constructing a cell from which a hologram can be reconstructed and an example of a Fraunhofer hologram that corresponds to Case A. Slit width and height as well as the cell size, are the adjustable parameters. From Brown and Lohmann, 1966, in Pribram, 1969b.

Holograms are thus not dependent on the physical presence of "waves" even though they are most readily described by the equations of wave mechanics. This independence of holography from physical wave production is an important consideration in approaching the problem of a neural holographic process. There is some considerable doubt whether "brain waves" as presently recorded form the substrate of any meaningful interference pattern organization for information processing, although they may indicate that some such process is taking place. The wave lengths recorded are, of course, considerably longer than those of light waves and can therefore be carriers of small amounts of information—even in the form of spatially interfering holographic patterns. The hypothesis proposed next therefore continues the theme of earlier chapters in emphasizing the role of junctional slow potential microstructures in brain function. These microstructures can be described either in statistical, quantal terms or in the wave mechanical language of convolutional integrals and Fourier transforms. The microstructures do not change their essential characteristics because we choose one or another description. Each language, each descriptive form, has its own advantages. For the problems of perception, especially those of Image formation and the fantastic capacity of recognition memory, holographic description has no peer. So why not apply its application to brain processes?

a neural holographic process

The essence of the holographic concept is that Images are reconstructed when representations in the form of distributed information systems are appropriately engaged. These representations operate as filters or screens. In fact, as we have noted, one derivative of the holographic process comes from a consideration of optical filtering mechanisms. Holography in this frame of reference is conceived as an instantaneous analogue cross-correlation performed by matched filters. In the brain correlation can take place at various levels. In more peripheral stations correlation occurs between successive configurations produced by receptor excitation: the residuals left by adaptation through decrementing form a buffer memory register to be updated by current input. At more central stations correlation entails a more complex interaction: at any moment input is correlated not only with the configuration of excitation existing at any locus, but also with patterns arriving from other stations. An example of this sort of complexity is shown in the experimental results described in Chapter 7 where the configuration of potential changes in the visual cortex was determined not only by the visual cues observed by a monkey, but also by the contingencies of reinforcement and the "intention" to make one or another response.

According to the holographic hypothesis, the mechanism of these correlations is not by way of some disembodied "floating field" nor even by disembodied wave forms. Instead, consider once again the construction of more or less temporary organizations of cortical columns (or, in other neural locations, other aggregates of cell assemblies) by the arrival of impulses at neuronal junctions which activate horizontal cell inhibitory interactions. When such arrival patterns converge from at least two sources their designs would produce interference patterns. Assume that these interference patterns made up of classical postsynaptic potentials are coordinate with awareness. Assume also that the analysis given at the beginning of this chapter is correct in suggesting that this microstructure of slow potentials is accurately described by the equations that describe the holographic process which is also composed of interference patterns. The conclusion then follows that information representing the input is distributed over the entire extent of the neural pattern just as it is over the entire extent of the physical holographic pattern. There is, however, considerable leeway in how one can currently conceive of this distribution and correlation process. The following exchange of ideas in the journal *Nature* gives a flavor of some tenable arguments:

> Our point of departure is Gabor's observation that any physical system which can correlate (or for that matter convolve) pairs of patterns can mimic the performance of a Fourier holograph. Such a system, which could be set up in any school physics laboratory, is shown in Fig. [8-10]. The apparatus is designed for making "correlograms" between pairs of pinhole patterns, and then using the correlogram and one of the patterns for reconstructing its partner . . . .
>
> [There] is [however] a slight embarrassment when one comes to consider how a discrete correlograph, with the reconstructive facility, could be realized in neural tissue. We will not dwell on this point, except to acknowledge that it was drawn to our attention by Dr. F.H.C. Crick, to whom H.C.L.H. is indebted for provocative comments. But it led us on to a further refinement of our model [Fig. 8-11] . . . . . In this form our associative memory model ceases to be a correlograph, having lost the ability to recognize displaced patterns, but its information capacity is now potentially far greater than before. . . .
>
> To summarize, we have attempted to distil from holography the features which commend it as a model of associative memory, and have found that the performance of a holograph can be mimicked and actually improved on by discrete non-linear models, namely the correlograph and the associative net . . . . Quite possibly there is no system in the brain which corresponds exactly to the principle on which it works and the quantitative relations which we have shown must hold if such a system is to perform, as it can, with high efficiency.
>
> [Willshaw, Buneman, Longuet-Higgins, 1969, pp. 960-62]

Willshaw, Buneman and Longuet-Higgins have proposed a nonholographic associative memory model for the brain [Willshaw, Buneman, and Longuet-Higgins, 1969, p. 960]. They also criticize the proposal made by myself [van Heerden, 1963, p. 393] and by Pribram [1966, 1969d] that the brain would be organized on the holographic principle. They say: "How could the brain Fourier-analyse the incoming signals with sufficient accuracy . . . ."

In a book on the subject [van Heerden, 1968] I discussed further how the brain could work physically very well as a three-dimensional hologram. If we have a three-dimensional network of neurones, in which each neurone is

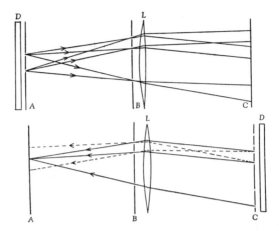

Fig. 8-10. Constructing a correlogram (upper figure), and reconstructing pattern (lower figure). D is a diffuse light source. L a lens and C the plane of the correlogram of A with B. Solid line indicates paths traversed during construction; dotted line indicates paths not traversed. From Willshaw, Buneman, and Longuet-Higgins, 1969.

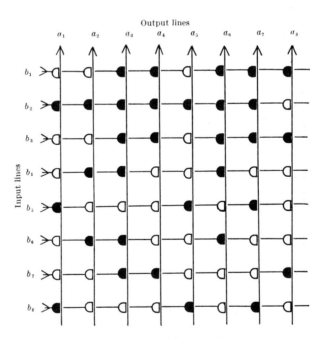

Fig. 8-11. The associative net discussed in text. Note that nodes can represent synaptic domains. From Willshaw, Buneman, and Longuet-Higgins, 1969.

connected to a few adjacent ones, and if a neurone in a certain layer, in receiving a signal, will send this on to a few neurones in the next layer, then signals will propagate in this network as a wave propagates in an elastic medium. If, moreover, the ability of the neurones to propagate received signals can be permanently enhanced by frequent use, then the network must act as a three-dimensional hologram, with a storage capacity of the order of the number of neurones present in the network.

For recognizing, we need a two-dimensional hologram for fast search, combined with a three-dimensional hologram which has a large capacity for storing information that is readily accessible [van Heerden, 1968]. This is still not sufficient, however, to explain the wonderful human capacity for recognizing. We can recognize a person, even one we have not met for a long time, at any distance and from many different angles. A fixed hologram memory would not be able to perform this operation. The flexibility needed can be provided by optical means: for example, a zoom lens can carry out a search to match the size of the image received to the image stored. It seems not too far-fetched to imagine that a neurone network has this flexibility. It could be realized by extended variable fields, analogous to those used in electron optics, to produce different gradients in the speed of propagation of the network by electrical or chemical means. This could effect a change in focal distance, or a rotation of the image, or small distortions, to achieve a clear, sharp recognition signal in the image plane.

Although the hologram principle is natural for a neurone network, it does not exclude the possibility that another model such as the correlogram of Willshaw, Buneman and Longuet-Higgins is actually realized in the brain. One has first, however, to show that such a model is reasonable. Their model, in the optical form they propose, seems to have a low storage capacity because of the diffraction of any kind of wave field (this is not irrelevant!). In the network model they propose, on the other hand, they do obtain the same storage capacity as the holographic model, but it seems to lack the flexibility for recognizing images which are displaced, of different size, or slightly distorted. One more aspect to be considered is the fact that three-dimensional holograms are capable of storing time dependent signals [van Heerden, 1963]. The recognition of speech, and our ability to speak or run or drive a car, is one more aspect of information processing in the brain which must be explained by any model.

P. J. van Heerden

van Heerden has discussed some of the differences between his holographic model of memory [1963] and a pair of non-holographic models that we put forward last year [Willshaw, Buneman, and Longuet-Higgins, 1969] . . . .

In its optical form the correlograph is, indeed, severely limited by diffraction and cannot be taken literally as a physical model for memory; nor did we intend that it should. But we felt that its logic, which is easy to appreciate, might possibly be realized in the nervous system. For instance, an associative net might be made to function as a correlograph by "tying together" certain of its switches. But there was no evidence that any such tying takes place and we therefore put forward the associative net as the more likely model. It could be simply realized, as we pointed out, by a system of neurones with thresholds and modifiable synapses; both these properties are known to occur peripherally in the nervous system [Eccles, 1957, 1964] and probably occur centrally as well [Burns, Bliss, and Uttley, 1968].

Although there is no conclusive neurophysiological evidence to support our theory against van Heerden's, the ability of parts of the nervous system to propagate waves according to Huygens's principle would be difficult to reconcile with the observed non-linearity of some neural responses, and the existence of a stable periodic source of excitation has yet to be demonstrated. We also feel that in any model of the brain it is of advantage to be able to modify synapses as well as nerve cells. The ratio of synapses to nerve cells in the cerebral cortex seems to be of the order $10^4 - 10^5$ so that the information that could be stored synaptically would be correspondingly higher [Cragg, 1967). As to the remarkable flexibility of the human perceptual apparatus, we feel that neither his model nor ours can be held to account for this in their present forms.

D. J. Willshaw

H. C. Longuet-Higgins

O. P. Buneman

I agree with the contention of Willshaw, Buneman and Longuet-Higgins, in their response to my communication [van Heerden, 1970], that the associative net they proposed [Willshaw, Buneman, and Longuet-Higgins, 1969] performs the specified function as well as the hologram. Two of the most striking capabilities of human memory, however, are not present in their network. The first is our ability to recognize a person we know, when he appears in our field of view, which may contain a hundred more people. The sudden flash of recognition we may feel, this absolute certainty of "this is him and it can be nobody else", is not just a subjective emotion, but is apparently evoked only by an extremely reliable and fast form of information processing in our brain. This function of recognizing is also performed by the two-dimensional hologram, as the appearance of a bright light point in the image plane of the optical arrangement, and the brightness and sharpness of the light point are a scientific measure of the degree of recognition.

The second capability is our ability, after recognizing a person, to recall quickly a considerable amount of the information we have about this person. In an optical arrangement, the recognition signal given by the two-dimensional hologram provides the instruction for generating total recall of the relevant information from a three-dimensional hologram . . . .

It is true that the scientific efforts to explain the capabilities of human intelligence as a theory of brain action are necessarily in a beginning state. There is little doubt, however, that we have the foundation for this theory. This foundation is information theory, the same theory which is used in radio, television, radar and photography. In information theory, recognizing, or speaking of the quantitative degree of two things being alike, is described by the correlation function of two time functions, or two images. The elaborate computation of the correlation function can be described mathematically as a filtering operation, but the computation of the matched filter required for this filtering operation is of course as involved as the original computation. The fact that the hologram performs this filtering function with 50 per cent efficiency, and that a neurone network with simple postulated properties can do the same, is due to the fact that accidentally and fortunately—or maybe it is in the nature of things—a propagating wave field carries out automatically this laborious computation demanded by the theory.

P. J. van Heerden

A neural holographic or similar process does not mean, of course, that input information is distributed willy-nilly over the entire depth and surface of the brain. Only those limited regions where reasonably stable junctional designs are initiated by the input participate in the distribution. Furthermore, for any effect beyond the duration of a particular input the more localized memory mechanisms described in Part I must be invoked. These can, however, be engaged in loci distributed in neural space once information has become dispersed. Retrieval from the more permanent memory store demands merely the repetition of the pattern (or essential parts thereof) which originally initiated storage. This capability to directly "address" content without reference to location, so readily accomplished by the holographic process does away with the need for keeping track of where information is stored.

What are some of the possibilities for making the junctional microstructure endure? Some more lasting property of protoplasm must be invoked to account for storage which can be of varying duration. Profound temporary interactions do occur between inputs separated by hours (as in the McCullough effect in which exposure to a set of colored bands influences subsequent observations of color) or in some individuals for days (as in the rare person who shows true eidetic capacities). And, of course, the longer range interactions that account for recognition and recall must also be taken into consideration. Conformational changes in macromolecules such as lipids or proteins and even longer lasting anisotropic orderings of macromolecular structure lend themselves to speculation: when similar in configuration, successive junctional microstructures may produce a cumulative residual effect by inducing ordering into previously disordered macromolecular chains or fibrils, or by increasing an existing order, so that the region thereafter responds more easily to a repetition of the same excitation. Early results of experiments performed on retinal tissue examined with the electron microscope show that such changes in molecular conformation can occur with excitation (Sjöstrand, 1969). Similar proposals not yet confirmed have been made by Lancelot Whyte (1954) and Ward Halstead (Katz and Halstead, 1950). Whyte suggests that:

> ... this cumulative medium- and long-range ordering of some of the protein chains throughout a particular volume of cortical cytoplasm is a kind of growth process of a pattern determined not by heredity but by activity, and involving the development not of a differentiated tissue but of an element of ordering in the molecular arrangement of an extended mass of cytoplasm. Here we are concerned with the *differentiation of particular vector directions* possibly parallel to the cortical surface in particular cortical layers. The templates of memory are not single localized molecular structures, but extended components of long-range order set at various angles to one another . . . . [However] the ordering will correspond only to the *statistically dominant pattern of activity* or simplest overall pattern common to the successive activity patterns. Moreover this tendency to select the dominant pattern will be reinforced by the fact that the simplest overall patterns will be the most stable, since their parts will mutually support one another. The random protein structures may thus act as a structural sieve taking a stable impress at first only of the simplest, most unified, and statistically dominant component in all the patterns of activity of a given general form . . . . In general [then] the development of the modification proceeds from a grossly simplified to a less simplified and more accurate record. This process of the development of a hierarchically organized modification corresponds to Coghill's 'progressive individuation' of behavior patterns during ontogeny, and may hold the clue to the self-coordinating capacity of cortical process. [Whyte, 1954, pp. 162–63]

These statements do not, of course, indicate all that is necessary to register wave forms. Conformational changes in macromolecules are apt to be reversible. A more permanent record probably demands such mechanisms as the tuning of "averaging circuits" in cortical columns and growth induced by the changes in membrane permeability consequent to and dependent on these macromolecular alterations. The "filter," "sieve," or "screen" of holographic patterns is composed not only of the lattice of membrane macromolecules making up the synapto-dendritic net, but also of a facilitation of all tendencies toward Image formation and the initiation of certain departure patterns of nerve impulses.

support for the hypothesis

One line of evidence in support of the holographic hypothesis comes from the studies on the development of visual perception in infants. Contrary to widely held views (e.g., Hebb), size and shape constancy do *not* emerge exclusively from a combination of prior and presumably more primitive perceptions (e.g., length of line, angle). Hebb's suggestion was based on the results of experiments and clinical observations in which subjects were reared under conditions of sensory deprivation. He assumed that experience was necessary for the proper *development* of receptor function. However, electrophysiological experiments (recall Fig. 7-12) show that the retinal and neural mechanisms for feature detection are already well developed in mammals (cats) at the time of birth. The effect of sensory restriction appears therefore to be either an *atrophy of disuse* or an *active suppression* of the sensory mechanism by an induced malfunction. As noted already, the situation is not too different in man. Bower (1966) performed experiments with six-week-old infants that show size and, to a large extent, shape constancy to be already present. In these experiments objects were placed so that actual size, distance, and retinal image (as calculated from actual size of figures observed) could be matched in various combinations. Complete and incomplete figures were used; flat, two-dimensional pictures of objects were substituted for the three-dimensional ones. Discriminations were taught by having the experimenter reward the infant with a peek-a-boo response. The test then elicited the learned response from the infant by substituting one of the matched stimuli for the original one. The results of these experiments demonstrated constancy only when distance cues were available or when one element of a figure moved while the rest remained stationary. Thus even in infants the visual system is innately set to register "the kind of information given by motion parallax and binocular parallax." What sort of built-in mechanism could handle parallax better than a holographic process which is constructed by a parallactic (interference effect) process?

Direct evidence that a Fourier-like parallactic cortical mechanism may be involved in Imagery is provided in experiments performed by Fergus Campbell and his associates (Blakemore and Campbell, 1969;

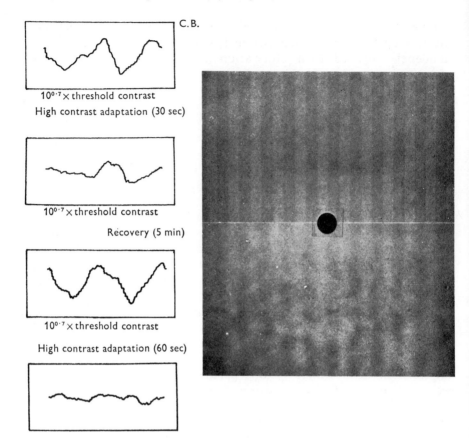

C. B.

$10^{0.7}$ × threshold contrast

High contrast adaptation (30 sec)

$10^{0.7}$ × threshold contrast

Recovery (5 min)

$10^{0.7}$ × threshold contrast

High contrast adaptation (60 sec)

Fig. 8-12. The effects of spatial adaptation on the evoked potential in man. A sine-wave grating pattern (12 c/deg.) was shifted in place by 180°, eight times per second, and the occipital potential evoked was summed 200 times on the Enhancetron to produce the records shown in boxes on the left. The stimulus was identical for each record. Each trace shows the potential for two phase shifts. The first record is for a low contrast grating (upper section of right hand panel), $10^{0.7}$ times the threshold contrast for this spatial frequency. C. B. then viewed a high contrast grating (lower panel) (1.5 log units above threshold) for 30 sec and the potential for the same low contrast grating was immediately re-measured. This second trace is clearly rather lower in amplitude than the first. After 5 min recovery the low contrast grating produced a record (3rd box) very similar to that of the original. The final record taken after 60 sec exposure to the high contrast grating has no distinguishable signal. The failure to record the potential was accompanied by subjective elevation of threshold. From Blakemore and Campbell, 1969.

Campbell, et al., 1968; Campbell, Cooper, and Enroth-Cugell, 1969; Campbell and Robson, 1968). These studies have shown that the cerebral cortex may be tuned to different ranges of spatial information. The experiments were performed on both cats and humans by presenting gratings of different coarseness and studying the effects of rotation on the visually evoked responses (man) and on the firing patterns of units in the visual cortex (cat). Neurons responded to a limited band of spatial frequency (four octaves) and prolonged viewing causes a depression of contrast sensitivity over a limited range of neighboring frequencies (Fig. 8-12).

The relationship between these experimental results and the Fourier hologram is best stated in the authors' own words:

In this study we have intentionally used the simplest optical stimulus . . . . The sine-wave grating is simple because it contains only one spatial frequency presented in one meridian. The most complex stimulus in Fourier terms is a single sharp disk of light for it contains a very wide band of spatial frequencies and they are present at all orientations. The 'bandwidth' of the individual spatial mechanisms revealed by adaptation is quite narrow (about 1 octave at half amplitude . . .). Therefore any complex pattern of light on the retina, containing a wide spectrum of Fourier components, will cause activity in many mechanisms. We should like to suggest that the pattern of responses from the family of mechanisms may serve to encode the spatial content of the particular retinal image and thus lead, in an unknown manner, to its identification . . . .

An advantage of a system based on frequency analysis might be that it simplifies recognition of familiar objects presented at unfamiliar magnifications. Consider a child who has just learned to differentiate the letters of the alphabet and suppose that it is asked to recognize letters presented at quite different magnifications. It does this readily even although it has never observed the letters at these specific magnifications. We know that if we are so close to an object that we cannot perceive it in entirety it cannot be readily identifed; 'we cannot see the wood for the trees.' Sutherland (1968) has lucidly reviewed the literature on size invariance and concludes 'that many species have the capacity to classify a shape as the same shape regardless of changes in size, at least over a considerable range, and that this capacity is innate.'

There must be a limited range of spatial dimensions which the visual system can handle with facility and speed. If it analyses the distribution of spatial frequencies in an object into independent channels covering its range of operation and then uses the ratios of these frequencies to identify the object, it would render the absolute size of the object redundant for the purpose of image recognition, for the relative harmonic content is independent of absolute size. Only the harmonic content would have to be stored in the memory system and this would require a much smaller store than if the appearance of every familiar object had to be learned at every common magnification. This generalization for size, and therefore distance, would greatly facilitate the process of learning to recognize images in our natural environment. This system might then be analogous to the auditory system where we can identify a musical interval (frequency ratio) independently of its position in the auditory spectrum . . . .

Such a mechanism for analysing spatial frequencies would be difficult to envisage if it had to operate simultaneously in two dimensions. It may well be significant that the visual system also transmits the input signal through a number of separate orientationally selective channels, each of which can then analyse the spatial frequency content of the object over a narrow range of orientations . . . . Although this arrangement would lead to a further economy in the size of the memory store it would also carry the penalty that no one would be restricted to recognizing familiar objects only if they were presented at the learned orientation.

Here is the Evidence

We cannot generalize for orientation as we can do so remarkably well for magnification. [Blakemore and Campbell, 1969, pp. 257–59]

Another line of evidence comes from an experience we have all shared. A great many more and much richer details can be recalled and re-imaged when we are given the appropriate context—for instance, when visiting a neighborhood we had lived in many years earlier, shops and doorways and living room furniture placements come to mind which only a few hours earlier seemed forever lost. What better mechanism can be operating than the associative recall provided by the holographic process?

The impetus to Imaging need not, of course, come from receptors. As I have noted and will discuss in detail in Chapters 17 and 18, arrival patterns can be produced in the input channels by excitation of the so-called association areas of the brain. Images assumed to be produced by this excitation can, as a rule, be readily differentiated from those initiated by receptor excitation—but under such special circumstances as temporary sensory deprivation the differentiation between internal and external production of Images breaks down resulting in the experiencing of illusions and hallucinations. The very fact that Imaging of this sort occurs, however, and that it displays similarities to the perceptual process, suggests that perception itself is to a large extent reconstructive. What mechanism other than the process of Image reconstruction by holography can be thought up to perform this function?

The major locus of reconstruction for visual Imaging is the striate area of the occipital cortex. Persons who have suffered bilateral removals of the occipital lobe are reported to totally lack visual Imagery (Konorski, 1967). Peripheral damage has no such result—in the auditory mode Beethoven is an excellent example of a peripherally deaf person who could still Image sufficiently to write his ninth symphony and the late quartets.

Further evidence congruent with the holographic hypothesis comes from experiments with electrical stimulation of the visual receiving area of the cortex in man (Brindley and Lewin, 1968). Such stimulation, which codes intensity only and is incapable of eliciting phase relationships, gives rise to punctate spots of light that look like "a star in the sky"—not lines or angles. When produced away from the point of regard, they may be slightly elongated, "like a grain of rice." The most peripheral perceptions are "cloud-like" and "about the size of peas at arm's length." They appear in a constant position in the visual field. By stimulation through several electrodes the patient can, however, be caused to see simple patterns. During voluntary eye movements the perceived spots move with the eyes; during reflex movement initiated by vestibular stimulation the perceived spots remain fixed in space. After very strong stimulation the visual perceptions sometimes persist for as long as two minutes. A fascinating set of observations which demand some mechanism beyond feature detection for the construction of the richly complex visual Images perceived in ordinary life.

Still another interesting line of evidence in support of a neural holographic process comes from studies of partial injuries to the occipital cortex. On the basis of a simple detector model no disturbance outside the scotoma produced by the lesion would be expected. But careful studies by Hans-Lukas Teuber and W. Stanley Battersby (Teuber, Battersby, and Bender, 1960) have shown that in the entire remaining field contours may fade more rapidly; fusion thresholds for flickering lights are reduced; and the perception of real and apparent motion is impaired. All of these phenomena are probably dependent on the inhibitory interactions which constitute the filter produced by the interference effects of the neural holographic process. A huge tear in such a filter would be expected to affect the quality, not the occurrence, of the Image produced by the remainder.

extensions and limitations

This account has been one-sided. Not only have I developed a single hypothesis, but I have singled out the visual mode for study and analyzed only its spatial, extensive quality in any detail. The hypothesis, with modifications, must hold for other sensory modes and other sensory qualities if it is to be more generally useful. For somesthesis the transposition is, as shown by Bekesy, relatively direct (recall Fig. 8-3) since the haptic sense is also seriously concerned with spatial image formation. Bekesy's model of the auditory process (1960) is so similar that work on its neural mechanism should prove not only feasible but rewarding. This similarity comes about because pitch (and therefore harmony) are, as S.S. Stevens (1951) has called it, dimensionally metathetic and thus related to neurological space. Too little is as yet known of the neurological processes involved in taste and olfactory perception to allow more than a guess that further inquiry will not yield data wildly inimical to the model proposed here. Preliminary transpositions to the gustatory mode made by Bekesy (1967) and unit analysis of neurons in the olfactory bulb by Lettvin (Gesteland, Lettvin, and Pitts, 1968) suggest, however, that the approach is reasonable.

Little can as yet be stated about qualities other than the more obviously extensive. Intuitively the hypothesis here presented fits the requirements of an opponens process color vision mechanism such as

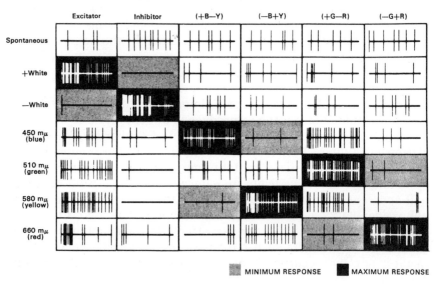

Fig. 8-13. Systematization of data recorded at lateral geniculate nucleus of monkeys demonstrating the opponens process of color vision. From R.L. DeValois and G.H. Jacobs, *Science,* 162, p. 539, November 1968, © 1968 by AAAS.

that proposed by Ewald Hering (1920; trans. 1964), and delineated experimentally by Leo Hurvich and Dorothea Jameson (1960). The work of Russell DeValois (DeValois and Jacobs, 1968; Fig. 8-13) on recording opponens color units in the visual system and that of Gunnar Svaetichin (1967) which provides clues about how the opponens process is constructed in the retina, bears out the possibilities of extending the model beyond pattern perception. These outlines are dimly viewed—yet at least outlines are before us where not so long ago only vague hobbits inhabited the land of neuromythology.

A more serious limitation to the holographic hypothesis is the current lack of quantitative data with which to specify the information processing capacity of the neural holographic process. As already pointed out earlier in this chapter there is considerable doubt whether "brain waves" as presently recorded form the substrate of any meaningful interference pattern organization for information processing, although they may be indicative that some such process is taking place. Because of their wave length these wave forms can carry only very small amounts of information—even in the form of spatially interfering holographic patterns. By contrast, the holographic hypothesis pursued here emphasizes the role of junctional slow potential "microwave" structures in brain function. Let me state once more, however, these microstructures can be described either in statistical, quantal terms, or in the wave mechanical language of convolutional integrals and Fourier transforms. The microstructures do not change their characteristics because a choice is made as to description. Each language, each descriptive form, has its own advantages. For the physical hologram, whether composed by the interference of light waves or by computer programming, the amount of information stored or processed is calculable from the quantitative description of the spatial phase relationships that determine the process. Experiments are sorely needed that spell out similar quantitative relationships for the interactions of cortical columns. The way has been paved by Rodieck's and Hartline's analyses of the interactions among receptor elements.

Despite these limitations, many hitherto paradoxical findings regarding brain function in perception become understandable when the holographic analogy is taken seriously. This does not mean that all brain function reduces to a holographic process—or that all the problems of perception yield to holographic analysis. The neural hologram is used to explain the psychological function of Imaging and the distributed memory mechanism in the brain. It does not follow that memory is distributed helter skelter all over the brain. The neural hologram deals with the facts of disruptions of the input systems. Its extension to other systems by extrapolation still does not mean that the systems get mixed up with one another. Memory mechanisms other than those that fit the holographic analogy must play a role—even in Imaging and certainly in recognition: the composition of these additional mechanisms has been detailed in Chapter 7 and will form the substance of several subsequent ones.

Altogether the holographic analogy fits comfortably into the system of elementary logic modules outlined in Part I. More important, the holographic hypothesis does not upset classical neurophysiological conceptions; it enriches them by a shift in emphasis from axonal nerve impulses to the slow potential microstructure that develops in post-synaptic, dendritic networks. At the same time, the holographic hypothesis enriches psychology by providing a plausible mechanism for understanding phenomenal experience. This permits consideration of components of psychological functions which become lumped together in a restricted behavioristic framework. Pattern recognition is a complex process in which feature analysis and the formation of a central representation of input are steps. In man, given the neural hologram, these steps lead to Image construction.

Science searches for explanatory principles, and psychological science is no exception. The success of the junctional slow potential microstructure in explaining some of the puzzles of perception and the success of a phenomenal concept per se in serving as an analytical tool in dissecting a behavioral operation into its functional components, merits follow-through. The next chapters will therefore continue along these guidelines and tackle another set of psychological functions, motivations and emotions, in terms of their phenomenal impressions, the feelings.

synopsis

Feature detection and analysis by neural units and by the logic they compose are insufficient to handle all of the phenomena of perception. An additional mechanism is available in the junctional patterns of neural activity. Superposition, i.e., spatial interactions among phase relationships of neighboring junctional patterns occurs, and such interactions can display Image forming properties akin to those of optical information processing systems—the properties of holograms.

feelings

the "world-out-there" and the "world-within"

From the energy configurations that excite some of our receptors we are able to construct a "World-Out-There." The excitations of sight and hearing we especially interpret as being distant from the receptors excited. Touch, taste, and smell do not ordinarily allow this attribution of distance—localization is to the receptor surface and thus establishes for us a boundary between what is out-there and in-here. Yet even with these receptor modalities we sense that we are touching, tasting, or smelling something apart from our own receptor reactions.

But there is another world: a "World-Within," a world of subjective feelings. In contrast to perceptions, subjective feelings are those phenomena, those ghosts which we immediately attribute to what is within the boundary, that bag we call the skin, which demarcates the "Us" from the "Other." *We* feel hungry or sleepy or sexy; *we* feel pain, happiness, or sadness; *we* feel contemplative or assertive. Are the processes that give rise to this inner world different enough from those already discussed to warrant the Cartesian dualism which has split the creative community into humanists and scientists for three centuries? The answer is a resounding no. This answer is based on evidence which makes our construction of an outer world understandable in terms of neural processes that engender projection and on the knowledge that we build up a "World-Within" when another, not altogether differently constituted, set of neural processes becomes engaged.

Clinical neurological experience tells us that the localizing of a perceptual Image is not a simple process. The paradoxical phenomenon of a phantom limb after amputation, for example, makes it unlikely that our experience of receptor stimulation "resides" where we are apt to localize it. The patient who asks the nurse to massage his toes because they are cramped, has not yet, and may never sense a loss of limb even though, as the nurse may unwittingly inform him, his foot has been sent to the pathology laboratory in a jar. Images are formed by the brain—why then do we locate an object where we do?

Bekesy has performed some critical experiments to answer this question. Using touch, which is not ordinarily interpreted as distant, he creates conditions under which this "distant" interpretation is made:

> Reflected light from an external object produces an image on the retina. The sensations exist only within our body, yet we localize the image outside the eye, even when we use only a single eye and look at an object far away. This localization beyond our perceptual system is of great importance for survival because it enables us to appreciate impending danger or objects of great necessity. This externalization is achieved without the slightest recognition of the optic image itself or the stimulation on the retina.
>
> The same conditions hold for hearing. The sensations are produced by the action of stimuli on the basilar membrane of the cochlea. The cochlea is deeply imbedded in bone, but we do not localize auditory sensations there but usually refer them to a source somewhere in the environment. However, as we have seen, this external reference does not seem to be true for hearing with earphones.
>
> This external projection has probably been learned early in life; certainly this is true for hearing and vision. But we have not acquired this kind of external projection for skin sensations, and so we have an opportunity to discover how stimulus projection in space is learned.
>
> For this study a pair of vibrators stimulate two fingertips [Fig. 9-1]. . . . Each vibrator is actuated by the same series of clicks, and their applied currents are varied to give equal magnitudes of sensation on each fingertip when the stimuli are presented separately. Also the setup includes a means of

vibrators

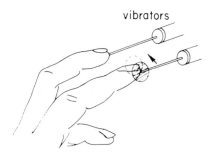

Fig. 9-1. Diagram of experiment described in text. In Békésy, 1967.

varying the delay time between the clicks of the two series. If a click is delayed for one finger more than 3 or 4 milliseconds, a person feels separate sensations in the two fingertips, as already described. If, however, the time between clicks is reduced to about 1 millisecond the two click series will fuse into one, and the vibratory sensation will be localized in the finger that receives each click the earlier. If the time delay is further decreased the sensation for a trained observer will move into the region between two fingers, and if then the time relation between the two click series is reversed the click will move to the opposite side . . . .

The interesting point in this experiment is that for the condition in which there is no time delay the vibrations are localized between the two fingers where no skin is present. If the fingers are spread apart the same effect is found, and when the amount of time delay is varied the sensation will move correspondingly in the free space between the fingers.

Even more dramatic than this experiment is the one in which two vibrators are placed on the thighs, one above each knee. Here the vibrators can stimulate large skin surfaces and produce strong vibratory sensations. By training an observer first to note the localization of the vibration when the knees are together, he can be made to perceive a sensation that moves continuously from one knee to the other. If the observer now spreads the knees apart he will again experience at first a jumping of the sensation from one knee to the other. In time, however, the observer will become convinced that the vibratory sensation can be localized in the free space between the knees, and he will be able to experience a displacement of the sensation in this free space when an appropriate time delay between one stimulus and the other is introduced. This experience is a very peculiar one.

This matter of the external projection of vibratory sensations seems to be strange and hard to believe, yet it is well known in many fields. Every well-trained machinist projects his sensations of pressure to the tip of a screwdriver, and it is this projection that enables him to work rapidly and

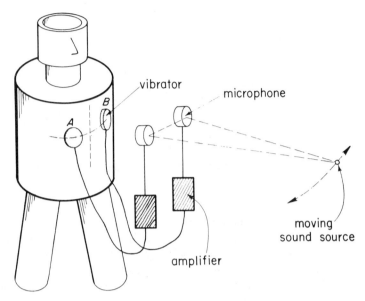

vibrator

microphone

B

A

moving
sound source

amplifier

Fig. 9-2. Equipment for study of the differences between auditory and vibratory localization. From Békésy, 1963.

correctly. For most people this projection is so common that they are unaware of its existence. The same type of projection occurs in cutting with a knife, and our adjustments of the blade make use of sensations projected to its edge.

I found the localization of sensations in free space to be a very important feature of behavior. To study the matter further I wore two hearing aids that were properly damped so that the sounds could be picked up by means of two microphones on the chest and then transmitted to the two ears without change in pressure amplitude [Fig. 9-2]. Stereophonic hearing was well established, but a perception of the distance of sound sources was lost. I shall not forget my frustration in trying to cross the street during rush hour traffic while wearing this transmission system. Almost all the cars seemed to jump suddenly into consciousness, and I was unable to put them in order according to their immediacy. I should probably have required weeks of experience to become adjusted to this new type of projection. A small change in the amplification of one side was enough to cancel the whole learned adjustment. [Bekesy, 1967, pp. 220–26]

These experimental results are, of course, not the full answer to the problem of how an organism constructs his "World-Out-There." Computations of constancies and of convergent series of transformations also allow extrapolations to be made from current receptor excitation. And other cues such as parallax and texture in vision aid the construction process. But Bekesy's observations considerably implement our ability to understand this hitherto unfathomable puzzle. They also provide a clue to the survival value of having two of everything arranged symmetrically in opposing halves of the body—there is obviously a good deal more to it than just carrying spare parts.

Imagine for a moment that we were bereft of all of these mechanisms which construct for us a World-Out-There. Try for instance to move around with ear plugs in place and shades covering your eyes. As in Bekesy's hearing aid experiment, life suddenly becomes more intimate: we are limited to a World-Within.

feelings as monitor images

This chapter will not expand further on feelings such as touch and taste which are referred to receptor surfaces. The mechanism of Image formation in these modalities is probably little different from that already encountered in vision. Rather, the present concern will be with the World-Within per se: the feelings of hunger and thirst, love and pleasure, discomfort and perturbation. The results of a great number of experiments and observations indicate that these feelings arise from excitations of receptors lying deep within the core of the brain, receptors which engage mechanisms in some respects similar, and in others considerably different, from those which give rise to perceptual images.

Feelings that "monitor" the World-Within share with other forms of Imaging the characteristic that the representation which generates them is one or another steady state produced by receptor events in a neuronal aggregate. The claim expressed in these chapters is that these steady states occur as representations consisting of configurations of junctional potentials. In the case of "monitor-feelings," the receptor events which govern the representation are patterned differently from those which govern perceptual Images. In addition, the organizations of neuronal aggregates in which the representations occur are different: feelings "monitoring" the World-Within are composed by multiply-interconnected neuronal aggregates, many of which are characterized by a vast number of short, fine-fibered, many-branched neurons. The microstructure of slow potentials in such an arrangement can be expected to differ considerably from that which occurs in flat sheets of horizontally connected cells cutting across parallel lines of nerve transmission.

At present we know little about the resultants of inhibitory interactions which take place in such networks; neurophysiology has completely ignored this area of study. But anatomical considerations alone preclude the clear separation between decrementing and lateral inhibitory processes that is so characteristic of sensory (and motor) channels. From these anatomical considerations we might conjecture that the decrementing and inhibitory interactions here blend into a device which governs the system somewhat like a gyroscope, but this conjecture needs neurophysiological testing at the unit level. Instead of orienting, habituation, and dishabituation, a "monitoring" of fluctuations in excitability with a tendency toward restitution to a mean ought to be discernible. Furthermore, the large number of synaptic junctions per unit volume in these neuronal aggregates makes them especially sensitive to chemical substances derived from the surrounding tissue and the blood stream and thus candidates for the role of receptor sites for monitoring the local concentration of neurohumors.

the core brain receptors

Over a century ago Claude Bernard (1865, trans. 1927) initiated a branch of neurophysiology concerned with the central nervous system's regulation of the organism's metabolic and

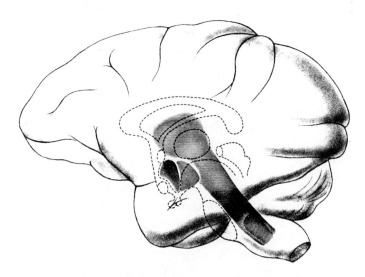

Fig. 9-3. Diagram of core brain within the outlines of the cerebral hemispheres. From Livingston, 1955.

endocrine functions. These now famous "picure" experiments, in which diabetes was produced by making small stab wounds in the brain stem, led to many others in which the body's vegetative functions, the *milieu interieur*, were disrupted by small holes or localized electrical stimulations in the brain stem (Fig. 9-3).

Thus changes in temperature, in the osmotic balance of tissue fluids, in the function of the pituitary and other endocrine glands, as well as in the glucose level of the blood were noted. As the organization of these neuronal aggregates was gradually worked out, it became evident that cell aggregates in the brain stem acted as receptor sites for the substances or variables being controlled. Specifically, it was found that hypertonic saline injected into the third ventricle immediately caused goats to drink voluminously (Andersson, 1953); heat applied to the base of the anterior extremity of the third ventricle immediately caused changes in the heat regulating mechanisms all over the mammalian body (Ranson, Fisher, and Ingram, 1937); just behind this area, injections of androgens and estrogens labeled with radioactive molecules resulted in differential uptake by brain cells which when stimulated will initiate sexual behavior (Michael, 1962; Davidson, Jones, and Levine, 1968; see also Fig. 9-4); similarly labeled glucose molecules are absorbed maximally by a group of cells still further back which control eating (see

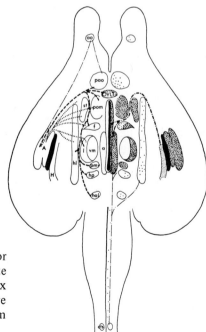

Fig. 9-4. Example of core brain receptor sites in rat brain: striped areas indicate uptake of labelled estrogen (female sex hormone) molecules. Lateral structure showing uptake is amygdala. From Stumpf, 1970.

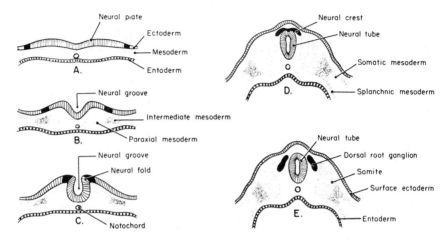

Fig. 9-5. Diagram of the formation of the neural tube which then develops into spinal cord and brain. From Truex and Carpenter, *Human Neuroanatomy,* 6 ed. ©1969 The Williams & Wilkins Co., Baltimore, Md.

Chapter 10; Mayër, 1963); and local changes in the partial pressure of CO_2 in the posterior brain stem dramatically alter the rate and depth of respiration (Meyer, 1957). All of these sensitivities are localized to structures fairly near the midline (third and fourth) ventricles of the brain stem.

The fact that this part of the brain contains receptors ought not to be too surprising. In embryonic development this midline part of the central nervous system is derived from the most dorsal part of the tissue that becomes the central nervous system. This tissue derives from the same origins as does skin: a crest of ectodermal cells on the back of the embryo becomes infolded to form a tube which encloses a space later to be filled with cerebro-spinal fluid (Fig. 9-5). At the head end of the embryo this space becomes the ventricular system of the brain. The lining of the space, the periventricular cells, are therefore akin to the ectoderm that forms the skin and some of the more specialized receptors, such as the retina. Thus the sensitivities of the periventricular structures are similar to those of the skin: temperature change, deformation, and changes in hydration are some of the major categories of stimuli to which both periventricular structures and skin are sensitive.

This sensitivity of the periventricular part of the brain was brought nome to me in dramatic fashion. One of the peculiarities of brain tissue is that *almost* everywhere it is insensitive to mechanical handling. Brain surgery is therefore performed in many instances under local anesthesia in order to save the patient the extra trauma and hazard of a general anesthetic. On one such occasion we were exploring the region of the fourth ventricle and, as customary in neurosurgery, we kept the brain moist by dropping liquid on the exposed parts. Ordinarily the liquid is made to simulate the concentration and composition of chemicals in the cerebrospinal fluid; on this occasion a rookie nurse had, in the purity of her approach, substituted distilled water. The moment the water hit the ventricle the patient suffered severe pain in the head, nausea, retching, and vomiting. The same reactions were produced by pushing or pulling lightly on the ventricle wall or using liquid which was cooler or warmer than body temperature.

In summary, then, the work of a century of neurophysiological experiment indicates that a series of specialized "monitor" receptors are located near the midline ventricular systems of the brain stem. These specialized receptors are the classical centers for the control of respiration, food intake, etc., that have interested physiologists and biochemists concerned with the neural regulation of the organism's metabolism and endocrine functions. These receptors function as "state" sensitive elements of a variety of servomechanisms—christened "homeostats" by Cannon (1929)—concerned with the regulation of appetitive-consummatory functions. Let us look now to some of the other components of homeostats.

biasing the homeostats

Immediately beyond the limits of the periventricular receptors lies a matrix of neural fibers spotted with neuronal aggregates and coursed occasionally by long nerve fibers. The anatomy of the midbrain reticular formation has been detailed by Alf Brodal (1958) and by the Scheibels (1958); its physiology is well documented in a symposium (Jasper, 1958) and by Horace Magoun (1958). What is often neglected, however, is the fact that an organization similar to that found in the midbrain extends upward from it into the forebrain along the midline ventricular system. Thus parts of the hypothalamus and midline thalamus and even the septal region share the attributes of the midbrain reticular formation. After all, the division of the brain into hind, mid, and fore portions is arbitrary. An equally valid, and, for the problem of homeostatic regulations, a more useful classification divides the brain into layers from inside out, much as in an elongated onion or celery stick. Characteristically, the core brain tissues are composed of fairly short, fine-fibered neurons which have vast dendritic networks (Fig. 9-6). Inputs con-

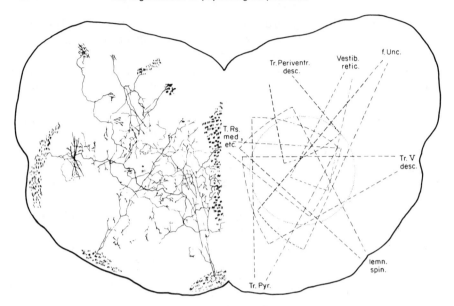

Fig. 9-6. Tranverse section through upper third of the medulla of the brain stem of a 10-day-old kitten, showing the convergence and overlapping of terminating afferent fibers in the reticular core. On the left, a small group of fibers are drawn directly from the microscope; on the right is a group of overlapping sectors. From Scheibel and Scheibel, 1967a.

verge on each nerve cell from many branches of the long classical projection tracts that originate in the various sensory receptors of the organism. Each neural element in the system is influenced by a variety of sensory modes as is indicated by changes produced in the electrical activity recorded with microelectrodes (Fig. 9-7). In addition, a reciprocal relation with the rest of the neuraxis exists, e.g., the cerebral cortex is activated when the core brain formations are electrically excited; conversely, cortical stimulation affects the activity of the reticular systems. This convergence of input and diffuseness of interrelations suggests that the most likely action of these systems is to influence the general state of excitability of the nervous system. This suggestion is supported by the finding that cortical rhythms are activated and deactivated by electrical stimulation of the core brain systems and by the fact that lesions and stimulations of these systems have been shown to be related to such psychological processes as the sleep-wakefulness cycle and alertness. Furthermore, the anatomical structure of these systems suggests that the graded response mechanisms characterizing the slow potential microstruc-

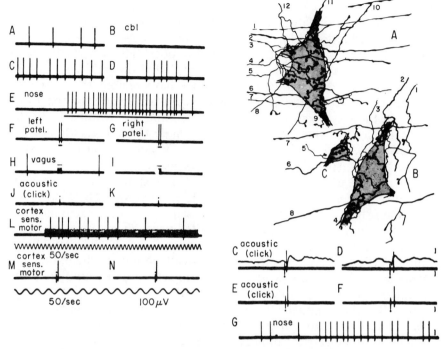

Fig. 9-7. Convergence of heterogenous afferents upon single elements of the brain stem reticular core demonstrated physiologically and histologically. Strips A through N and C through G illustrate patterns of extracellularly derived spike discharges from two elements of bulbar reticular formation. A: spontaneous discharges; B: inhibition by cerebellar polarization (anterior lobe, surface positive); C: rebound following cessation of polarization; D: return toward normal spontaneous pattern; E: driven by nose pressure; F and G: driven by patellar tendon taps bilaterally; H and I: unaffected by short bursts of vagal stimuli; J and K: unaffected by clicks; L: driven by repetitive cortical stimulation; M and N: driven after a brief latency by single shocks to cortex (note expanded time base beneath these last two records). Strips C, D, E, and F show another unit that is sensitive to nose pressure and can also be driven by clicks.

Cells A, B, and C are bulbar reticular elements in 10-day-old kitten whose synaptic scale of terminating afferents is partially shown. Horizontal-running fibers such as A, 1 through 7, and B, 6 through 8, may belong to long spinoreticular and reticulo-reticular components while B, 1 through 4, represent sensory collaterals and cerebelloreticular terminals. From Scheibel and Scheibel, 1967a.

ture are dominant and not the transmission of signals. Synapses and dendrites are abundant; fibers are, for the most part, short and fine so that conduction velocity of an impulse is slow and its amplitude small. As noted in Chapter 1, the slow potential microstructure is especially sensitive to changes in chemical environment. As we shall shortly see, a great number of studies have related the action of neural transmitters and psychopharmacological agents to the functions of these systems. But first let us examine the significance of the reticular core to the problem of the "homeostatic" regulation of the organism's *milieu interieur,* a significance which stems from proximity to the specialized periventricular receptors.

Within the core brain is located a set of systems that is especially effective in regulating the homeostatic mechanism. The history of this important discovery gives some insight into unexpected happenings that can turn into fantastic scientific discoveries.

Two investigators at McGill University, James Olds and Peter Milner (1954), were preparing to electrically stimulate the brain stem reticular core of rats while these animals were learning to solve problems. They implanted electrodes with the stereotaxic apparatus into what they thought would be the appropriate placement in the rat's brain. In preliminary "shakedown" trials they noticed that whenever the electrical pulse was turned on, the rat would run to a particular spot. This puzzled and piqued the interest of the investigators. After repeating the observation many times, they wanted to automate the procedure in order to study this "repetition compulsion" in detail at leisure. They therefore arranged the situation so that the rat would find in the corner a lever which when pressed, would turn on the pulse. The rat quickly learned to press repetitively and so the technique of self-stimulation of the brain was born.

Olds then carefully mapped the sites in the brain from which the effect could be obtained. The stereotaxic technique had not led the experimenters where they had thought it would—the placement was far anterior to the location aimed for. But the site hit so fortuitously—the median forebrain bundle in the region of the septum—has remained one of the prime areas for obtaining the effect. The remainder of the self-stimulation system spreads backward from this location and seems to encompass the sites of the core-brain receptor mechanisms already detailed in this chapter (Olds, 1961; Fig. 9-8).

Many experiments have been performed using the self-stimulation technique and many interpretations of the effect have been given, ranging from simple hedonistic declarations that the pleasure centers of the brain have been discovered to cautious behavioristic state-

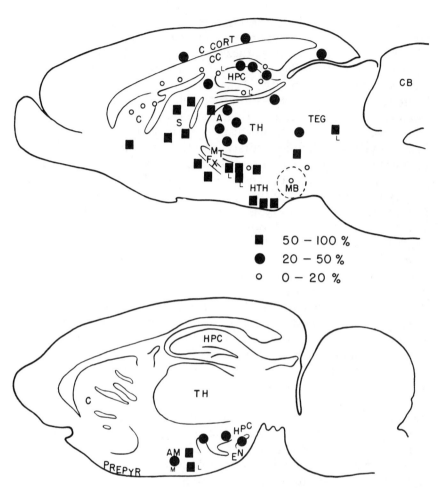

Fig. 9-8. Medial (upper diagram) and lateral (lower diagram) sagittal sections of the rat brain showing loci of different rewarding effects with self-stimulation. The squares and circles indicate the percentage of bar-pressing produced during a 6-hour test period. Key: *A*, anterior thalamus; *AM*, amygdala; *C*, caudate nucleus; *CB*; cerebellum; *CC*, corpus callosum; *C CORT*, cingulate cortex; *EN*, entorhinal cortex, *FX*, fornix; *HPC*, hippocampus; *HTH*, hypothalamus; *MB*, Mammillary body; *MT*, mammilothalamic tract; *PREPYR*, prepyriform cortex; *S*, septal region; *TEG*, tegmentum; *TH*, thalamus. The medial section (upper) is near the midline; the lateral section (lower) is 2 to 3 mm. more lateral. The letters *M* (medial) and *L* (lateral) near a given indicate that it is above 2 mm. medial or lateral to the plane shown. From Olds, 1961.

ments concerning the reinforcing properties of the process. My own view is based in part on reports given by an occasional human patient who has been implanted in these sites, and on the anatomical and behavioral fact that the locations for effective self-stimulation and for the control of appetitive behaviors such as eating are essentially identical. On this evidence I interpret self-stimulation of the brain to momentarily change the setting, the bias of the core homeostatic mechanisms so that the organism does in fact have the feeling of being temporarily hungry, thirsty, and the like and then quickly feels momentary satiety only to repeat the cycle once more. The particular feeling stimulated depends on the core-brain receptor system closest to the site chosen for self-stimulation and leads to the related activity when opportunity is given for this to occur (Olds, 1955). Therefore the self-stimulation process would be something like repeatedly adjusting and returning to its original location the setting device on a home thermostat in a room that is already warm. The furnace turns on briefly, only to go off again as the setting is returned to its baseline.

Electrical manipulations of bias are not the only ones that have been made. As noted, a series of studies using minute injections of chemicals has also produced appetitive behaviors. Again the sites of chemical stimulation are identical with those which produce electrical self-stimulation and the specific effects observed depend on the proximity of one or another core-brain receptor system to the site. These experiments show that at least two distinct biasing processes can be activated: one is aminergic and is heavily concentrated in the midbrain, the other is cholinergic and concentrated in the more forward portions of the core-brain. Since aminergic and cholinergic chemicals act as synaptic transmitters, their special role in biasing appetitive mechanisms needs explanation.

the neurochemistry of sleepiness and mood

The effectiveness of chemicals in the core-brain is related to the type of neurons making up this part of the central nervous system. As noted, these neurons have for the most part relatively short fine fibers which branch richly and so make contact with many neighbors. Slow potentials characterize junctions among neurons. Thus any portion of the central nervous system which has fine branching fibers and is rich in junctions will characteristically be sensitive to those influences to which slow potentials are responsive. Among these, of course, are the chemical influences—especially those that are involved in junctional transmission.

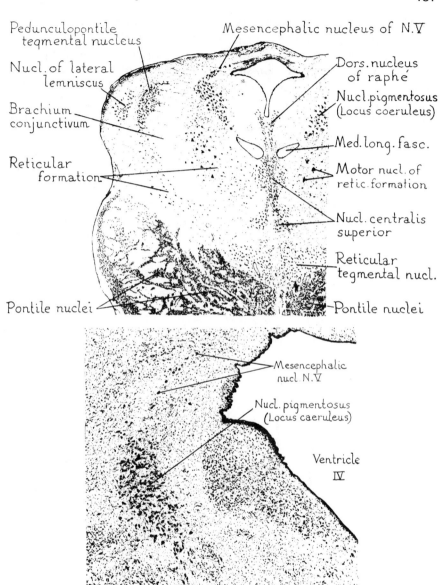

Fig. 9-9. Sections through brain stem showing the nuclei of the median raphe (a serotonin indole-aminergic structure) and the locus ceruleus (a norepinephrine catechol-aminergic structure) which have been involved in studies of ordinary and Rapid Eye Movement (REM) sleep respectively. From Strong and Elwyn, *Human Neuroanatomy.* © 1943 The Williams & Wilkins Co., Baltimore, Md.

Much of the impetus for examining these biochemical biases has come from inquiries into the site of action of psychopharmacological drugs and from the study of the processes responsible for sleep. Two types of aminergic mechanisms have been identified in the core-brain (see Fig. 9-9). The nuclei of the median raphé (seam) of the midbrain have been found to be especially sensitive to serotonin (an indole amine), one type of aminergic transmitter; this chemical is involved in "ordinary" sleep. The other aminergic site is the locus ceruleus which has been found to be especially sensitive to norepine-

TABLE II - CLINICAL RESULTS WITH αMₚT IN AFFECTIVE ILLNESS

PATIENTS' CLINICAL STATE	IMPROVEMENT	NO CHANGE	WORSE	TOTAL
MANIC	5*	1	1	7
DEPRESSED	0	0	3	3

a   *Two of the patients who improved showed relapse with placebo substitution.

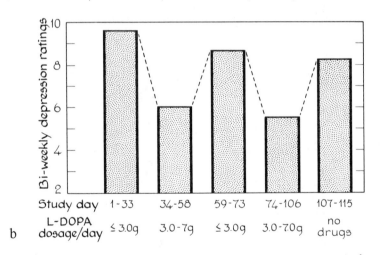

b

Fig. 9-10. (A) Clinical results in treating manic-depressive symptoms with alphamethylparatyrosine (αMPT), a substance which inhibits brain catecholamine synthesis. (B) Response of depression to high doses of L-DOPA, a precursor of norepine-phrine, a catechol amine. Chronologic depression ratings of one patient as related to the dose of L-DOPA administered. From Bunney, et al., 1969 and Brodie, et al., 1970.

phrine (a catechole amine) and involved in "paradoxical" forms of sleep in which much active dreaming occurs. So it appears that we feel sleepy when the sleep receptor sites in the core-brain become stimulated by the accumulation of aminergic substances. But this is a very active field of research; our ideas about the regulation of the accumulation of these substances and their special effectiveness at these particular sites continue to change rapidly. So far only some of the most general aspects of the neurochemical control of sleep have been clarified (Jouvet, 1967).

Even less well understood, but also under active investigation, are the mechanisms that give rise to the feelings we usually group under the rubric "mood." Again, research results suggest that core-brain receptor sites and the same chemical substances (i.e., the indole and catachole amines) are responsible for such feelings as depression and elation (see, for example, Fig. 9-10). Aggressiveness, on the other hand, appears to be stimulated by cholinergic mechanisms (King and Hoebel, 1968). Thus the essentially passive, energy conserving feelings of sleepiness and alertness and of depression and elation may well be aminergically determined while the more active feelings of assertiveness are cholinergically regulated. What then controls the necessary balance between aminergic and cholinergic processes? Chapters 10 and 15 address this question.

But it is still too early to tell just how many basic chemical biasing mechanisms will be found and what their relation to one another and to various moods and behaviors may prove to be. Specific chemicals and sites are being sought in many laboratories. The discovery and effectiveness of antidepressant and tranquilizing drugs have spurred this effort and the drugs themselves have provided keys to the type of mechanism involved.

synopsis

The organization of junctional processes by receptor stimulation is perceived as distant from the body surface when certain conditions of bilateral symmetry are met. The sum of such perceptions constitutes our World-Out-There. When these conditions are not present we do not perceive objects and occurrences; instead we construct a World-Within on the basis of our subjective feelings. A great deal is known about one class of feelings which is related to a set of receptors that lie deep in the central core of the brain. This class includes hunger and thirst, sexiness, sleepiness, and mood.

appetites and affects

hunger and thirst

Perhaps the simplest way to portray the involvement of the brain in the production of feelings is to trace how some of the experimental evidence on particular feelings, for instance, hunger and thirst, has accumulated.

Some years ago, when the physiological basis for feelings was thought to be determined by visceral structures outside the nervous system, research explored the hypothesis that the contractions of the stomach produced hunger. Stomach contractions were observed directly through an opening made in the abdomen of animals or occasionally through an accidental opening which occurred in man. Stomach contractions were also measured indirectly by having a human subject swallow a deflated balloon which was inflated when it was in place in the stomach. The balloon was attached by a tube to a measuring device. Correlations were thus established between the contractions and reports of subjective feelings of hunger.

In like manner observations on mouth and throat dryness can be correlated with the feeling of thirst. These observations, in the realm of common experience, are somewhat easier to make.

But how were the contractions of the stomach and the dryness of the mouth initiated? Changes in the composition of the circulating blood were suspected. In experiments on hunger, blood taken from starving dogs was injected into the veins of sated ones whose stomach contractions were being monitored. The injections produced contractions whereas control injections of blood taken from sated animals did not (Luckhardt and Carlson, 1915). Diluting or concentrating the blood with intravenous injections of hypotonic or hypertonic solutions of water assuaged or enhanced thirst and stopped or started drinking.

But where did the chemical or osmotic composition of blood exert its action? The answer to this question took a number of years to tease out. As already noted, it was discovered early that damage to certain parts of the brain stem core of animals led to the excretion of large amounts of sugar in their urine. Damage to other nearby structures led to obesity. Were these core brain locations the site of action of the hunger producing chemical? Were changes in the amount of sugar circulating in the blood responsible for the observed contractions of the stomach and the feeling of hunger? Closer scrutiny was required.

Researchers combined the sugar molecule with others that could be easily identified once they became imbedded in the brain. A substance, gold thiogluconate, was found to be an effective tracer in locating the areas in the brain which selectively absorbed the glucose molecule. And these locations fit to a considerable extent those which, when damaged, produced disturbances in the abnormal excretion of sugar and in eating (Mayër, 1963).

As in any experimental program which engages the scientific community for decades, discrepancies and disparities in results arose and many of these paradoxes, though not all, became resolved as the simpler story became more complicated. Thus substances in addition to sugar probably play critical roles in the regulation of eating: e.g., fats and proteins are involved, but just how must still be worked out.

The discovery of the receptive site for thirst was more dramatic. A small tube was inserted into the brain stem core of goats and a small amount of concentrated salt solution was injected (Andersson, 1953). Immediately the goats began to drink gallons of water. Anatomical studies showed that the critical core-brain area involved was highly vascular and especially suited to sensing the concentration of electrolytes in the blood.

In the case of thirst, the relationship between the core brain and a

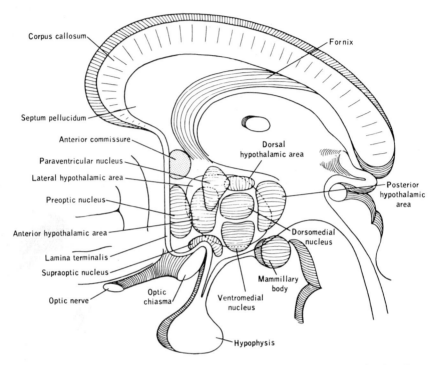

Fig. 10-1. Three-dimensional reconstruction of the hypothalamus. From *A Functional Approach to Neuroanatomy,* House
and Pansky. Copyright 1967 by McGraw-Hill Book Company.

part of the pituitary gland is of great importance in the regulation of
water balance; many other core-brain mechanisms share this type of
special relationship with the pituitary, and, in fact, many of these
relationships appear to be effected by *secretions* from core-brain cells
which reach the "master gland" via a network of veins that connects
the hypothalamus with the pituitary (see Fig. 10-1). Further, the
locations of brain cells sensitive to the chemicals involved in the
regulation of hunger and thirst are most likely *distributed* in a system
within the core brain rather than being concentrated in a single
"center," although nodes in the system can be identified.

The mechanism by which the receptive cells work their regulative
effect turns out to be much more interesting than was at first
suspected. As already noted, destruction of one nodal location in the
system (the ventromedial area of the hypothalamus) results in
obesity. Rats with such lesions eat and eat. They appear unable to
stop eating once started. (They also drink a good deal, but this may

be related to their need to dilute the eaten food for digestion.) Thus, the destroyed area does not so much indicate hunger as it does satiety to the organism. And, indeed, when electrical records are made by probes located in this "satiety" location, the cells are found to be active when there is a large difference between the amount of sugar circulating in the arteries and that circulating in the veins of the blood stream going to and from the brain; the cells are not active when this difference in the concentration of blood sugar is small (see Figs. 10-4, 10-5).

stop and go mechanisms

But definitive as these results were, they left the production of hunger—the original puzzle—unsolved. Not until some experiments were undertaken in which I played an inadvertent role did clarification come.

I was working on the analysis of the functions not of the brain stem, but of the temporal lobe of the hemispheres of the brain and

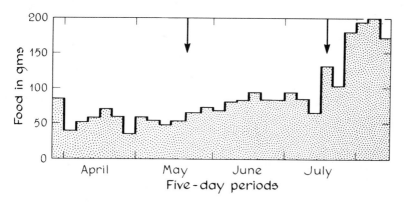

Fig. 10-2. The effect of bilateral amygdalectomy on the food intake of a monkey on an ad libitum diet. Arrows indicate surgery, first the resection of one amygdala, then the other. From Pribram and Bagshaw, 1953.

had found that the disturbances in eating (Fig. 10-2) produced by large removals of this lobe could as well be initiated by removing only a small part on the medial surface of its pole—the amygdala, a limbic system structure usually classifed as one of the basal ganglia (Fig. 10-3). My experiments were performed with monkeys, whose eating behavior is especially difficult to measure. Monkeys store food in cheek pouches; they peel and crumble food offered them and throw edibles about when sated. Still, preliminary quantitative results showed a doubling of food intake after amygdalectomy.

My colleagues in the department of physiology at Yale who were skilled in the production of obesity in rats by making lesions in the hypothalamic "satiety" mechanism, and John Brobeck, in particular, became interested in the problem and assigned Bal Anand, a postdoctoral fellow who had come from India to study with him to work on it. The three of us laid our plans: I was to make surgical lesions while they inserted probes in the amygdala to destroy it with electric current. We set up situations which we thought would tell us whether the eating disturbances were due to a change in gustatory sensation (noted by the relative intake of bitter and sweet solutions and of a mixture of sawdust and axle grease from a fatty mash similar in consistency and appearance and readily available to them) or whether some more basic disequilibration of metabolism was responsible (rectal temperatures and weight were regularly measured as was the activity of the animals housed in activity wheels).

Our patron saint in these explorations must have been Robert Burns. All of our elaborate and painstaking measures could have been dispensed with: the results of the experiments were dramatic and observable—literally—to the naked eye. First, over half of my rats died, not from surgery but *before* it because they drank so much bitters and ate so much axle grease and sawdust that they became violently ill with quinine poisoning and diarrhea. Wild rats had been reported to know what was good for them (and my surviving ones did, they never again touched the lethal stuff)—but specially bred laboratory white rats obviously had not properly read the literature. And, even though I found that indeed after amygdalectomy the rats returned to drinking bitters and eating axle grease and sawdust, I did not feel like carrying out the experiment to its predictable termination. Also, since the experiment failed to answer any of the questions relevant to the problems we were investigating we never reported it.

My colleagues Anand and Brobeck fared even worse—or perhaps much better, depending on viewpoint. Almost all of their rats died after the stereotaxic surgery—again not from the direct effects of surgery, however, but because the animals *stopped eating and drinking altogether.* Now this result was the opposite of what I had found in my monkeys, although *temporary* post-surgical aphagia and adypsia (cessation of eating and drinking) had often occurred. At this

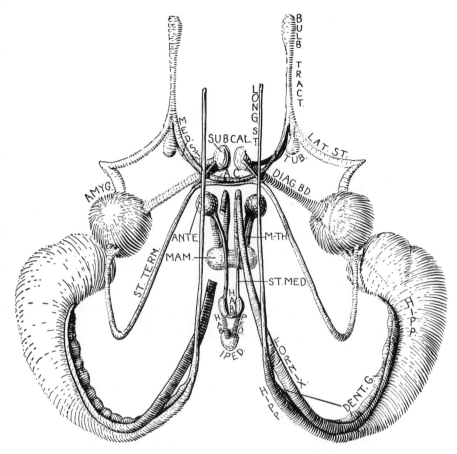

Fig. 10-3. Reconstruction showing a few of the relationships between limbic (amygdala and hippocampus) and core (hypothalamic) structures. From Krieg, 1966.

point, almost a year after we had begun the experiments, we were not altogether encouraged by what we had found. So, though disheartened, Anand (who soon had to return to India) undertook the drudgery of making the anatomical analysis of the lesions he and Brobeck had produced.

And now came the final surprise. The stereotaxic instrument had produced damage not at all where it was directed—i.e., the amygdala—but more toward the middle of the brain, between the amygdala and the hypothalamus! (Fig. 10-4)

Thus what is now known as the far-lateral hypothalamic feeding

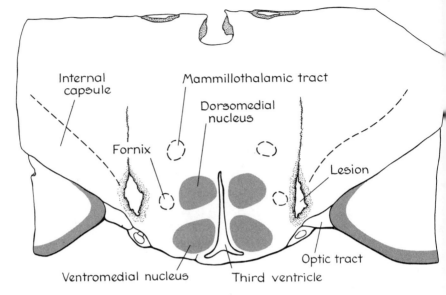

Fig. 10-4. Diagram of section through rat's hypothalamus locating the far lateral "feeding centers" with black lesioned areas. Redrawn after Anand and Brobeck, 1951.

mechanism (or, for short, the Anand-Brobeck center) was discovered (Anand and Brobeck, 1952). Anand, carefully extending his research over the years, showed that the satiety and feeding mechanisms were reciprocally coupled: when the satiety center showed activity as recorded with small electrodes, the feeding area became inhibited. When the satiety mechanism was quiescent (as in the case when blood sugar levels were low), the feeding mechanism was disinhibited and active (Anand, 1963; Fig. 10-5).

The far-lateral hypothalamic feeding and drinking mechanism turns out to be composed not of cell masses, receptors, sensitive to physico-chemical excitation. Rather, it serves as a crossroads of tracts from various parts of the brain which connect peripheral and central stations concerned in the initiation and cessation of eating and drinking. The details of the organization of this system are as yet not worked out. As already noted, however, a good deal is known about the relationship of the feelings of hunger and thirst and processes such as contraction and filling of the stomach, dryness of the mouth, etc., which make up the peripheral portions of the system. Much less is known directly about the central mechanisms involved. But a beginning (Brobeck, 1963) has been made.

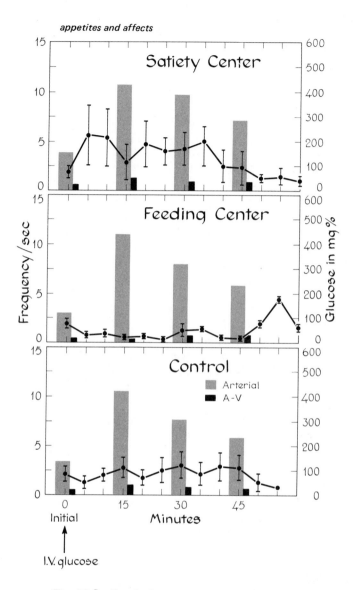

Fig. 10-5. Graph showing separately the mean of the frequencies of unit discharges recorded from the satiety center, the feeding center and the control regions, and correlating these with the arterial blood glucose levels and the amount of glucose utilization (A-V difference). The changes in the frequencies of discharges from the satiety and feeding center cells appear to correlate better with the amount of glucose utilization than with the absolute level of arterial glucose. Redrawn after Anand, 1963.

feelings and facts

The amygdala, which initiated our experiments, is one of the structures sending fibers into the far-lateral hypothalamic crossroads. Its function in regulating eating and drinking has been thoroughly pursued. Although minute quantities of certain chemicals (which have aminergic or cholinergic effects) injected into the hypothalamic satiety mechanism can start or stop eating and drinking (depending on the chemical), similar injections into the amygdala produce no such effect. If eating or drinking are already underway, however, then injections of these same chemicals will alter the amount of food eaten or water drunk (Grossman, 1966; Fig. 10-6b). A beautiful quantitative relationship between amount of injection and amount of ingestion of water has been established (Russell, et al., 1968; Fig. 10-6a) and the curve which displays this relationship is reminiscent of many threshold curves generated by psychophysical experiments performed in the visual and auditory modes. Thus the psychological processes of perception and of feeling have been shown to share a good many characteristics.

This congruence is probably not fortuitous. I once had the opportunity to examine some patients in whom the medial part of the temporal pole—including the amygdala—had been removed bilaterally. These patients, just as their monkey counterparts, typically ate considerably more than normal and gained up to a hundred pounds in weight. At last I could *ask* the subject how it felt to be so hungry. But much to my surprise, the expected answer was not forthcoming. One patient who had gained more than one hundred pounds in the year since surgery was examined at lunch time. Was she hungry? She answered, "No." Would she like a piece of rare, juicy steak? "No." Would she like a piece of chocolate candy? She answered, "Umhumm," but when no candy was offered she did not pursue the matter. A few minutes later, when the examination was completed, the doors to the common room were opened and she saw the other patients already seated at a long table eating lunch. She rushed to the table, pushed others aside, and began to stuff food into her mouth with both hands. She was immediately recalled to the examining room and the questions about food were repeated. The same negative answers were obtained again, even after they were pointedly contrasted with her recent behavior at the table. Somehow the lesion had impaired the patient's *feelings* of hunger and satiety and this impairment was accompanied by excessive eating!

As yet we understand little of how this impairment comes about. Nevertheless, this example points clearly to the folly of believing that

Fig. 10-6. (A) Relations between change in water intake and dose level of carbachol (cholinergic) stimulation of the amygdala, at three levels of water deprivation. The abscissa is plotted in moles x 10^{-11} in order to avoid negative log units. From Russell, et. al., 1968. (B) Effects of adrenergic and cholinergic stimulation of the hypothalamus of satiated rats on rate of bar pressing for food and water rewards on a 30 sec variable-interval schedule. Control levels were determined during a 1 hr. period preceding each stimulation. Redrawn after Grossman, 1962.

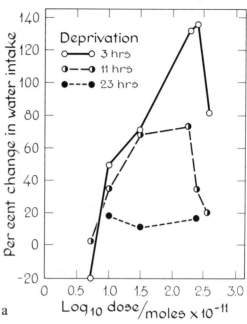

a

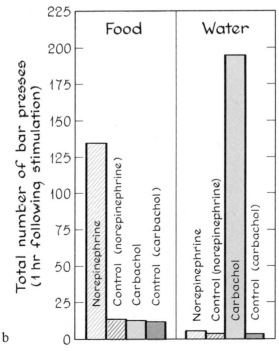

b

a direct match exists between observations of any particular type of behavior and introspectively derived concepts. Are we to say that the patient *felt* hungry because she ate ravenously despite her verbal denial? Or are we to take her statements at face value and seek elsewhere for an explanation for her voracious eating? The paradox is resolved if, as in earlier chapters on perception, we consider the behavioral function to be composed of several processes, one of which is the feeling state reported verbally.

At the hypothalamic level a similar paradox has plagued investigators. As already noted, when lesions are made in the region of the ventromedial nucleus of the hypothalamus, rats will eat considerably more than their controls and will become obese. But this is not all. Although rats so lesioned ate a great deal when food was readily available, they worked less for food whenever some obstacle interfered (Miller, Bailey, and Stevenson, 1950; see also Fig. 10-7). It was also found that the more palatable the food, the more the lesioned subject would eat (Teitelbaum, 1955), giving rise to the notion that the lesioned animals did not show greater "drive" to eat but were actually more "finicky" than their controls. Recent experimental results obtained by Krasne (1962) and by Grossman (1966) added to the paradox: electrical stimulation of the ventromedial nucleus stops both food and water intake in deprived rats and chemical stimulation of the cholinergic mechanism produces foot stamping (in gerbils,

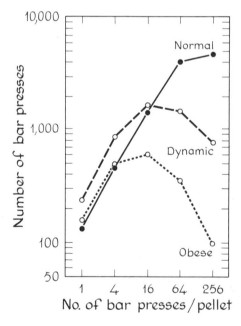

Fig. 10-7. Mean number of bar presses (per 12 hr. period) of normal, obese hyperphagic, and dynamic (non-obese) hyperphagic animals as a function of the number of bar presses required to obtain each pellet. From Teitelbaum, 1957.

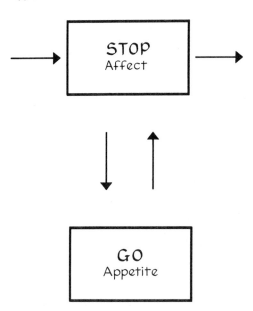

Fig. 10-8. Stop and Go mechanism in TOTE terms.

Glickman, personal communication) and fighting if provoked (King and Hoebel, 1968). Grossman summarizes these results with the succinct statement that medial hypothalamic manipulations change affect not appetite. But we are once again faced with our earlier dilemma. If the medial hypothalamic mechanism does not deal with motivation, how does eating, drinking, etc., come about? The data hold the answer. The ventromedial and lateral hypothalamic regions form a couplet, the lateral portion serving as a feeding, a "go" mechanism (which, when ablated, will produce rats which tend to starve), and the medial portion contains the "stop" mechanism (Fig. 10-8). The paradox is resolved by the hypothesis that processes ordinarily involved in taking the organism "out of motion" also generate affects or feelings of e-motion. Thus an important distinction between motivation and emotion becomes clarified: the term "motivation" can be restricted to the operations of appetitive "go" processes (such as those converging in the lateral hypothalamic region) that ordinarily result in behavior which carries forward an action, and the term "emotion" to the operations of affective "stop" or satiety processes of reequilibration.

But more of this in the next chapter. Note here, however, that the explanations—the only explanations with which scientists can make sense of the data—are made in terms of the changes in feelings, appetitive (motivational) and affective (emotional), produced by the lesions. These changes in feelings are inferred from observed neuro-behavioral evidence—but more (e.g., the neural data) than just the behavior itself must be kept in mind if sense is to be made of the experimental results.

synopsis

Experiments detailing the functions of the core-brain receptors produced a series of puzzling paradoxes which were not resolved until descriptions of the results were couched in the subjective language of feelings. For each of the receptor functions a "go" motivational and a "stop" emotional mechanism has been delineated. "Go" processes are expressed as appetites and "stop" processes as affects.

interest, motivation
and emotion

modifiers of homeostats

The fantastic success and promise given by the neuro-chemical approach to the specification of many of the feelings which make up our "World-Within" has unfortunately blinded most physiologically oriented scientists to some problems which remain. This chapter deals with these problems. In the days when physiology was primarily concerned with sensory and with humoral mechanisms, it was easy to claim that perceptions stemmed from an elaboration of sensory processes and that feelings were exclusively the elaboration of humoral mechanisms. Unfortunately this view has continued into the present despite the fact that a rich harvest of new neuro-behavioral data makes it untenable today.

The issue is this. Observers of, and experimenters with, the human scene repeatedly find inadequate a neuroendocrine-based approach to appetites and affects, the subjective experiences we call feelings. The thrill of discovery, the disappointment of failure, the joy of sensing, the gloom of separation—these experiences seem distant from the core homeostats just described.

197

A type of experiment initiated by Stanley Schachter (Schachter and Singer, 1962) helps to delineate the problem. Four groups of students took an examination. In one early experiment, two groups took it in a socially hostile, two in a socially friendly, environment. In each setting, one group received an injection of adrenaline, the other a control injection of normal saline solution. The students related their experiences. The hostile setting bred hostility, the friendly setting produced friendly feelings, as expected. The effect of adrenaline, however, was unexpected. The drug produced an enhancement of *both* friendly and hostile feelings. Whatever the physiological state produced by the injection, its *label* was determined by the *setting*—by the student's social environment and not by the injected drug.

Schachter's more recent experimental results (Schachter, 1968) support the earlier ones. The control of hunger (as manifested in eating) is now under scrutiny. Schachter finds that two classes of variables—internal and external—determine when eating occurs. Most eating takes place when internal drive and external opportunity coincide. By his usual ingenious (and sometimes somewhat fiendish) techniques, Schachter has dissociated the occasions when neurohumoral stimuli are maximal from those when opportunity beckons: He has shown that the obese among us rarely fail to heed the call of opportunity (e.g., when a plate of cookies is available while they are answering a questionnaire; the answers given are, of course, irrelevant to the experiment—it's the number of cookies consumed that is of interest) regardless of humoral state; the more usual response of the average person is to forego food "unless it's time to eat."

"Unless it's time to eat." This phrase capsulates the first of the issues I want to emphasize. You are prepared to eat, predisposed to eat, by the workings of the homeostatic mechanism. But this mechanism is tuned by prior experience; its bias is adjusted to operate around a setpoint by experience much as the behavior of the home heating plant is determined by setting the thermostat. Coming in from a tennis match you are often thirsty and gulp water to just the amount necessary to assuage the thirst. You stop drinking much before the amount of dilution of the blood required to produce satiety has taken place. Experiments with dogs have shown that such quantitative gulping is exquisitely "tuned" to the amount of water needed (Adolph, 1950; Fig. 11-1). Modification on the basis of experience is clearly involved in the operation of the system—even when the system is humorally operated. For the obese, modification is also involved, but, instead of humoral stimuli, gustatory, olfactory, and even visual stimuli initiate the motivation. And, lest you think

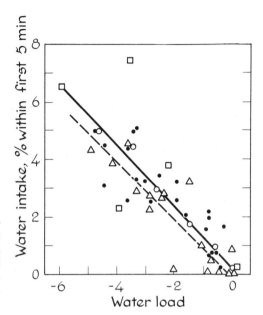

Fig. 11-1. Type of experiment discussed in text which shows that the amount of immediate drinking when opportunity arises is proportional to the amount of dehydration. Symbols indicate individual dogs. From Adolph, 1943.

the motivation of the obese is so completely different from that of the normal you and me, go on a trip (preferably on an unlimited budget) to include, say, an ocean voyage, Munich beer parlors (during the Octoberfest), Viennese coffee houses, and Provencal restaurants. Then—if you dare—weigh in on your return. Especially if you are over 35. Thus, once modified by experience the core homeostats of the brain are under the control not only of humoral but also of sensory receptor stimuli.

Students of animal behavior have also been concerned with this problem of the sensory control of motivation and emotion. The multiplication of drive names, of which "curiosity" and "incentive" are the most ubiquitous, attests to the need for a wider base of data (than the neurohumoral) for understanding "motivation and emotion."

"The time to . . ." indicates what this base might encompass. Experience builds within the organism a set of expectancies, neuronal models of the events experienced. Until recently a term such as "expectancy" had little hard neurological fact to support it. This situation has changed radically with Sokolov's classical demonstrations that orienting and dishabituation occur whenever a repetitiously experienced configuration of input is changed along any of its parameters. The behavioral (eye movements, head and body orientation), the neuroelectric (EEG, low-voltage fast-activity in isocortex and theta activity in the hippocampus), and visceral (GSR, change in heart and respiratory rates) responses have been extensively used to investigate the neurology of novelty (orienting, dishabituation) and of habituation. These studies suggest that some form of modification of servomechanisms such as homeostats and of TOTE logic elements in sensory systems is ubiquitous in the brain.

A whole category of feelings turns out to be related to the more or less harmonious interactions that occur among servomechanisms simply because all take place within the same brain. How these interactions become organized has been touched on in Chapters 7 and 8 and forms the substance of Chapters 14, 15, and 16. At this point we need only review the fact that the interactions occur through the organization of logic elements into temporary microstructures which are characterized by the patterns of junctional slow potentials that are involved. The stability-lability of such overall organization is a dimension which can be and has been extensively studied in terms of the orienting reaction and the course of its habituation (Lacey and Lacey, 1958; Lacey, et al., 1963). We recognize it readily when in everyday life we characterize a person as stable or unstable or when we admit we feel upset.

arousal as uncertainty

What initiates this disequilibration, this upset? Evidence shows that even the initiating process is not simple. Feelings of "interest," of motivation (appetites) and emotion (affects), stem from perturbations resulting when the organism faces novelty— novelty created by a continually changing World-Within immersed in an ever different World-Out-There. Studies performed in my laboratory, using brain lesions, have succeeded in isolating at least two components of the orienting reaction: one component indicates searching and sampling, the other component is manifest when a novelty is registered. Only after such registration does habituation occur.

This research result came about as follows: Some years ago we showed that easily observed effects of removal of the temporal lobes of the brain on temperament and personality resulted from the removal of the amygdala, the temporal lobe structure regulating appetites discussed in the previous chapter (Pribram and Bagshaw, 1953; recall Fig. 10-3, p. 187). Further analyses showed that the amygdala was involved in a variety of behaviors which we labeled as the four F's, an extension of Cannon's "fight and flight" reactions that occur when parts of the hypothalamus are electrically stimulated (Pribram, 1960b). Our four F's included, in addition to Cannon's, feeding and sexual behavior. The close anatomical linkage between the amygdala and hypothalamic structures made this result reasonable and acceptable until I became dissatisfied with just a descriptive correlation between brain anatomy and behavior and tried to understand the mechanism of operation of this relationship.

Had I been satisfied to pursue behavior per se I would have next asked, as others have, whether different parts of the amygdala served feeding, fighting, fleeing, and sexual behavior. An essentially negative answer was obtained when experiments (whether ablation or stimulation) were addressed to this question. But what I wanted to know concerned the psychological process, the commonality, that characterized the four F's, so that a single lesion (even of a somewhat complex anatomical formation) could alter, at one stroke, all of these diverse behaviors. The concept, "instinct" (Beach, 1955), though plausible, failed to satisfy for a number of reasons—e.g., social determinants crucially influenced the effects of amygdalectomy on fighting (Fig. 11-2)—as did a variety of forms of the concept "drive," which would have been a natural because of the strong connections between amygdala and hypothalamic mechanisms. However, as already noted, such drive concepts also failed to account for the effects of hypothalamic damage and stimulation. I therefore decided to take an opposite approach to the problem and ask whether behaviors which in no apparent way were innately based or drive controlled would be affected by amygdalectomy.

The experiments performed went far afield from the four F's. In collaboration with Jerome Schwartzbaum (Schwartzbaum and Pribram, 1960), with Muriel Bagshaw (Bagshaw and Pribram, 1965) and with Eliot Hearst (Hearst and Pribram, 1964a, 1964b), I undertook transfer of training experiments. In one procedure the monkeys were asked to discriminate the lighter of two intensities of grey; then, on test trials, the lighter grey of the pair was matched to a still lighter grey. Normal control monkeys chose the lighter of the test cues; amygdalectomized monkeys responded to the test trials as if they constituted an entirely new problem—i.e., they performed at the chance level (Fig. 11-3). The other transfer task consisted of training monkeys to discriminate the larger of a pair of painted squares and then testing to see whether they would chose the larger of a pair of circles. The control subjects did; the amygdalectomized monkeys did not. In addition, stimulus generalization was analyzed

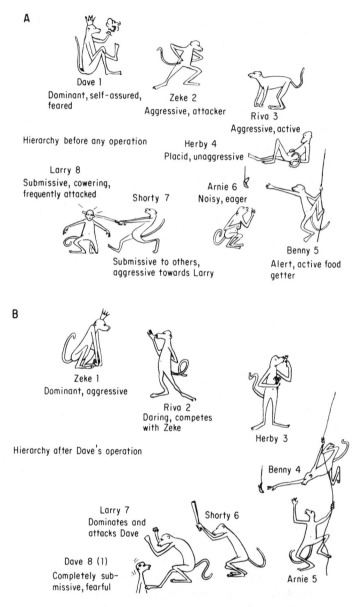

A

Dave 1
Dominant, self-assured, feared

Zeke 2
Aggressive, attacker

Riva 3
Aggressive, active

Hierarchy before any operation

Herby 4
Placid, unaggressive

Larry 8
Submissive, cowering, frequently attacked

Arnie 6
Noisy, eager

Shorty 7
Submissive to others, aggressive towards Larry

Benny 5
Alert, active food getter

B

Zeke 1
Dominant, aggressive

Riva 2
Daring, competes with Zeke

Herby 3

Hierarchy after Dave's operation

Benny 4

Larry 7
Dominates and attacks Dave

Shorty 6

Dave 8 (1)
Completely sub-missive, fearful

Arnie 5

Fig. 11-2. A: dominance hierarchy of a colony of eight preadolescent male rhesus monkeys before any surgical intervention. B: same as A after bilateral amygdalectomy had been performed on Dave. Note his drop to the bottom of the hierarchy. C: same as A and B, except that both Dave and Zeke have received bilateral amygdalectomies. D: final social

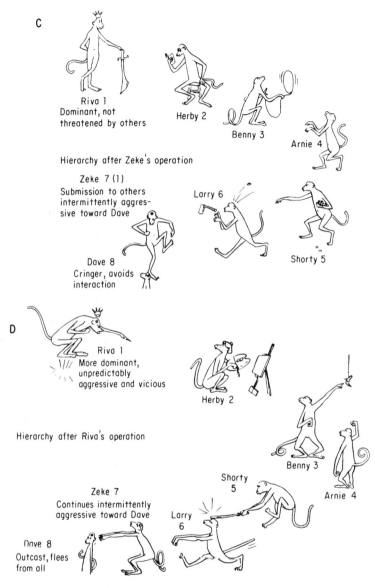

C

Riva 1
Dominant, not
threatened by others

Herby 2

Benny 3

Arnie 4

Hierarchy after Zeke's operation

Zeke 7 (1)
Submission to others
intermittently aggres-
sive toward Dave

Larry 6

Dave 8
Cringer, avoids
interaction

Shorty 5

D

Riva 1
More dominant,
unpredictably
aggressive and vicious

Herby 2

Hierarchy after Riva's operation

Benny 3

Arnie 4

Shorty
5

Zeke 7
Continues intermittently
aggressive toward Dave

Larry
6

Dave 8
Outcast, flees
from all

hierarchy after Dave, Zeke, and Riva have all had bilateral
amygdalectomies. Note that Riva fails to fall in the hierarchy.
Minimal differences in extent of locus of the resections do not
correlate with differences in the behavioral results. The
disparity has been shown in subsequent experiments to be due
to Herby's nonaggressive "personality" in the second position
of the hierarchy. From Pribram, 1962.

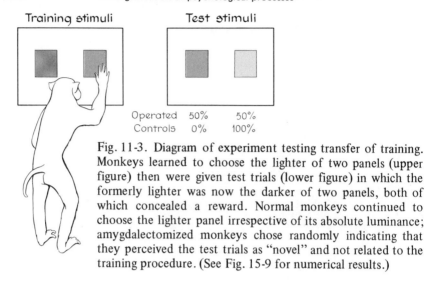

Fig. 11-3. Diagram of experiment testing transfer of training. Monkeys learned to choose the lighter of two panels (upper figure) then were given test trials (lower figure) in which the formerly lighter was now the darker of two panels, both of which concealed a reward. Normal monkeys continued to choose the lighter panel irrespective of its absolute luminance; amygdalectomized monkeys chose randomly indicating that they perceived the test trials as "novel" and not related to the training procedure. (See Fig. 15-9 for numerical results.)

in an operant conditioning situation in which the rate of lever pressing was contingent on the illumination of the testing box. On this problem amygdalectomized monkeys did not differ in response rate from the controls when the illumination was varied in steps from the initial training stimulus. (This surprising dissociation between transfer and generalization is interesting in and of itself but is irrelevant here.)

The tasks were chosen because they seemed reasonably remote from hypothalamic influence. Since amygdalectomy affected performance in both transposition experiments, one of my conclusions was that the amygdala influences processes other than those ordinarily ascribed to the hypothalamus.

A clue to what this process might be came from an observation made while testing the monkeys on the transposition task. As noted, the amygdalectomized subjects neither transposed nor did they choose the absolute cue. Instead they treated the test trials as completely novel situations, performing initially at chance (Douglas, 1966; Schwartzbaum and Pribram, 1960).

Pursuing this observation (Bagshaw and Benzies, 1968; Bagshaw and Coppock, 1968; Bagshaw, Kimble, and Pribram, 1965; Bagshaw and J. Pribram, 1968; Kimble, Bagshaw, and Pribram, 1965), we showed that amygdalectomy did indeed alter monkeys' reactions to novelty. Behavioral (and some components of EEG) habituation to novelty were markedly prolonged. On the other hand, the visceral indicators (GSR, changes in heart and respiratory rates) of orienting to novelty were erased by the lesions (without impairing the response mechanisms per se; Fig. 11-4). These results suggest that orienting to

novelty proceeds through two hypothetical stages: the first, characterized by behavioral orienting reactions, "samples," scans the novelty; the second, characterized by visceral reactions, leads to the
"registration" of the novelty and so to its habituation (Pribram,
1969c). Thus I interpreted the deficit in fighting, fleeing, feeding,
and sexual behavior on the basis of a difficulty in the process of
registration which is necessary to the temporal organization of behavior. A test of this interpretation predicted that delayed alternation behavior (alternating between two identical food boxes which
were baited right-left-right-left, etc., on succeeding trials; Pribram,
Lim, Poppen, and Bagshaw, 1966) would also become impaired and
this prediction was borne out.

With these results a much greater span of functions attributable to
the amygdala are encompassed. And this is not all. Reference to the
psychological process of registration helped explain an until then
inexplicable observation (Miller, Galanter, and Pribram, 1960,
Ch. 14). The patient referred to in Chapter 10 on whom a bilateral
amygdalectomy had been performed a year earlier had gained a great
deal of weight. She seemed to present a golden opportunity to find
out directly what she experienced to make her eat so much. Her
answer was always that she experienced little—she did *not* feel, i.e.,
monitor and register, that she was inordinately hungry. Such a lack
of registration is a commonplace in clinical epileptic seizures originating from abnormalities around the amygdala, abnormalities which

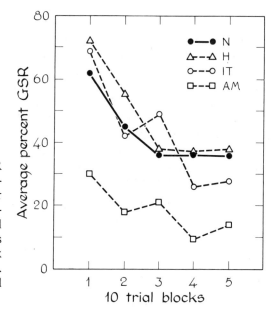

Fig. 11-4. Curves of % GSR response to the first fifty presentations of a tone beep for a normal (N) and three experimental groups with bilateral resections of hippocampus (H); inferotemporal cortex (IT); and amygdala (AM). From Bagshaw, Kimble, and Pribram, 1965.

also produce the famous *deja vu* (inappropriate feeling of familiarity) and *jamais vu* (inappropriate feeling of unfamiliarity) phenomena. Thus monitor Images can be said to characterize *feelings* about the World-Out-There much as perceptual Images characterize its attributes.

These experiments and their analysis make it relevant to consider a second major view held currently of how motivational and emotional feelings are produced, viz., that feelings of interest, the appetites and affects, depend on the mechanism of arousal. The experimental results just mentioned raise the questions: when does arousal (which is measured by the same techniques and the same criteria as those used in the amygdala studies) lead to registration and habituation, and when does arousal lead to disruption? The classical answer given (Lindsley, 1951; Hebb, 1955) has been that the amount of arousal determines its outcome. What can be added now is that on the basis of the evidence obtained in the studies of the orienting reaction, amount of arousal is shown to be dependent on organization, on the configuration of the expectancies, of the brain state challenged by the novel input. "Amount of arousal" is properly understood, therefore, as amount of match and mismatch between configurations, an amount of organization or disorganization, not an amount of excitation which is altered (see Hebb, 1949; Luria, 1960). Since a measure on organization is involved, "amount" can be expressed as information and uncertainty. Amount of information or uncertainty expresses the number of yes-no statements that are needed when the question is posed as to whether two items of an organization are the same or different. Uncertainty is the obverse of information; the term "uncertainty" is used retrospectively, the term "information," prospectively: a specified number of "bits" (binary yes-no statements) of information will reduce the uncertainty of a system by that number of bits. Thus I might quip that this new view of arousal theory has built into it a measure of uncertainty.

The "amount" referred to by arousal or activation theorists has, according to this analysis, been to some extent misidentified. Amount of arousal, amount of activation, is not some quantitative change in intensity, in energy *level* in the central nervous system, but a change in the equilibration, the organization as measured by the amount of *uncertainty* (and thus the amount of information) characterizing the system. At the neural unit level "arousal" is accompanied in the brain stem reticular formation (see Huttenlocher, 1961) and at the cortex (Burns, 1968, Ch. 5) by a change in pattern, not in overall amount of firing. Even the original definition of arousal as EEG activation is based on the observation that low-

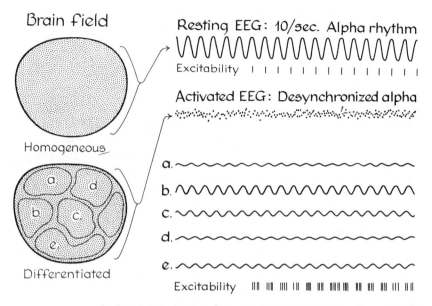

Fig. 11-5. Hypothetical brain fields, illustrating type of EEG assumed to be associated with each. Resting alpha at 10/sec. characterizes the "homogeneous," or relaxed, condition. A desynchronized, activated EEG is associated with a "differentiated" state of brain function. The activated EEG is characteristic of attention and problem-solving, and, in general, more efficient perception and performance. According to the concept that an excitability cycle is associated with the waxing and waning phases of the waves, it is evident that alternating periods of excitability and unexcitability could occur only 10 times per second in the case of the resting EEG, whereas almost continuous excitability is represented in the case of the desynchronized EEG resulting from a differentiated brain field. Redrawn after Lindsley, 1961.

voltage fast-EEG activity occurs and that such activity indicates desynchronization. As noted by Lindsley (1961) this suggests that during desynchronization neural elements become functionally independent of each other and thus available to function as separate information processing channels. It is this enhanced separation which can be described as an increased amount of organization or in information measurement terms, an increased uncertainty (Fig. 11-5).

A corollary of this view would suggest that arousal represents a state where the independence of the activities of neuronal aggregates makes for freedom to "resonate" with others which, though spatially distant, have common characteristics. Thus distributed information becomes more easily addressed in the arousal state.

This is as far as the arousal—the uncertainty mechanism—can take us. But this is not all there is to arousal. For example, in an experiment designed to study the effects of restrictions on early experience we found that behavioral *in*activity was accompanied by increased autonomic lability (Konrad and Bagshaw, 1970). But before the relationship between uncertainty and the control of behavior can become clear we need to return once again to servotheory. The Schachter results are not yet accounted for: the augmentation of this or that feeling by adrenaline can be handled by the quantitative change produced by the drug in the uncertainty process; the specification of feelings as hostile or friendly, etc., still need explanation.

cortical control and the cybernetics of coping

The specificities of feelings suggest that there is more to motivation and emotion than quantitative disequilibration and uncertainty, more than the disruption of the psychological process, certainly more than just a hypothalamic mechanism. The diversity of feelings of interest suggests the operation of a variety of processes engaged in coping with changes in equilibrium, *in elaborating specific types of control to meet specific expectancies* (see Zimbardo, 1969).

One road open to the organism in coping is to do something to, to act on his environment. As described more fully in Chapter 16, whenever a servosystem becomes stabilized, new sensitivities develop and new techniques are adduced to handle these new sensitivities. For example, when thermostats were initially introduced into homes, the occupants for the first time became aware of the chilling effect the cooling of the outside walls produce at sunset because of the radiation of body heat to those walls. Outside wall thermostats were therefore introduced, adding variety to the control of heating in houses. This spiraling aspect of the functions of control mechanisms is neglected in the more usual formulations of the biological homeostatic process and in the arguments levied against biological servotheory.

But action is not the only way in which an organism can achieve variety in control. The possibility exists that he may cope by exerting self control, i.e., he may make internal adjustments with his neurological system, adjustments that will lead to reequilibration without recourse to action. My thesis will be that it is these internal adjustments that are felt as emotions.

We now have good neurophysiological evidence that such internal adjustments are not only possible but are also commonplace. A large number of experiments have been done to show that the organism's input channels and even the sensory receptors themselves, are subject to efferent control by the central nervous system. A recent series of studies performed in my laboratories demonstrated corticofugal (cortico → subcortical) influence, originating in the so-called association areas, as far peripherally as the cochlear nucleus and optic tract (Dewson, Nobel, and Pribram, 1966; Nobel and Dewson, 1966; Spinelli and Pribram, 1966, 1967; Spinelli, Pribram, and Weingarten, 1965; Spinelli and Weingarten, 1966; Weingarten and Spinelli, 1966). Changes in click- and flash-evoked electrical activity were shown in these locations and even the size and shape of receptive fields of units in the visual system could be altered by stimulation of the cortex (see Fig. 11-6).

The flash- and click-evoked electrical response data are of special interest here. When a double click or a double flash is used to evoke a neural response, the amplitude of the second of the pair of responses

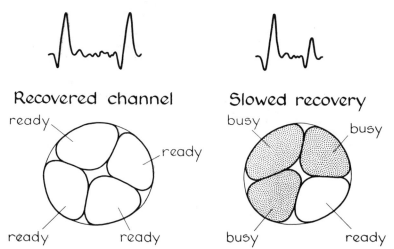

Fig. 11-6. Interpretation of the meaning of slowing of the recovery of an afferent channel after stimulation. Tests are made by presenting pairs of stimuli separated by varying intervals and plotting (see Fig. 11-7) the amplitude of the second response evoked as a function of the amplitude of the first. When the second response is comparatively small, large portions of the afferent channel are assumed to be still busy processing the effects of the first stimulus (shown in lower part of the figure). Note similarity to Fig. 11-5.

serves as an indicator of the duration over which a part of the system is occupied in processing the first of the pair of inputs. A depression in the amplitude of the second of the pair of responses thus indicates a longer recovery—a longer processing time for a signal within the channel. Such an increase in processing time effectively desynchronizes the channel to repetitive inputs: fewer fibers are available for processing any given signal in the series. Prolongation of recovery thus reduces redundancy, the number of fibers carrying the same

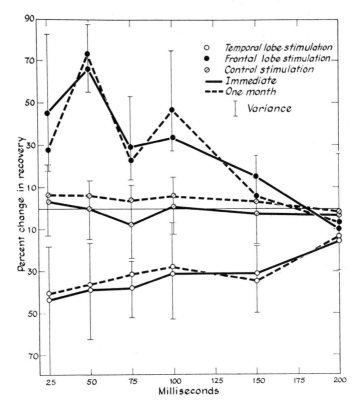

Fig. 11-7. The change produced by cortical stimulation in recovery (see Fig. 11-6) of a response in an afferent channel. Cortical stimulation of 8 Hertz was maintained continuously for several months. Control stimulations were performed on the parietal cortex. Records were made immediately after the onset of stimulation and weekly thereafter. The initial recovery functions and those obtained after 1 month are shown. Vertical bars represent actual variability of the records obtained in each group of four monkeys. From Spinelli and Pribram, 1967.

signal, in the channel. Thus at any moment more information, a greater number of different signals, can be processed—provided the system has sufficient reserve redundancy to handle inefficiency due to noise—and there is good evidence that this is so (Attneave, 1954; Barlow, 1961). Our experiments showed further that stimulation of certain parts of the cortex of the temporal lobe (not the amygdala but the infero-temporal area) reduces redundancy, while stimulation of another part of the cortex (the frontal) enhances redundancy in the visual system (Fig. 11-7). These opposing effects operate essentially either to "open" the organism to his environment, allowing the processing of a greater number of different signals, a greater amount of information to go on at any moment, or, conversely, to "close down" the input channels so as to restrict processing to a more limited number of different signals, a more limited amount of information.

The results of these experiments suggest that the organism has at least two ways in which he can internally adjust to, control his uncertainty, neither of which entail behavioral action. One way is to increase the rate with which he processes information, the other is to decrease that rate. One mechanism "opens" the organism to input, the other restricts input. Coping by way of internal control can thus be attempted in at least two ways: either through enhanced monitoring of the external environment or by minimizing the external and focusing on internal configurations.

experience and expression

We must now try to meet head on some of the problems posed by this new neurology for explanations of motivation and emotion. Perhaps the clearest approach is to resort to that old-fashioned trilogy and ask what the difference is between perception, action, and motivation-emotion. There is now ample evidence that when an organism *perceives*, he is forming an internal representation of his environment. Miller, Galanter, and I in *Plans and the Structure of Behavior* (1960) argued that when an organism *acts* he is making an external representation of his Plans, the neural programs (complex codes) in his brain. Edward Tolman (1932) and Fred Skinner (1938) had earlier pointed out that an act is to be defined by its outcomes, that the operant conditioner's "responses" were the marks of behavior left on the paper fed through the cumulative recorder. These marks can now be identified realistically as external representations of an organized neural operation constructed to meet the requirements (test) of deprivation and other physiological states and the expectations of the organism set up by the schedules of cues and reinforcers. (To social scientists and humanists, of course, the concept of Act as a representation is certainly familiar.)

To turn to motivation and emotion within this framework suggests the obvious observation that motivation and emotion express relationships between perception and action. The relationships manifested appear to be the following.

When the variety of perceptions exceeds to some considerable extent the repertory of action available to the organism, he feels "interested" and is motivated to, i.e., attempts to, extend this repertory. Whenever this attempt fails, is nonreinforced, frustrated, or interrupted, the organism, of necessity, feels emotional, i.e., the coping mechanisms of self-regulation, self-control come into play. Further, on the basis of previous experience, emotion is likely to occur when the probability of reinforcement from action is deemed low.

The converse situation produces a relatively "flat" motivationless and emotionless state. When the repertory of actions exceeds the variety of current perceptions a curious course of events is initiated. The constructed external representations that become composed by the actions comprise a larger and larger share of the organism's perceptions until a means-ends reversal takes place: "The medium becomes the message." This situation occurs only when the organism restricts his perceptions to a limited, relatively "closed system" part of his universe. To deal with this inversion, i.e., to produce interest, he must "open" himself to variety—in today's language he must take a "trip." The current popularity of consciousness-expanding drugs and encounter groups is therefore a corollary of our technologically overproficient society.

The suggestion is that ordinarily interests, feelings of motivation (appetites) and emotion (affects), occur when the organism attempts to extend his control to the limits of what he perceives. To the extent that this attempt appears (on the basis of trial or experience) feasible at any moment, the organism is motivated; to the extent that the attempt appears infeasible at any moment, the organism becomes of necessity emotional, i.e., he relies on self-regulatory mechanisms— either to participate in the uncontrollable or to prepare for another attempt. Motivation and emotion must go hand-in-hand. But motive implies action, the formation of an external representation; e-motion, on the other hand, implies the opposite, i.e., to be out of, or away from, action. To be emotional is to be, to an extent, "possessed." Motivation and emotion, action and passion, to be effective and to be affective, these are the organism's polar mechanisms for attaining control when he perceives more than he can accomplish.

Those terms by which we label feelings of interest can serve as well for emotions as for motives, though a distinction remains: thus "being in love" refers to emotion, "loving" to motivation; fear the emotion, has its counterpart in fear the motive; and being moved by music can be apposed to being moved to make music. Emotions and motivations are ordinarily gracefully interdigitated. But when either the passive or the active expression of the interest becomes prepotent, maladaptation is likely to occur: too much emotion leads either to disruption or to rigidity. Emotion is, however, not to be avoided. Too closely motivated action leads to a narrowness of purpose and a poverty in values (see Chapters 15 and 16).

Finally, a word about the behavioral expressions of emotional feelings. According to my analysis, expressions of motives are acts, while expressions of emotions indicate that an internal process of control is operative. In a social environment (or to the organism himself) such expressions serve as communicative signals which can be usefully read and taken into account in further interactions. Such affective signals signify the interests of the organism as clearly as do his actions—they suggest, however, that action at the moment, for one reason or another, is infeasible.

At this point the neurobehavioral approach gives way to other methods for the study of feelings. The neuropharmacologist, neuroendocrinologist, and neurochemist are busily researching moods; the psychoanalyst has been deeply concerned with the signal aspect of affect; the social scientist is thoroughly versed in uncertainty; the ethologist has detailed the social significance of emotional expression in behavior; and the behavior therapist deals daily with the problem of control.

The view of motivational and emotional feelings presented here— the results of Image-constructing cortically regulated states which monitor and control the relationships between sets of biased homeostats, logic elements processing information derived not only from the core receptors but from sense organs as well—hopefully gives a new reach to the way we understand our psychological world.

synopsis

Experiments performed on man show that the production of appetites and affects is not limited to the core-brain mechanisms. Appetitive and affective interest is more generally aroused whenever the interrelationships among neural logic structures anywhere in the brain are disturbed. A cybernetic theory of motivation and emotion develops from neurophysiological experiments that detail the control on these relationships exerted by the brain cortex.

part 3

the neural control and modification of behavior

"In a more advanced account of a behaving organism 'historical' variables will be replaced by 'causal.' When we can observe the momentary state of an organism . . . [and] when we can generate or change a state directly, we shall be able to use it to control behavior."

B. F. Skinner, 1969, p. 283

"Instead of repeating constantly that reinforcement leads to control, I would prefer to emphasize that reinforcement can lead to . . . [achievement based on] competence. And . . . I would prefer to speak of . . . commitment [as] a function of the rewards associated with achievement . . . ."

G. A. Miller, 1969, pp. 67–68

movements

"The singleness of action from moment to moment. . . is a keystone in the construction of the individual whose unity it is the specific office of the nervous system to perfect" (Sherrington, 1947). "The neurological problem is in large part, if not entirely, the translation of the afferent pattern of impulses into the efferent pattern. . . all skilled acts seem to involve the same problems of serial ordering, even down to the temporal coordination of muscular contractions. . ." (Lashley, 1951). This part of the book is heir to these words of wisdom that define the issues which must be dealt with in any neurophysiological treatment of the organization of behavior. The problem is this. Because of the way in which motor systems are organized (Figs. 12-1, 12-2) only one step of an action can be performed at a time. Yet when you or I sit down to write, or type, or speak, or play the piano, we have stored in our brains a considerably detailed representation of how the entire action is to be achieved. The evidence for such a stored representation comes from "slips of the tongue" in speaking or "slips of the fingers" in musical

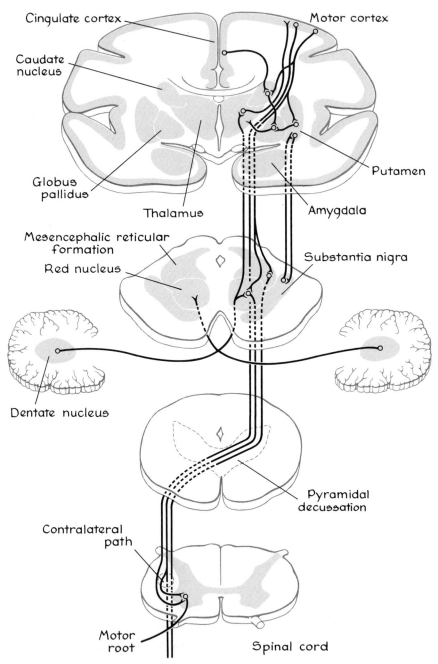

Fig. 12-1. Diagram of essential connections of the motor system.

performances, inversions in the order of words in a sentence or letters in a word, the flexibility in the arrangement of the order in which thoughts are expressed on different occasions and the like. The problem is thus not completely unfamiliar. The question is what type of transfer function is involved when one representation is transformed by virtue of neural operations into another. This problem has already been met in earlier chapters.

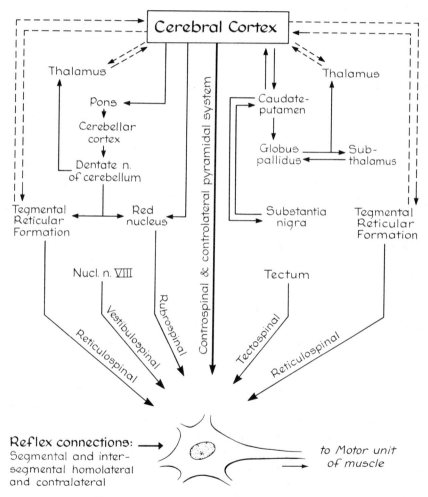

Fig. 12-2. A few of the many descending systems influencing the activity of the "final common path," the motor neuron. Modified from Ranson and Clark, 1959. Compare with Fig. 12-1 for anatomical location of structures referred to.

Chapters 3, 4, 7, and 8 discussed the formation of representations, states, in the brain as a function of receptor and input system processes. We saw that the formation of such representations depends on processing a set of like elements whose distinctive pattern resides in the order in which they occur into a set of distinctive elements each of which labels uniquely the pattern represented. Our example was the "talking" to a computer whose controls are binary, i.e., whose switches can only be put into an up or down position. Perceiving the differences between arrays of U U D D D U U D D U U D proved difficult—encoding into octal or decimal notation made conversation with the computer possible. But equally important, and relevant to the problems of this chapter, is that decoding of octal (or decimal) into binary must take place before the operator can act on the computer. The operation of decoding is the inverse of what was required for encoding; now a set of distinct elements must be degraded into a pattern composed of like elements. This is the problem of the serial ordering of behavior; this is the problem of the singleness of action from moment to moment.

The modifications in pattern must operate on the spatial as well as temporal characteristics which produce the peripheral code. The composer's symphony must be simultaneously decoded into the bowing of a string and its stoppage; the configuration of the cerebral organization must be transformed into spatially and temporally organized patterns of nerve impulses which instruct the steady state contractility of the vocal cords to modulate the plosions of air through them. Even in a simple flexion of a forepaw the pattern of signals must be so generated that the remainder of the organism holds steady while reciprocally contracting and relaxing his flexors and extensors. Viewed in this fashion *the organization of behavior, its serial ordering, is due not to the chaining of movements but to the differentiation, the decoding, of an already formed spatial configuration.*

In many ways the problem of behavior is thus the inverse of the problem of Image. Where an Image is a representation within the organism of its environment, a behavioral Act is a representation in the environment of something within the organism. Acts are achievements in the sense that building a nest or writing a book accomplishes in the external world something the organism had planned, was disposed or set to do. How an Act becomes organized makes the substance of this part of our study.

Return once again to the model of the production of speech which introduces this book. The sentence "I love you" produced by the machine is an Act. True enough, only the peripheral vocal instrument was modelled—i.e., electronic hardware was substituted for the unique vocal apparatus. The adjustments of the instrument had to be made by a human operator using his brain. Nonetheless, the instrument focuses on the fact that the generation of even as complex an activity as the vocalization of a sentence can be accomplished by appropriate modification of two basic processes. How then are these modifications managed?

My thesis is that the organization of action is to a large extent the management of receptors embedded in the contractile tissue of muscle (muscle spindles) or in the tendons that attach muscles to bones and joints. These receptors react not only to the contractions of muscle, whether produced by external forces or by nerve impulses originating in the brain (via a system of efferent fibers labeled alpha because of their large diameter) but also to excitations reaching them directly via the gamma efferent fiber system. The immediate organization of movement is therefore dependent on a process that involves receptors, afferents from those receptors to the spinal cord, efferents from there to contractile muscles, *and to receptors.* (refer to Figs. 5-2, 5-6).

Whenever this process produces an invariant response to stimulation, we identify the process as a reflex. In this chapter I will first note some interesting problems concerning the operation of reflexes which are raised by the presence of central control over receptors. I then go on to detail the management of muscle receptor function by brain mechanisms.

the servo control of muscle contractors

Because of the presence of direct central nervous system control over receptor function by way of the gamma system of efferent fibers, the neural organization of the reflex can no longer be conceived as an arc, a simple stimulus-response sequence. Rather, abundant evidence proves that receptors are controlled by the central nervous system—especially those receptors sensing muscle contraction. These central controls act as feedback and feedforward processes in what is essentially a biasable servomechanism. The evidence has become so overwhelming that Ragnar Granit, one of the foremost students of motor as well as of sensory mechanisms, was wont to remark recently that:

> . . . as far as motoneurons are concerned, the essential problems no longer center around reflexes, though reflexes are still the helpful tools they always have been in this field. The essential problems concern the biasing or setting of the various mechanisms by the aid of which motoneurons are made to operate, reflexly or otherwise. There is biasing of them by the neuromuscular

intrafusal [muscle spindle] machinery of the gamma loop, by internuncial systems, and neurohormones operating on the alpha and gamma motoneurons from higher stations . . . . [Granit and Kellerth, 1967]

A great deal was learned about the servocontrol of movement from an experiment which, in the style of the neurobehavioral method, produced a paradox.

If a muscle is maintaining a contraction by the discharge of motor impulses from the spinal cord, then a shock delivered to the motor nerve will superimpose a twitch on the tension record. During the twitch it is observed that the discharge of motor impulses to the muscle is interrupted [Fig. 12-3]. This is

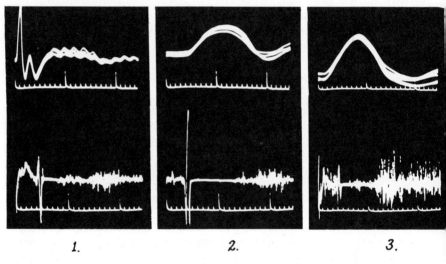

1.   *2.*   *3.*

Fig. 12-3. Silent periods in the human soleus muscle recorded with a needle electrode (lower records). A hinge fitted beneath the heel of the subject and tension in the ankle extensors (upper records) recorded as the downward pressure at the toe. Time: 10 and 100 msec. Five superimposed records in each picture. 1: silent period during a tendon jerk elicited by a tap in the Achilles tendon. Contact of the hammer with skin triggers tendon. Contact of the hammer with skin triggers sweep. 2: during a reflex contraction set up by a shock to afferent fibers in the popliteal fossa. 3: during a twitch in the lateral part of gastrocnemius set up by a stimulus over that muscle. Note that soleus itself is not excited by the stimulus. Time marker (bottom trace in each record) indicates 10 and 100 msec. By courtesy of Merton, from Granit, 1955.

the silent period. It is a reflex effect [for discussion of evidence, see Merton, 1951] and is believed to be due to the stoppage of discharge from muscle spindles during the twitch. It is this discharge which normally excites the stretch reflex and when it is withdrawn the motoneurones become silent. The interpretation of the silent period in the language of servo theory is this: the shock breaks into the servo loop and interpolates an extra motor volley that causes the muscle to shorten; the negative feedback mechanism therefore operates to cut off the spinal motor discharges until the muscle is restored by relaxation to its former length. It must be noted that negative feedback not only tends to neutralize the effects of changes in load or interpolated volleys, but also to make the performance of the muscle independent of fatigue or changes in synaptic excitability, in exactly the same way that a feedback amplifier is insensitive to changes in supply voltages or in the gain of the valves. Stability is only required in the feedback element: in the amplifier, a feedback network of stable resistors; and in the muscle, sensory organs which do not fatigue. It is known from Matthew's work that muscle spindles have these properties . . . .

To return to the proprioceptive mechanism of the silent period, the reason the muscle spindles interrupt their discharge during the twitch is that they are attached "in parallel" with the main muscle fibres. When the muscle shortens, the strain is therefore taken off the spindles and they no longer discharge. This "in parallel" arrangement of the spindles is the key to the whole theory. Its great significance is that it enables them to signal information about length, whereas if they were "in series" they could only respond to tension. A mechanism, such as the stretch reflex servo, which is so obviously concerned with maintaining length and not tension, must necessarily have receptors which record length. [Merton, 1953, pp. 248-59]

There are, of course, other receptor-effector relationships that control muscle contraction. There are receptors in tendons and in joints—and stretch of the skin around the muscle and joints is not to be neglected as a source of information for controlling movement. But more is known about the gamma loop than about the other mechanisms and the innervation of muscle spindles is most likely the fundamental upon which the other mechanisms build (See Fig. 12-4).

Gamma fibers have been found to be of two different kinds. One type of responsive fiber shows a constant frequency of discharge when the muscle is maintained at a constant length. The other type, by contrast, shows a decrease of frequency of discharge occurring on the completion of the dynamic phase of stretching. P.B.C. Matthews (1964) suggests in the conclusion of an extensive review on the subject that this double γ innervation of each muscle spindle "provides relatively independent control of the 'bias' and of the

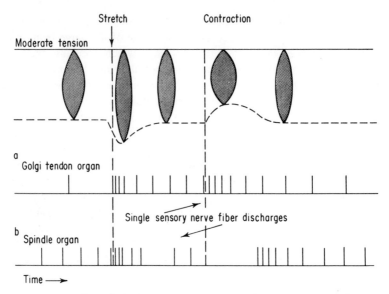

Fig. 12-4. Response patterns of sensory nerve fibers from Golgi tendon organ (a) and a spindle organ (b) to stretch and contraction of a muscle. Note that spindle organ (which operates by way of γ loop) shows response both to stretching and to length of muscle. See text and Fig. 12-5 for dissociation of these effects. After Granit, 1955, from Thompson, *Foundations of Physiological Psychology,* Harper & Row, 1967.

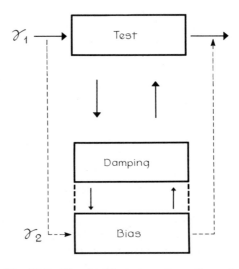

Fig. 12-5. The double innervation of muscle spindles diagrammed in TOTE terms.

'damping' of the servo loop," since each type of control has been shown to be separately manipulable by central stimulation (Fig. 12-5).

This analysis is important in two respects. First it focuses on the fact that any but the simplest muscle twitches must be governed by the patterns of signals which reach the muscle receptors, either exclusively or at least in concert with those which reach the contractile elements in muscle. Evidence (see next sections) suggests that parts of the brain—e.g., the basal ganglia, the anterior portion of the cerebellum—function to gang together the direct contractile α and the indirect receptor controlling γ discharges so that such concert can be achieved.

Second, management of the reflex servomechanism can be readily visualized as taking place at the receptor surface. There is therefore no need for a piano keyboard type of mechanism by which impulses from the brain bear the message: contract now this, now that, muscle fibril to this or that extent. Rather, the existing state of contraction of the muscle fiber sets the state variable of its receptor. The arrangement of nerve impulses interacts with this state to alter the bias of the servo and thus the muscle contraction. The brain must still send spatially and temporally arranged signals, but the messages in these signals need not be coded in accord with the contraction or relaxation they are to produce since this information already resides in the receptor state variable. The next chapter details the messages that such a code must contain.

To summarize: Neurophysiological evidence has given meaning to the anatomical presence of direct afferent connections from spinal cord to muscle receptors. At the most fundamental level, the organization of even the simplest reflex becomes not a stimulus→CNS→ response arc but a servomechanism, a test-operate-test-exit (TOTE) sequence. When reflexes become integrated by central nervous system activity into more complex movements, integration cannot be effected by sending patterns of signals directly and exclusively to contractile muscles, playing on them as if they were a keyboard. Such signals would only disrupt the servoprocess. In order to prevent disruption, patterns of signals must be transmitted to the muscle receptors, either exclusively or in concert with those reaching muscle fibers directly. Integrated movement is thus largely dependent on changing the bias, the setting of muscle receptors.

readiness to respond

An analysis consonant with the view presented in these chapters has been suggested by Fred Mettler (1967). He recognizes first, a "tonic background for movement: the canvas ... on which movement is depicted." It is "within" a framework of afferent impulses that some "potentially dominant" brain process "has to manifest itself." This "canvas," this state, is constituted of the sum of the peripheral servomechanisms which control muscle contractions.

Next, Mettler recognizes "associated movements [the topic of this section], the large color masses against which the details are painted . . . ." These massive regulations of muscle tonus devolve on the basal ganglia, the most forward structures of the brain stem. Finally, "upon and within this background of static and broadly moving forces, the cortex is responsible for the focus and intensification as well as for alterations in the velocity of movement in progress and the rate at which it is activated and stopped."

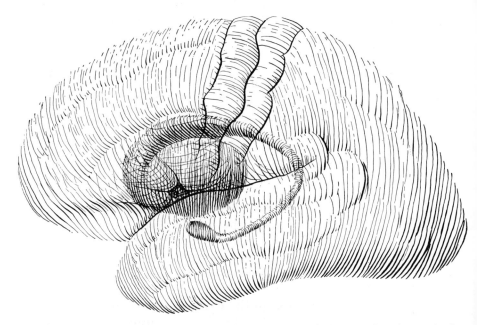

Fig. 12-6. The location of the basal ganglia within the cerebral hemispheres of the brain. From Krieg, 1966.

The state aspect of muscle function is called its *tonus*. Tonus is, however, not just the amount of spasticity or flaccidity of the contractile tissue. Rather, tonus is the state of readiness of the entire neuromuscular apparatus—the precondition for action.

The central circuits especially involved in the regulation of tonic muscular activity are those involving the basal ganglia (Fig. 12-6) and

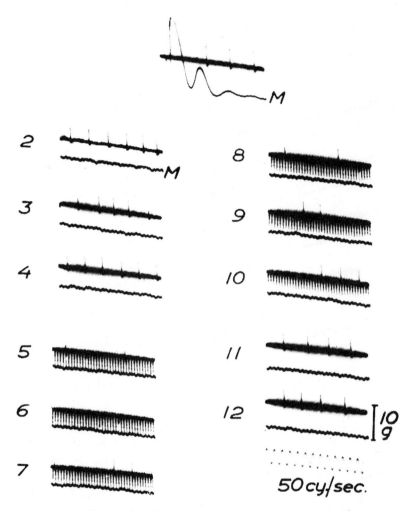

Fig. 12-7. Inhibition of muscle spindle discharge from anterior lobe of cerebellum. Upper traces in each record show spindle discharge extending upward from trace, stimulus artifact extending downward. Lower traces in each record are myograms. Decerebrate animal. Gastrocnemius. Initial tension 66 g. Myograph at maximum sensitivity (see record 12) except in 1, in which (clonic) contraction to single shock to the gastrocnemius nerves demonstrates silent period. 2-4: controls before stimulation; 5-10: during cerebellar stimulation at 140/sec. with 1-msec. shocks for 26 sec.; 5-7: after 18-20 sec.; 8-10: after 24-26 sec.; 11-12: immediately after cessation of stimulation. Note drop in spindle frequency from about 20/sec. to an irregular discharge frequency of about 5/sec. Granit and Kaada, 1952, in Granit, 1955.

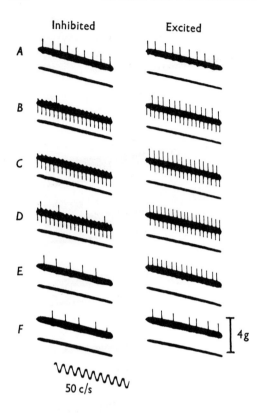

Inhibited   Excited

A
B
C
D
E
F

50 c/s

4g

Fig. 12-8. Recording from spindle in soleus muscle. Effect of stimulation of the inhibitory and excitatory loci in basal ganglia and other brain stem structures. As in Fig. 12-7, upper traces of each record indicate spindle discharge extending upward and stimulation artifact extending downward from trace. A: base-line; B: first record during stimulation (note shock artifacts); C: during stimulation; D: last record before cessation of stimulation; E, F: immediately afterward. Myograph record on lower trace: initial tension 55 g. Cat under chloralose and dial. Eldred, Granit, and Merton, 1953, in Granit, 1955.

the anterior portion of the cerebellum (Fig. 12-10). Lesions of these structures markedly alter the state of readiness of the muscular apparatus: removals of the anterior cerebellum lead to flaccidity, loss of muscle tone; lesions of the basal ganglia to a completely flat, expressionless facial appearance, the Parkinsonian mask, and tremors in the extremities when they are not moving. Phylogenetically these brain structures became developed when vertebrates first adapted to moving on land. They are therefore intimately involved in postural adjustments—which constitute, of course, a readiness to respond, the background state from which discrete action can take off.

The regulation of muscular activity by the basal ganglia and anterior cerebellar circuits has been extensively investigated but has not as yet become completely clarified. For the most part, the γ system seems to be primarily involved although, as already mentioned, the ganging of a and γ outflow also plays an integral role. The critical characteristics of the system depend in large part on the proportions and time course of the reciprocal relationships established between a and γ activities and on the spatial coordination of recurrent patterns of signals in the system (Figs. 12-7, 12-8). These characteristics are not easy to determine in experimental situations in which anesthetics are usually given, thus rendering the natural postural mechanisms useless. Nonetheless, present knowledge suggests that modulations of states of readiness in the muscular apparatus are performed by the basal ganglia—anterior cerebellar circuits, primarily by damping the ongoing cyclicities inherent in the peripheral negative feedback mechanism, the servo which characterizes the reflex. This damping probably takes place by spatially coordinating, locking, and ganging together the reciprocal activities of the various servomechanisms. By these mechanisms flexibility is introduced into the tonic background state of the motor system.

the fact of voluntary movement

Servocontrol has another aspect. Sometimes the servomechanism is not only outcome-informed but becomes preset to a new level, prior to an activity which demands its stabilizing influence. These feedforward processes (Fig. 12-5) are ubiquitous in the motor system and are labeled as voluntary, willed, or intended movements and actions. The problems involving volitional activity are far reaching in any attempt to understand the neural control of behavior; a good beginning to understanding comes from studies of the gamma system. Let us return for a moment to Merton:

Now what happens during voluntary shortening? It is easy to make a voluntary contraction, taking off from the steady level, which rises faster even than the maximal twitch. The rate of rise of the small twitch corresponds only to a leisurely rate of increase of voluntary effort. This raises a very interesting problem, for if the servo goes on working in the same way as before during such increasing contractions, it will clearly tend strongly to oppose them. Immediately after voluntary shortening begins, the strain would be taken off the spindles, and the resultant cessation of excitatory afferent impulses would depress the motoneurones... powerfully as... when the shortening was produced by a small motor-nerve stimulus. This is really equivalent to saying that extra motor discharges produced by excitation of the motoneurones in the spinal cord should have the same effect in the servo loop as impulses excited further round the loop in their axons by an electric shock. In either case, the servo should react strongly to offset their mechanical effects. If these inferences from the experiment are valid, it follows that during shortening the resistance offered by the servo must be either overcome or removed.

... the need for excitation of the main motoneurones connected to the intrafusal muscle fibres by descending impulses in the spinal cord has disappeared. The excitation all goes to the small motoneurons [spindle receptors] and the servo makes the main muscle follow. Shortening thus involves just the same mechanism as a steady contraction, namely a servo for keeping the muscle in step with its spindles, and it is therefore under the stabilizing influence of feedback in just the same way. Excitation applied to the main motoneurones is seen to be wrong in principle because it is just the sort of interference a feedback loop is designed to neutralize. The loop is best activated by altering the bias on its null-detector.

This hypothesis is to some extent supported by recent experiments on the small nerve supply to mammalian muscle. In particular Hunt (1951) observed that in reflex contraction the discharge of motor impulses to the intrafusal muscles [spindle receptors] preceded the appearance of activity in the main motor units. [Merton, 1953, pp. 251–53]

Voluntary movements are therefore, as a rule, initiated by action on the intrafusal muscle spindles. An exception to this rule occurs, however, when movements are suddenly initiated. Because of the relatively small diameter of the γ fibers and the length of the pathway, conduction time is too slow to account for sudden muscle contractions. Such movements will, however, be relatively simple and control quickly taken over by the γ system.

The direct pathway to main motor neurons is not to be completely dismissed, therefore. A limited amount of preprogramed ("contract-relax") information can be sent through this pathway provided the starts and stops are kept temporally separated by a sufficient interval to let the γ servo make an adjustment. Studies by Joseph Berman and his colleagues (Taub, Bacon, and Berman, 1965) have shown both the extent and the limitations of such preprograming. Berman prepares a monkey whose spinal cord has been completely de-afferented by sectioning the dorsal root along its entire extent. This procedure breaks the servo loop. Yet these monkeys can still make conditional responses (gross limb flexions) after de-afferentation. In man, such de-afferentations undertaken in now abandoned efforts to relieve pain and other sensory disturbances have produced severe restrictions on skilled movements performed with that extremity.

In summary, reflex and integrated movement, whether initiated by an environmental or by a central event, is largely managed by biasing the muscle spindle receptors of the γ servo loop. The central control of movement, therefore, resolves itself into the central control of receptor processes, a problem with which we became familiar in Part II and which will be spelled out in even greater detail in Part IV. Let us now just note the paradox—a particularly cruel one for a practitioner of a restricted behaviorism: *even the observable response mechanism contains in its makeup a centrally controlled receptor process.*

a fast time prediction mechanism

Given the fact that voluntary movement takes place, the question is how? Part of the problem lies in the proper formulation of the feedforward concept and part in the delineation of preprogramming processes that can compute the outcome of a series of movements before that outcome is materialized.

Recall that Chapter 5 pointed out that feedforward processes need

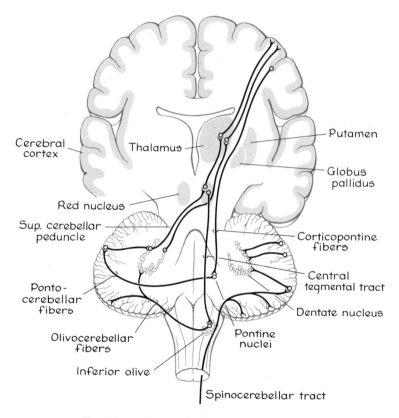

Fig. 12-9. Midline section through brain and brain stem to show location and major connections of cerebellum. Modified from Krieg, 1966.

only "a rough sketching out of the operations to be performed." Once the sketch is available, the ordinary feedback servocircuits can take over to smooth out the roughness. One neural system appears, on the basis of neuroanatomical and neurophysiological evidence, to be ideally constituted to serve the sketching function, and neurobehavioral evidence indicates that in fact the function is carried out by this system. Its nidus is the phylogenetically newest part of the cerebellum, a fascinating structure that demands a short detour to view the panorama it presents (Figs. 12-9, 12-10).

As noted, the anterior cerebellum developed in response to the evolutionary landing of marine vertebrates. Before this occurrence the cerebellum functioned mainly as an extension of the vestibular control mechanisms. Fish maintain orientation with reference to their own bodily axis; movement takes off from this baseline.

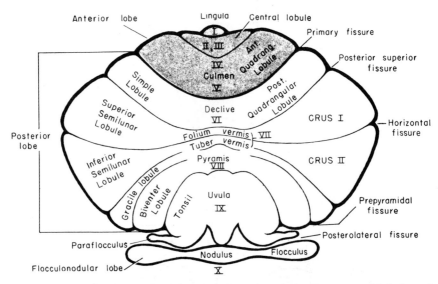

Fig. 12-10. Schematic diagram of the fissures and lobules of the cerebellum (Larsell, 1951; Jansen and Brodal, 1958; Angevine; et al., 1961). Portions of the cerebellum caudal to the posterolateral fissure represent the flocculonodular lobule (archicerebellum), while portions of the cerebellum rostral to the primary fissure (shaded) constitute the anterior lobe (paleocerebellum). The neocerebellum lies between the primary and posterolateral fissures. Roman numerals refer to portions of the cerebellar vermis only. From Truex and Carpenter, *Human Neuroanatomy*, 6 ed. © 1969 The Williams & Wilkins Co., Baltimore, Md.

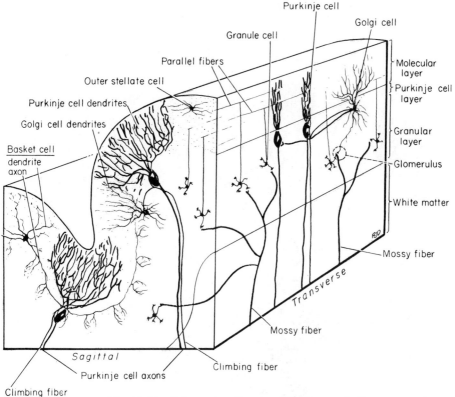

Fig. 12-11. Schematic diagram of the cerebellar cortex in sagittal and transverse planes showing cell and fiber arrangements. Compare with Fig. 12-12 which shows these arrangements in cross section. From Truex and Carpenter, 1969. *Human Neuroanatomy,* 6th ed. © 1969 the Williams & Wilkins Co., Baltimore, Md.

Amphibia and other landed creatures find an additional baseline: the ground under them, "under" being determined by gravitational forces. New postural uprights become useful and the anterior cerebellum develops. Finally, primates free themselves to some extent from the gravitational baseline by manipulation and adopt arboreal habitats and erect posture. Now the cerebellar hemispheres become dominant. In man, damage to these hemispheres produces incoordination, a marked overshooting of targets, and a jerkiness in carrying out intended movements.

Fortunately for neurophysiology, the cerebellar hemispheres are remarkably homogeneous structures (Fig. 12-11) and therefore relatively simple to analyze. Their major connections are: (1) through

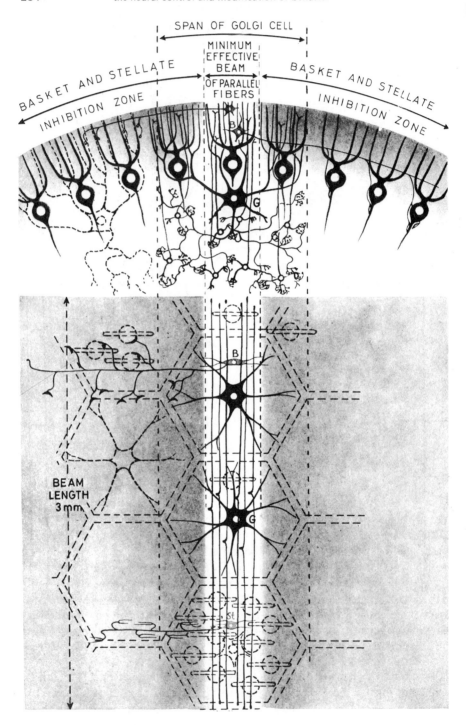

SPAN OF GOLGI CELL

MINIMUM
EFFECTIVE
BEAM
OF PARALLEL
FIBERS

BASKET AND STELLATE

INHIBITION ZONE

BASKET AND STELLATE

INHIBITION ZONE

B

G

BEAM
LENGTH
3 mm

B

G

St

Fig. 12-12. Diagram illustrating the extension of inhibitory fields (shadowed areas) in the case that a narrow beam of parallel fibers be excited. The upper part of the diagram is a transverse section of the folium and the lower part a view at the folium surface from above. It is assumed that there is a "minimum effective beam" of simultaneously excited parallel fibers, which is more likely to stimulate a row of Purkinje, stellate, and basket cells. Golgi cells having a much larger dendritic spread would be more likely to be excited by broader bands of simultaneously excited parallel fibers. Effective stimulation of the Golgi cells would then in turn tend to stop—as a negative feedback—all mossy input. Thus the Golgi cell system can be considered as a "focusing" device restricting—or giving preference to—granule neuron (parallel fiber) activity in relatively narrow bands. From Eccles, Ito, and Szentagothai, 1967.

the spinal cord from and to movement sensitive structures, and (2) from and to the cerebral cortex (Fig. 12-9). Because of these connections the cerebellar hemispheres can operate as a comparator, matching signals from the cerebral cortex with those derived from the periphery.

The nature of this comparison process is what becomes so interesting in the light of recent exquisitely detailed anatomical and physiological analysis (See Fig. 12-12). The cerebellar hemispheres have a cortex that is made up of "rectangular lattices" reminiscent of the columnar structures found in the cerebral cortex—except that all the cerebellar lattices are practically identical. Further, the lattices are so constructed that after one or two synapses all inputs into the cerebellum are transformed into inhibitory interactions. Such a fantastically developed inhibitory mechanism must serve a purpose:

This exclusive transformation of all inputs into inhibition with at most two synaptic relays gives the cerebellum a 'dead-beat' character in its response to input. There is no possibility of the dynamic storage of information by impulses circulating in complex neuronal pathways such as occurs within the cerebral cortex and along the various circuits between it and the basal ganglia. Within at most 30 msec after a given input there will be no further evoked discharges in the cortical neurones.

... what the rest of the nervous system requires from the cerebellum is presumably not some output expressing the operation of complex reverberatory circuits in the cerebellum, but rather a quick and clear response to the input of any particular set of information. [Eccles, Ito, and Szentagothai, 1967, p. 311]

The rapid wipe-out of the contents of a register suggests that rapid successions of comparisons are computed. This is not a usual characteristic of feedback servos in which a state must be maintained long enough to become informed by the consequences of its output. Theodore Ruch in the *Handbook of Experimental Psychology* (1951) already gauged the problem correctly—much before the presently available evidence was gathered:

> The cerebral-[neo]cerebellar circuit may represent not so much an error correcting device as part of a mechanism by which an instantaneous order can be extended forward in time. Such a circuit, though uninformed as to consequences, could, so to speak, 'rough in' a movement and thus reduce the troublesome transients involved in the correction of movement by output informed feedbacks. (Ruch, 1951, p. 205)

The power of the cerebellum, i.e., the size of the register, is such that the roughing-in need not be all that sketchy. In fact, a momentary state similar to those produced by the cerebral cortex is composed on the background of spontaneous activity:

> Thus, we must envisage that, even under conditions of minimal sensory input, there is a state of dynamic poise in the level of activity of the various types of cerebellar neurones .... The negative image of the integrated output from the cerebellar cortex is, as it were, formed by a process analogous to sculpturing stone. Spatio-temporal form is achieved from moment to moment by the impression of a patterned inhibition upon the 'shapeless' background discharges of the subcerebellar neurones, just as an infinitely more enduring form is achieved in sculpture by a highly selective chiselling away from the initial amorphous block of stone. [Eccles, Ito, and Szentagothai, 1967, pp. 6, 10]

I will say more about this state and its counterpart in the cerebral cortex in Chapter 13. Here we need only know that the feedforward sketch can be conceived to constitute the equivalent of a rapid computation of the end point of a convergent series. The hologram analogy of Image formation suggests that a Fourier transform is involved—but again more of this in the next chapter. In any case, the results of the computation are almost immediately available to both the peripheral muscular servos and to the cerebral motor cortex by way of the cerebellum's connections. In engineering man-

machine interfaccs, such fast time computations of expected outcomes have recently proved extremely useful guides (Kelley, 1968).
The brain-behavior interface apparently learned this lesson long ago.

synopsis

The neurological problem of the organization of behavior is, in
many respects, the inverse of the construction of Images (percepts
and feelings). Because of the ubiquitous presence of feedback (and
feedforward) in the nervous system, the control of movement is
effected not directly by signals to the contractile muscle fibers, but
by signals to the receptors that gauge muscle contraction. The muscle
receptor thus becomes part of a tunable loop (a TOTE servomechanism) whose setting determines the muscle's reaction to
environmental change. In short, the neural regulation of behavior
turns out to be effected by the regulation of receptor processes, not
by the direct control of muscle contractions.

actions

the motor cortex

The detailing of behavior falls to the cerebral motor cortex. This cortex located in the precentral gyrus of the hemispheres (Fig. 13-1) has connections to the basal ganglia and with the cerebellum. What then is the function of this motor cortex? For a century arguments have raged over the nature of the organization of the central motor system. Some (Woolsey and Chang, 1948) maintain that anatomically a point-to-point representation of muscles and even slips of muscles exists in the motor region, that the motor cortex is the keyboard upon which all other cerebral activity—and indeed all willed action—plays. By contrast others (e.g., Phillips, 1965) have pointed out that the receptive fields of neighboring cortical units cover a wide sample of muscles although most of those recorded at any one location relate to a particular joint. Consonant with this observation is the fact that electrical excitations of the motor cortex produce movements, integrated sequences of muscle contractions, and that the movement produced by a particular excitation depends in part on the state of the brain and the position of

238

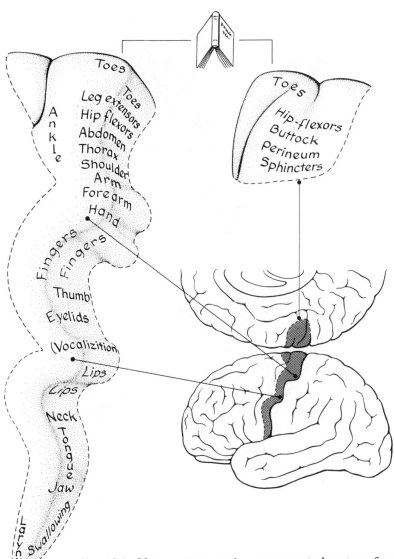

Fig. 13-1. Motor representation on precentral cortex of man. (c) Diagram of surface of left cerebral hemisphere, showing location of precentral gyrus. (a) Precentral gyrus isolated, enlarged, and viewed from the same aspect as in (c). (b) Medial aspect of the precentral gyrus. Actually there is considerable overlapping and variation in individual cases but the order is constant. From data on electrical stimulation of precentral cortex and observations of the resulting movements obtained by Foerster, Penfield and Boldrey and others. Redrawn after Krieg, 1966.

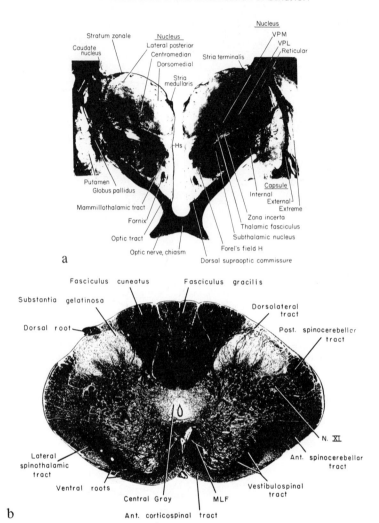

Fig. 13-2. (A) Photograph of transverse section through the thalamus, hypothalamus, and basal ganglia at the level of the optic chiasm. HS indicates the hypothalamic sulcus in the wall of the third ventricle. VPM and VPL refer to the ventral posteromedial and ventral posterolateral nuclei of the thalamus. Weigert's myelin stain. (B) Photograph of transverse section through uppermost portion of spinal cord of 1-month infant. Weigert's myelin stain. Note similarity of location and configuration between dorsal horn of spinal cord and dorsal thalamus; also between ventral horn and basal ganglia (and subthalamus). From Truex and Carpenter, *Human Neuroanatomy,* 6 ed. ©1969 The Williams & Wilkins Co., Baltimore, Md.

the limbs to be influenced by the stimulation. The interpretation made of these neurophysiological data has always been that movements, not muscles, were represented in the motor areas.

Some years ago I reexamined this controversy by repeating many of the critical experiments and extended the observations by using some additional techniques (Pribram, et al., 1955-1956).

The results of these experiments and observations showed that the motor regions of the cortex were critically involved in the control of neither individual muscles nor specific movements. Rather, the motor cortex seemed to play some higher order role in directing action—action defined not in terms of muscles, but of the achievement of an external representation of a psychological set or Plan. This result led me to suggest that the central motor mechanism is akin to the sensory systems, that damage to the motor cortex produces "scotomata of action," using the analogy of the scotomata, the holes, in the visual field produced by damage to the visual cortex.

The evidence for this view continues to accrue. Initially I had to face an anatomical paradox. The input to the motor cortex arrives via the dorsal thalamus, a brain stem structure which lies (as its name implies) dorsally and is therefore homologous with the dorsal parts of the spinal cord which receive what Bell (1811) and Magendie (1822) found to be the "sensory" part of the peripheral nerves (see Fig. 13-2). Why should the motor cortex be so closely tied to an otherwise sensory structure?

This anatomical paradox was dramatized during the course of some experiments in which electrical potential changes were evoked in the cortex by electrical stimulation of peripheral nerves. Quite by accident one morning such potential changes were observed to be evoked in the motor cortex. At first these observations were too radical to believe—in fact, as it turned out, though they had been made by others, no one had thought to report them—except once a footnote mentioned them as possible artifacts. But it became evident from our experiments (Malis, Pribram, and Kruger, 1953; Fig. 13-3) and those of others (Albe-Fessard, 1957; Penfield and Boldrey, 1937) that indeed input does arrive at the motor cortex from the periphery, that it is routed through the dorsal thalamus, that it does not come by way of any hitherto identified sensory areas such as the somatosensory cortex which lies adjacent to the motor, and, in fact, that this input was independent of the cerebellum. Further, the input originated not only in those nerve fibers that innervate muscle but also in those that connect exclusively with skin.

Evidence from other observations and experiments also emphasized the sensory nature of the motor cortex. Monkeys and men who

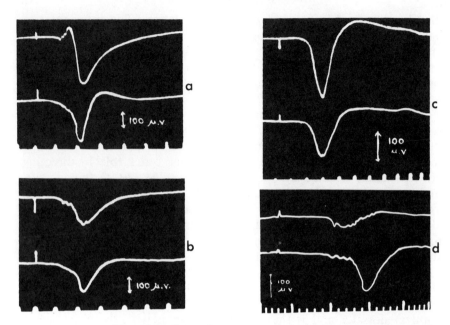

Fig. 13-3. Cortical responses evoked by sciatic nerve stimulation before resection of postcentral cortex and cerebellum. Upper trace, postcentral; lower trace, precentral. Time: 10 msec. B: Same immediately after resection of both cerebellar hemispheres. C: Same following additional resection of anterior lobe of cerebellum. D: Same after additional resection of both postcentral gyri. Note that postcentral record now registers only white matter response. From Malis, Pribram, and Kruger, 1953.

had suffered removals of this cortex were able to make any and all movements provided the circumstances were "right": war veterans whose hands had been paralyzed for years by motor cortex injury, would under duress, such as the outbreak of a fire in their ward, rotate door knobs with that hand. Monkeys after motor cortex removals were examined by slow motion movies and shown, although clumsy in performing the skilled sequence of opening latches on boxes containing peanuts, to make exactly the same hand and finger movements without undue difficulty while climbing the wire mesh sides of their cages or while grooming. Only some Acts, some achievements were difficult, and the difficulty had little to do with the specific movements required (Pribram et al; 1955-1956). How then is the motor cortex involved in transforming movement into action?

an image-of-achievement

The ready answer to the question of how movement becomes transformed into action is that a sort of Imaging process must occur in the motor cortex and that the Image is a momentary Image-of-Achievement which contains all input and outcome information necessary to the next step of that achievement. To test this hypothesis it is necessary to show that just as the visual cortex encodes events other than visual (a right or a left panel press and success and error), so the motor cortex must encode events other than movement. The likelihood that this encoding will take place is great, since one large part of the input to the motor cortex is derived from the cerebellar cortex, a structure shown to be rich in connections from all of the sensory receptors.

But just how can the cortical surface become the locus of a momentary Image-of-Achievement? How might input from the peri-

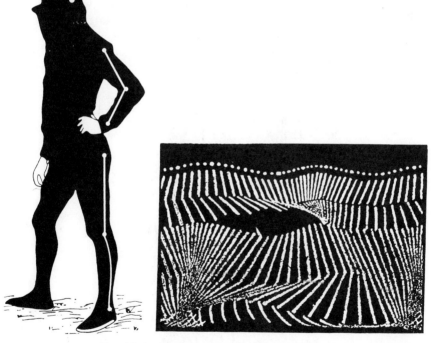

Fig. 13-4. A: Subject in black costume with white tape. B: Cinematograph of walking. Movement is from left to right. The frequency is about 20 exposures per sec. Reprinted with permission from N. Bernstein, *The Co-ordination and Regulation of Movements.* © 1967 Pergamon Press Ltd.

pheral structures involved in movement be organized to anticipate the outcome of that movement rather than simply to serve as a record of the components of the movement? A classical experimental analysis performed during the 1930s by Bernstein (1967) in the Soviet Union helped to answer this question. Put together with current knowledge of the importance of γ efferent control over movement, this crucial and very puzzling aspect of the organization of action begins to unravel. How then does the organism construct a pre-Image of the consequences of his behavior?

Bernstein's analysis was made from cinematographic records of performances such as walking, running, hammering, filing, or typing. Human subjects were dressed in black costumes outfitted with white dots to mark the various joints of the limbs (Fig. 13-4). The film strips would therefore be composed of a continuous pattern whose wave form could be analyzed mathematically. For instance, Bernstein found that any rhythmic movement could be represented by a rapidly converging trigonometric series and that the next step in such movements could be predicted "to an accuracy of within a few millimeters in the form of a sum of three or four harmonic oscillations, the so-called Fourier trigonometric sums" (Fig. 13-5).

The fact that these activities could be represented in mathematical terms that can be characterized as a "temporal hologram" immedi-

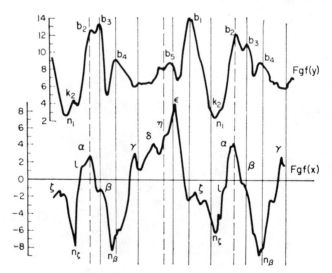

Fig. 13-5. Force curves at the center of gravity of the thigh in normal walking. Above: vertical components. Below: horizontal components. Reprinted with permission from N. Bernstein, *The Co-ordination and Regulation of Movements.*   © 1967 Pergamon Press Ltd.

ately leads to the realization that their brain representation might also be organized by this sort of transformation rather than the usually assumed keyboard control mechanism. Thus the pattern of events in the motor cortex could be conceived to reflect some sort of holographic transformation, some sort of projection of prior external forces present in the field of action. Bernstein summarizes this view:

It is clear that each of the variations of a movement (for example, drawing a circle large or small, directly in front of oneself or to one side, on a horizontal piece of paper or on a vertical blackboard, etc.) demands a quite different muscular formula; and even more that this, involves a completely different set of muscles in the action. The almost equal facility and accuracy with which all these variations can be performed is evidence for the fact that they are ultimately determined by one and the same higher directional engram in relation to which dimensions and position play a secondary role . . . . We must conclude from this that the higher engram, which may be called the engram of a given topological class, is already structurally extremely far removed (and because of this also probably localizationally very distant) from any resemblance whatever to the joint-muscle schema [which is represented in the parietal cortex; damage to this cortex produces "astereognosis," the inability to identify the position and whereabouts of the affected extremity]. It [the higher engram] is extremely geometrical, representing a very abstract motor image of space. This makes us suppose—for the time being merely as an hypothesis though it forces itself upon us very strongly, that the localizational areas of these higher-order motor engrams have also the same topological regulation as is found in external space or in the motor field (and that in any case the pattern is by no means that which maintains in the joint-muscle apparatus). In other words there is considerable reason to suppose that in the higher motor centres of the brain (it is very probable that these are in the cortical hemispheres) the localizational pattern is none other than some form of projection of external space in the form present for the subject in the motor field. This projection, from all that has been said above, must be congruent with external space, but only topologically and in no sense metrically. All danger of considering the possibility of compensation for the inversion of projection at the retina. . . and many other possibilities of the same sort are completely avoided by these considerations. It seems to me that although it is not now possible to specify the ways in which such a topological representation of space in the central nervous system may be achieved, this is only a question of time for physiology. It is only necessary to reiterate that the topological properties of the projection of space in the C.N.S. may prove to be very strange and unexpected; we must not expect to find in the cortex some sort of photograph of space, even an extremely deformed one. Still, the hypothesis that there exist in the higher levels of the C.N.S.

projections of space, and not projections of joints and muscles, seems to me to be at present more probable than any other. [p. 49]

As we shall see shortly, Bernstein's prediction that topological properties of space are represented in the motor cortex turned out to be in error. Instead the forces exciting muscle receptors are represented. But this does not detract from Bernstein's overall insight that properties of the environment, not configurations of muscles and joints, become cortically encoded.

the motor mechanism

As noted, Bernstein's observations suggest that constancy can be achieved in action regardless of the particular movements or the amount of contraction of any particular muscle or muscle group. In fact the action can be performed just because movements become attuned to the "field of external forces" involved at the moment. As already noted in the discussion of the gamma efferent servo, load changes on the system are compensated by the mechanism so that the state of readiness remains constant. Thus constancy takes into account the adjustments and compensations to external forces, and the representation includes these parameters. In fact, a great deal of the central neural mechanism is involved only in these adjustments and compensations; the central representation must therefore be constructed of, as it were, a "mirror image" of the field of external forces. (Note how similar this conclusion is to the one reached in Chapter 12.)

Specific evidence that indeed the neurons of the motor cortex, especially those giving rise to its output, are sensitive to the forces acting on muscle contraction comes from another elegant series of studies. In these experiments Edward Evarts (1967; Fig. 13-6) trained monkeys to manipulate levers which were loaded with various weights to oppose their movement. Once the monkeys had learned to move the lever, unit recordings were made, while they performed the task, from neurons located in their motor cortex. The experiments showed that these neurons were activated *before* external evidence (myographic recording) of the initiation of movement occurred. Careful analysis showed the electrical activity to be a function of the amount of force needed rather than the amount of displacement of the lever. Further, the units reacted most to the *change* of force required, although some activity relating to the required force-magnitude could not be ruled out (Fig. 13-7).

The conception that the motor cortex anticipates parameters of

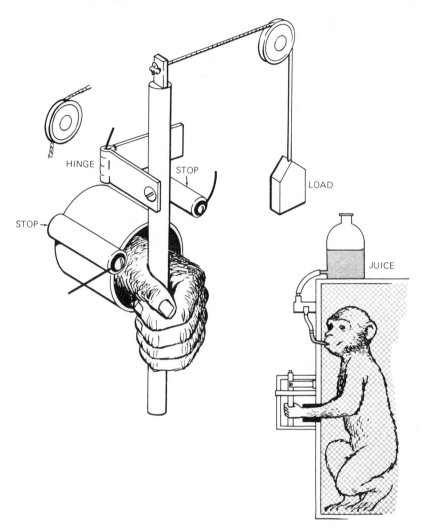

Fig. 13-6. Behavioral testing device for recording motor effect on cells in precentral cortex. The monkey's left hand protrudes from a tube in a lucite panel attached to the front of the home cage. In order to receive a fruit juice reward, the monkey is required to grasp the vertical rod attached to a hinge and to move it back and forth. The monkey is required to move the handle through the arc between the stops. Breaking contact with one stop and making contact with the other must be achieved between 400 and 700 msec, and the previous movement in the other direction must also fall within these time limits in order to operate a solenoid valve which delivers a reward. From Evarts, 1968, in Milner, 1970.

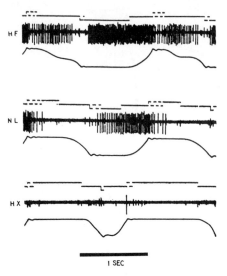

Fig. 13-7. The activity of a unit in the motor cortex of a monkey under the condition portrayed in Fig. 13-6. The activity of the unit is shown at each of three load conditions. The three loads employed are 400 g opposing flexion (shown at the top), 400 g opposing extension (shown at the bottom) and no load opposing the movement (shown in the middle). It may be seen that the unit became much more active with a load that opposed flexion and therefore required increased flexor force. Conversely, the unit was almost totally silent during periods when the movement was 'carried out with a heavy load opposing extension. From Evarts, 1967. From: *Neurophysiological Basis of Normal and Abnormal Motor Activities,* p. 225. Edited by M.D. Yahr and D. P. Purpura. © 1967 by Raven Press, New York.

force is critical. Because reflexes are constituted of servomechanisms, their central representations are constructed not of records of muscle length or tension, but of the parameters of adjustment and compensation to the changing external forces involved in the activity. The convergent properties of these transformations allow this representation to form an Image not just of the prior and current changes of environmental forces acting on the system but, by virtue of the cerebellar fast-time computation, of the changes that will be engendered by the continuation of the activity.

The motor cortex is thus conceived as a sensory cortex for action. It participates in the spatial modulation of states of readiness via its connections with the basal ganglia and in the fast-time computation of states-of-achievement via its participation in the cerebellar circuit. The formation of the resulting Image is dependent, as elsewhere in the cortex, on what we have come to call the neural holographic representation, "a highly selective channeling of activity in the horizontally running intracortical networks which excite and inhibit the corticofugal neurons" (Phillips, 1965). That this motor representation is indeed similar in many respects to those formed in the sensory regions of the brain cortex can be ascertained from studies of the receptive fields of units. These experimental results (Welt, et al., 1967; Fig. 13-8) show that "sensory convergence into the motor (sensory) cortex is superimposed on topographically uniform output organization in radial arrays, the diameter of which is estimated to be

Receptive Field Type	Antidromic Latency in msec, Mean ±s.d.	Adequate Stimulus	Antidromic Latency of Subgroup in msec, Mean ±s.d.	No. of Cells
Fixed Local	1.99±1.03 S.E.=0.17 (N=40)	Hair Touch Pressure Joint	2.57±1.08 1.88±1.07 1.72±0.92 1.69±0.65	11 11 10 8
Fixed Wide	1.94±1.19 S.E.=0.22 (N=30)	Hair Touch Pressure Joint	1.45±0.93 1.94±1.24 2.75±0.77 3.13±1.15	14 9 4 3
Labile	1.45±0.59 S.E.=0.16 (N=18)	Hair Touch Pressure Joint	1.40±0.42 1.48±0.38 1.58±1.01 1.27±0.34	3 8 4 3

$N = 88$

(From: *Neurophysiological Basis of Normal and Abnormal Motor Activities*, p. 278. Edited by M.D. Yahr and D.P. Purpura. © 1967 by Raven Press, New York.)

Fig. 13-8. Receptive field types and antidromic latencies of motor cortex cells. Antidromic latencies of 88 cortical cells, grouped by receptive field types, were compared in a simple randomized design. The "labile" group differed from both "fixed" groups at better than 1% by a t-test on the assumption of equal group variances. s.d.: standard deviation; S.E.: standard error of mean; N: number of cells. See text for the similarity between the role assumed for the labile cells and directionally sensitive cells in Werner's cortical list structures (Fig. 7-7) based on the TOTE conception. From Welt, et al., 1967.

0.1 to 0.4 mm. Thus, neurons with fixed local receptive fields provide a radially oriented framework [a reference system] for common peripheral inputs . . . . Interspersed with these cells having local fields, constituting three-fourths of the total, there were neurons with wide, stocking-like, or labile fields that overlapped with the local fields" [p. 285]. Here for the motor cortex is the evidence which for the visual cortex is still needed.* What remains to be done is the analytical step performed so beautifully by Rodieck for his data on the retina: to show quantitatively just which transformation accurately describes the peripheral-cortical relationship.

In summary, the neural control of behavior is achieved largely through an effect on receptor functions. At the reflex level, receptor sensitivity to the imposition of load initiates and guides an adaptive

*This evidence has now been obtained (Spinelli, Pribram, and Bridgman, 1971).

counter-process in the servomechanism. The sum of such adaptations constitutes the background tonic steady state against which new adjustments occur. Large-scale adjustments such as changes in posture are controlled by the basal ganglia-anterior cerebellar (extra-pyramidal) system of the brain, while more discrete movements such as typing or playing the piano are regulated by a fast-time extrapolatory computation carried on by the neocerebellar system. The precise mechanism of these central controls has yet to be worked out, but we know enough to ascertain that patterning of the peripheral servomechanisms is involved, and that this patterning is achieved by changing the mechanism's bias. Finally, the conception of the functions of the cerebral motor cortex of the precentral gyrus has radically changed. This part of the brain cortex has been shown to be the sensory cortex for action. A momentary Image-of-Achievement is constructed and continuously updated through a neural holographic process much as is the perceptual Image. The Image-of-Achievement is, however, composed of learned anticipations of the force and changes in force required to perform a task. These fields of force exerted on muscle receptors become the parameters of the servomechanism and are directly (via the thalamus) and indirectly (via the basal ganglia and cerebellum) relayed to the motor cortex, where they are correlated with a fast-time cerebellar computation to predict the outcomes of the next steps of the action. When the course of action becomes reasonably predictable from the trends of prior successful predictions, a terminal Image-of-Achievement can be constituted to serve as a guide for the final phases of the activity.

The model that emerges from these researches differs considerably from the conception of the motor cortex as a keyboard upon which the activities of the rest of the brain (and/or mind) converge to play a melody of movement. Rather, patterns of know-*how* here become encoded and make possible effective Acts, the external representations of brain processes.

The next chapters discuss the manner in which these external representations become modified over successions of Acts. And the final part of this book also looks to action by examining Acts serving the communicative process.

synopsis

Of several brain processes that organize behavior, one holds special interest. This process involves the junctional mechanism of cerebral motor and cerebellar corteces and constructs an Image-of-Achievement by means of a fast-time calculation which extrapolates a projection from the immediately preceding changes in force exerted on muscle receptors. This Image-of-Achievement, therefore, encodes environmental contingencies (e.g., forces), not patterns of muscle contraction. The Image-of-Achievement regulates behavior much as do the settings on a thermostat: the pattern of the turning on and off of the furnace is not encoded on the dial, only the set-points to be achieved are. Simplicity in design and economy of storage result.

competence

behaviorism, stimulus, response, and reinforcement

In the previous chapters we distinguished between movement and action. Movements, i.e., patterned muscular contractions, provide the postural set, context, or matrix within which behavioral Acts are formed. The neural mechanism controlling action is composed of information derived from environmental contingencies such as fields of forces, not by the specifics of the length of this or that muscle or the position of joints. A fairly large variety of potential movements can thus carry out any specific action. To paraphrase Granit's statement concerning reflexes (quoted in Chapter 12): the essential problems therefore no longer center around movements per se, though movements are still the helpful tools they have always been. The essential problems concern the biasing or setting of the various servomechanisms by the aid of which motoneurons are made to operate. And these biases are set in large part by the environmental forces operating in the behavioral situation.

Suddenly the question posed by the neurophysiologist has a familiar ring to the psychologist. The specification of the environmental contingencies that determine action is what the behaviorist has been studying; he has attempted to forge his views from an analysis of the *environmental arrangements that come to acquire meaningful relationships through the offices of organisms.* He has rightly seen that *stimuli, responses, and reinforcers can all be defined as environmental and not organismic*—though they demand a behaving organism to define them. Why then, shouldn't psychology become reduced to "the study of behavior"?

There is more to the relationship between stimulus, response, and reinforcement than meets the behavioristic eye. Though the focus of interest varies, the behaviorist has, with few exceptions, formulated the relationship as a chainlike sequence. Stimulus → Response → Reinforcement, is, to be sure, the order which an observer sees occurring. As soon as it is realized, however, that the brain of the organism *makes* this order occur, the apparent chaining is seen to be the result of a considerably more complex interaction.

Take, for instance, the fact that reflex organization is not an S–R arc, but a servosystem. This fact has an important consequence on the definitions of stimulus and response. The usual Newtonian and Sherringtonian chaining of agent and reaction becomes complicated by the introduction of feedback and feedforward operations. Two courses are open: to ignore the internal complexities of the system, or to account for them and deal effectively with the necessary alterations. For the most part, behaviorists have ignored the new complexity. But they can't avoid the problem that stimulus can be defined only by the response elicited, and, conversely, that response can be defined fully only by the conditions that provoke it. In other words, the behaviorist's stimulus and response mutually imply each other. This dilemma can be resolved only when the reciprocity between S and R is recognized. S ⇌ R is not just so neurologically but logically as well. A mathematical set and its partitions provides a sophisticated statement of this reciprocity (Estes, 1959). The elements of the set are conceived to be stimuli; the partitions on these elements correspond to responses (Fig. 14-1). Or in more familiar terms, the objects classified are stimuli; the process of classifying constitutes response. This resolution of the S–R dilemma demands, however, the exercise of strict discipline in how one talks about one's data. Much of the confusion of tongues in current psychology comes from the failure to fully recognize this reciprocal relationship between stimulus and response—in physiological psychology, especially, major controversies rage between those who

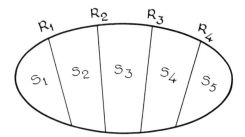

Fig. 14-1. A set is partitioned by responses (R_r) into stimuli (S_s).

describe their data in stimulus language and those more comfortable with the response mode. And, of course, confusion is frequently perpetrated by mixing languages.

According to this logically and neurologically derived view of the S–R relationship, descriptions should be anchored either in stimulus language or in response language, but not both. Confusion is compounded because the words used in each language are the same, though their meanings are differently derived. Most of the subdisciplines of psychology have avoided the confusion by locking into one or another analytic mode. Thus perceptual psychologists and psychophysicists use the stimulus mode of expression: response mechanisms are defined by their stimulus organizing properties. By contrast, operant conditioners and cognitive psychologists use response language: stimuli are defined by their response-eliciting characteristics. Two complementary frames of reference are thus created and physiological data are sometimes referred to one, sometimes to the other frame (Fig. 14-2). A muddle results when the frame of reference is not clearly identified. In accordance with these precepts, Part II, which deals with subjective experience, was framed in the stimulus language of sensory psychophysics and perceptual psychology. For Part III the response language of operant conditioning and cognitive psychology is more appropriate, since it more directly addresses behavior.

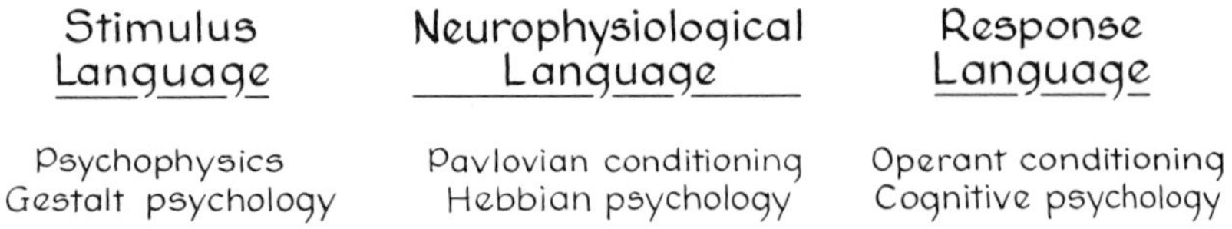

Stimulus Language	Neurophysiological Language	Response Language
Psychophysics	Pavlovian conditioning	Operant conditioning
Gestalt psychology	Hebbian psychology	Cognitive psychology

Fig. 14-2. Examples of stimulus, response, and physiological "languages" used in psychology.

Perhaps most interesting to analyses performed in behavioral terms is the objectivity attained in the definition of reinforcement when the S → R or reflex arc concept is replaced by servotheory. The agent in the servomechanism is the test—a match or mismatch between spatial representations, the ongoing "state" of the servo and the energy configurations impinging on that state. Thus what psychophysicists have called the "proximal" stimulus is dependent on the states of the system exposed to the input: the cognitive psychologist's "sets" and "expectancies." Parallel considerations make the reinforcing properties of events depend critically on a match between the state which produces the behavior and that which is produced by it. This chapter and Chapters 15 and 16 examine, therefore, various neurophysiological and neurobehavioral contributions to the study of the reinforcement process, the mechanisms by which modification of behavior takes place. For we must now really come to grips with the temporal organization of behavior.

contiguity and context

Aside from its very basic contribution to investigative technique, the behavioristic approach has so far made its greatest additions to knowledge in the analysis of behavior modification. But even here the focus has been restricted. Only those changes that are directly produced by manipulations of the guides and goads, the cues and incentives to action, have been studied. Learning produced through challenge of the emotional process involved in self control has hardly been recognized by experimentalists. And configural and transformational types of learning have not received adequate attention from behaviorists (Pribram, 1970). Nonetheless, from a body of experiments, mostly performed on animals, has come a limited behavior theory that needs now to be grounded in brain facts. This is the restricted goal before us.

The behaviorists' dictum is that behavior modification takes place by virtue of reinforcement. What, then, is reinforcement? The purists among behaviorists state that the question does not concern them: they are interested only in describing the environmental contingencies that produce reinforcement (Skinner, 1969). Note, however, that even by this dessicated definition, reinforcement must be some sort of *process*. This process must be taking place within the organism and is thus accessible to physiological inquiry.

Behaviorists concerned with the nature of the learning *process* have produced a long history of often tortuous reasoning and experimentation and have come up with two major viewpoints. One viewpoint, generally known as the contiguity position, suggests that learning results whenever coincidence is established by the repetition of occurrences. The other view, held by drive and expectancy theorists, maintains that some state change within the organism must take place for learning to be achieved. As we shall see, the simple "contiguity-only" viewpoint becomes untenable when one considers what is taking place in the brain.

Contiguity theorists split into two categories: those who speak stimulus language and those who are response oriented. Both believe that behavior is guided simply by sets of stimuli sampled probabilistically, weights being assigned the probabilities (Estes, 1959). Stimulus theorists assign weights from experimental data, i.e., essentially from computed correlations among stimuli; response theorists emphasize that the weights accrue by virtue of the very occurrence of the behavior which therefore becomes "its own chief guide" (Guthrie, 1942).

The fundamental questions posed by these approaches to behavior modification through simple contiguity are: (1) can learning take place at all in the absence of action (an environmental outcome reinforcing behavior), and, if it can, (2) what is contributed to learning when action takes place?

We already know that learning can take place in the absence of action. When experimentally controlled signals are repetitiously presented to an organism in a situation that remains constant, the organism habituates.

During the 1960s habituation has received significant attention from neurophysiologists and psychophysiologists, and as a result, our conception of the process has altered radically. Let us briefly review once again the critical experiment performed in Moscow by Eugene Sokolov (1963). A tone beep of specified intensity and duration was presented at irregular intervals to a subject whose electroencephalogram, galvanic skin response, and plethysmographic record were recorded (recall Fig. 3-1). At the onset of such an experiment characteristic changes in these traces appear. These changes, known as the orienting reaction, accompany behavioral alerting. As the experiment proceeds, these indices of orienting become progressively more attenuated until the beep of the tone no longer seems to have any effect. The subject has habituated. Then Sokolov reduced the intensity of the tone without changing any of its other characteristics. Immediately the electrical traces from the subject signalled another orienting reaction. Sokolov reasoned, therefore, that habituation could not be simply some type of fatiguing of sensory and neural elements. Rather, the central nervous system must set up a process against which it matches incoming sensory signals. Any *change* in signal results in the orienting reaction. Sokolov tested this idea by habituating his subjects anew and then shortened the tone beep. The orienting reaction occurred at the moment the shortened beep ended. The electrical traces showed alerting to the unexpected *silence.*

Ample evidence has verified the occurrence of the self-adapting mechanism we have come to know in this book as a filter or screen through which and against which incoming signals are matched. The screen may be thought of as a coded representation of prior signals generated by organism-environment interaction; it is gradually built up; it is subject to alteration by signals of mismatch (i.e., a partial match); it leads to "expectancies" of environmental occurrences by the organism (see Fig. 14-3). The neural composition of this self-adapting mechanism has already been detailed, and Bruner (1957) has spelled out the conceptual issues for psychology of this experimental validation of an expectancy process in a paper on "perceptual readiness." Here I will pursue the meaning of the results in terms of "tissue readiness" or "competences" in the brain of the organism, using the term much as the embryologist does when he describes the developing organism.

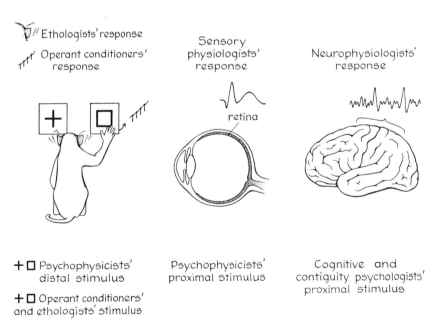

Fig. 14-3. Some meanings of "stimulus" and "response" in various languages.

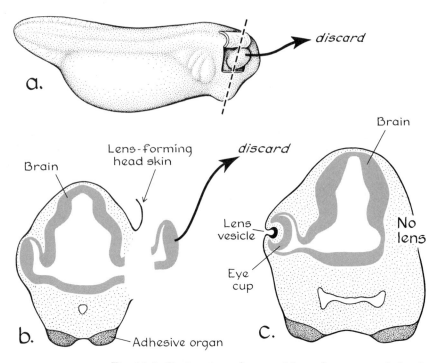

Fig. 14-4. Extirpation of eye vesicle to demonstrate induction of lens by the eye: B is a section through A in Plane X-Y; C, same as B, several days later. Redrawn from Hamburger, 1961.

The biological concept that tissue must be competent in order to differentiate comes from a series of studies that attempt to delineate how differentiation is initiated and controlled, i.e., how tissue development is induced. In essence, induction is a chemical conversation between a competent tissue and extrinsic organizing properties which guide its flowering. An early experiment, the classic example, is that of the determination of the lens by the eye vesicle. Contact between this vesicle with the overlying epidermis stimulates the latter to form a lens in the region of contact. If the eye vesicle is removed, the epidermis fails to differentiate a lens (Fig. 14-4).

This experiment raised a whole set of problems which generated a direction of research in experimental embryology bearing a striking resemblance to current explorations in experimental psychology and ethology. The first and logical assumption was that the inductor acted merely as a trigger; that, in the classical example, the head skin is already "predisposed" to form a lens and that it requires only a signal to start. Two lines of evidence disproved this concept of

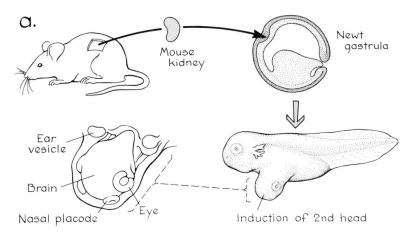

a.

Newt gastrula

Mouse kidney

Ear vesicle

Brain

Nasal placode   Eye

Induction of 2nd head

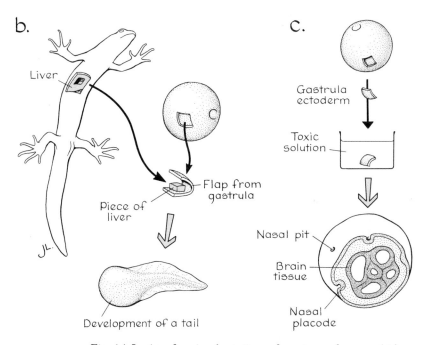

b.

Liver

Flap from gastrula

Piece of liver

Development of a tail

c.

Gastrula ectoderm

Toxic solution

Nasal pit

Brain tissue

Nasal placode

Fig. 14-5. A: after implantation of a piece of mouse kidney into a newt gastrula a brain flanked by nasal placodes, eyes and ear vesicles is induced; B: a piece of newt liver implanted into a jacket of gastrula ectoderm exposed to a toxic solution differentiates into a brain vesicle and several nasal placodes. Redrawn from Holtfreter and Chuang in Young, 1957.

induction. First, the optic vesicle was shown by transplantation to induce a lens in skin other than head skin—for example, flank skin. Second, the area of head skin which normally forms a lens was shown by other transplantation experiments to be *polypotential* and therefore definitely not "pre-determined" for lens formation *only*. If the region of the head epidermis which normally forms the lens is combined with an ear inductor, for example, it will respond with ear formation; if combined with a nose inductor, it will form a nose (see also Fig. 14-5).

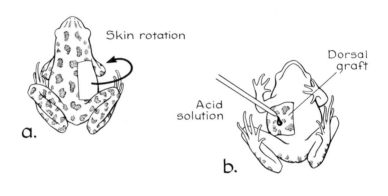

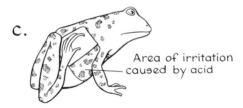

Fig. 14-6. The effects of rotating patches of frog larval skin. Such grafts develop their innate pigment patterns after metamorphosis, as shown in the dorsal and ventral views of adult animals. Following the rotation, the interrupted nerve fibers in the dorsal roots of the spinal nerves regenerate into ventral skin, and vice versa. When the skin grafts are stimulated, behavioral responses are dorsoventrally reversed. That is, the central competence engaged by the inducing sensory axons entering the grafts is appropriate to the local skin area rather than to the general topography of the body surface and the central nervous system topology which represents it. Redrawn after Sperry, in Edds, 1967.

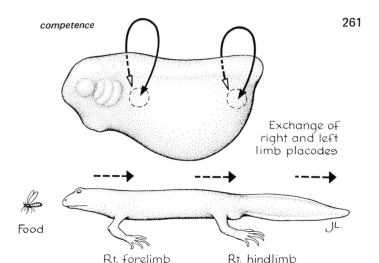

Exchange of
right and left
limb placodes

Food

Rt. forelimb   Rt. hindlimb

Fig. 14-7. The complementary motor experiment to the one shown in Fig. 14-6. The limb transplants behave (e.g. during swimming) as if they were in their original location. If the right limbs are transplanted to the left, they still behave as right limbs despite the new innervation. The resulting behavior can be maladaptive as shown here where the animal is forced to swim away from food rather than toward it. Again the central competence induced is specified by the peripheral tissue. These results are difficult to account for in terms of ordinary neural connectivity. My explanation (Pribram, 1961, 1965) is that spatio-temporal patterns of nerve impulses become the codes that identify the peripheral tissue. Such spatio-temporal patterns become decoded centrally in the developing nervous system regardless of the pathways by which they are transmitted. The patterns are specific to the peripheral structure because each peripheral innervation is characterized by a specified fiber size spectrum which determines speed of nerve impulse conduction (Quilliam, 1956; Thomas, 1956). Modified from Weiss, 1950, and Hamburger, 1961.

To these facts must be added those which show that the reacting tissue must be "ready" or "competent," i.e., in the proper state of responsiveness, to allow induction to become effective. For example, tissue which is already "launched" toward a different destination, will fail entirely to respond. Further, inductors were found to be insensitive to species differences. An inductor can be effective on tissues which belong to a different species, genus, or even order. The suggestion is, therefore, that inductors are made up of chemicals common to many organisms (more of this in a moment). These chemicals apparently determine the overall character of the induced structure while the hereditary equipment of the cells of this structure determines its detailed form. For example, when the flank skin of a frog embryo was induced to form head structures by salamander tissue into which it was transplanted, the embryo had a salamander head with the horny jaws and other features of the frog (see also Figs. 14-6, 14-7).

A long series of chemical experiments has currently culminated in the view that the ribonucleic acids (RNA) are most likely, and perhaps uniquely responsible for the inductive effect (see Niu, 1959), though ribonucleoproteins and steroids have not been entirely ruled out. For the most part ribonuclease (RNAse) destroys the inductive effect, although the problem remains that RNAse has other effects on the induced tissue which may disrupt its differentiation. More direct evidence, however, comes from demonstrations of the inductive effect of RNA extracted from different organs. Not only has this been accomplished, but RNA isolated from different sources was shown to be capable of inducing the recipient tissue to differentiate into different specific structures. These experiments suggest that there are many species of RNA in an organism and each has a specific function.

To sum up, contiguity theorists assume that behavior modification results whenever stimulus events occur simultaneously or when such simultaneously occurring stimulus events are generated by responses. The facts of habituation show that the contiguity theorist's "stimulus" must be conceived as a "proximal" stimulus; a stimulus event arises from a partial match between input and a central state which, in turn, has formed by the prior occurrence of partial matches between central states and input from environmental events. Thus, at any moment in time, the central state must be competent, ready to provide the context in which stimuli arise. Contiguity of stimuli is therefore to be seen not as some vague, haphazard, and probabilistic "association," but as a biologically determined process that organizes a context-content relationship. If this is so, stimulus contiguity theory and expectancy theory become "brothers under the skin"—in the central nervous system. Thus, simple, haphazard contiguity per se as the agent in learning does not exist and must be replaced by a biological concept based on competences: sets of occurrences (basically innate, though they become modified by experience) are encoded as central states which become competent to process subsequent occurrences as stimuli.

This process of behavior modification resembles embryogenesis which is dependent on the inherited and inherent properties of the genetic constitution of the organism that are evoked by the inductive capacity of the milieu in which the cells grow. The inductive capacity is itself specific, but in a somewhat different sense than is the genetic potential. The genetic competence is individual-, species- (and genus- and order-) specific. Hereditary factors proscribe commonalities with the past and future while assuring variation within any single generation. Inductors, on the other hand, are nonspecific with respect to individuals, species, and so forth. They are relatively simple chemicals—RNA—common to all living organisms. Inductors thus provide the existential commonality which allows the possibility of modification of the competences of a single generation according to the exigencies of the moment.

contiguity and consequence

The second question raised by the contiguity approach was: what, if anything, is contributed to learning when action takes place? This question can now be reformulated by asking whether the habituation paradigm applies not only to stimulus repetition but more generally to manifestations of overt behavior. Although no definitive answer can be given—and work is badly needed in this area—the suspicion has been voiced that habituation and behavioral extinction have factors in common. For instance, David Premack (Premack and Collier, 1962), in an analysis of the nonreinforcement variables affecting response probability, finds it necessary to state that:

> There are at least several reports of unconditioned responses failing to show complete recovery following repeated elicitation. Although the topic has been little investigated, in one of the few pertinent studies, Dodge (1927) reported a partial but apparently irreversible decrement in both latency and magnitude of no less than the unconditioned patellar reflex. Further, the biological literature on habituation contains several cases in which presumably unconditioned responses, having undergone decrement with repeated elicitation, failed to return to initial latency .... The question is ... whether some degree of irreversible decrement is not more widely characteristic of behavior than is customarily assumed. [p. 15]

That behavior is regulated by a process similar to that which controls sensory processes, makes these observations likely to be correct and readily understandable. The really puzzling problem is why behavior does not always decrement. A tentative and superficial answer is that, in the normal course of events, an "override" on habituation and extinction must take place and that one of the functions of reinforcement is to produce this override. An experiment by Stephen Glickman and Samuel Feldman (1961) illustrates that in fact such an override occurs. These investigators were interested in finding out whether the activation of the EEG which results from stimulations of core brain structures would habituate as does orienting (or arousal) when external stimulation becomes repetitive. They found that EEG activation produced by core brain stimulation does habituate unless the electrode happens to be in the areas from which the self-stimulation effect is obtained (recall Fig. 9-8). Repetitive excitation of these loci, perhaps by continuously setting and resetting bias as suggested in Chapter 10, acts as an override on the habituation process.

To summarize the problems posed by contiguity theorists: Neither "stimulus sampling" nor "behavior as its own guide" in and of itself provide adequate answers to the problem of behavior modification, probably because these theories have failed to note the importance of the temporal organization of the learning process. Organisms do not respond to just *any* occurrences that happen simultaneously, contiguously. Their behavior is guided by the *previously established competence of the brain to organize stimuli,* including those consequent to behavior. Stimuli are thus neurally determined events, "sampled" on the basis of a central competence (a neural "set") which in turn is determined by *prior* experience and by other central events. An organism's behavior is not only stimulus produced, but, by virtue of the self-adapting properties of the screening process, on occasion also stimulus inducing (i.e., productive of orienting). This happens whenever the outcome of behavior partially matches the central competence that inititated the behavior. In such circumstances, reinforcement takes place and behavior becomes its own guide.

An interesting experiment performed by E. Roy John (John and Morgades, 1969) illustrates the point that organisms do not respond appropriately just because occurrences happen simultaneously. Three cats were trained to press one lever when a light flickered at two cycles per second, and another lever when the flicker rate was eight cycles per second. The electrical activity evoked in the lateral geniculate body of the visual system was recorded. The waveshapes of the elicited electrical responses clearly differed for each stimulus condition once the animal was performing the discrimination satisfactorily. In a fourth untrained control animal these differences did not appear. When a cat made an error, when it failed to respond correctly on any trial, *the differences in the electrical record also disappeared* for that trial. Note also that John concluded that some sort of dynamic (in the conceptual framework of this book, perhaps a neural holographic) process must therefore be responsible for the differences observed to correlate with the correct response:

> In differentially trained animals the waveshapes elicited at any electrode position by the two differentiated stimuli were clearly different. These differences were observed from responsive ensembles anywhere within the mapped regions. Thus, neural ensembles which reported the presence of the discriminated signals were broadly distributed throughout extensive regions and consistently displayed two different patterns of response to the two different stimuli. Analysis showed that the information contained in the averaged response pattern of any of these local ensembles was sufficient to discriminate between the two peripheral signals. Multiple unit ensemble responses displayed impressive stability suggesting an invariant mode of discharge to a particular stimulus. In contrast, single unit activity was extremely variable with many different response patterns displayed to the same stimuli. These findings suggested that the firing pattern of extensive neural ensembles constituted a far more reliable source of information on which to base differential response than did the firing patterns of single cells.
> Striking similarity in the waveshape of electrical responses was observed between different brain structures in a trained animal. Gradient analysis revealed these similar responses to be extensively distributed with no evidence for volume conduction. The dynamic nature of this phenomenon was illustrated by the collapse of similarity in trials resulting in behavioral error or on presentation of novel stimuli. These findings suggest that similarity of electrical activity in different brain regions reflects the operation of an endogenous process established during learning and is not passively produced by the action of the physical stimulus itself. [John and Morgades, 1969, pp. 205–6]

This view of the reinforcement process is beginning to be recognized even by behaviorists. Thus a recent review (Perkins, 1968) holds that the concept of "attractiveness" brings together a number of otherwise disparate findings. For instance, "all classical conditioned responses may be described as preparatory responses by which it is implied that these responses increase the characteristic attractiveness of the stimulus situation at the time of unconditioned stimulus presentation." Others have used the words "desirableness," "incentive value," or "impellance," and I have here used the term "interest" as the subjective counterpart of "attractiveness," but the conception common to all of these formulations is that the reinforcing process does its work by appealing to, and in turn inducing changes in, some prior state, some competence within the organism.

the competent brain

What then are these competences that guide behavior? They are hierarchically organized mechanisms (logic modules) of servoprocesses, programs, or Plans set to achieve an environmental effect, an Act. Chapters 12 and 13 detailed the neurological organization of competences involved in actions such as hammering a nail; an anatomical substrate of point-to-point correspondences between muscles and brain cortex becomes organized into a representation that controls whatever movements are demanded by the environmental "terrain" or "field of forces" so as to achieve an effect. The achievement has become encoded in the representation, a state, the junctional slow potential microstructure, by computing a fast-time extrapolation of modulations of recurrent regularities that appear in the series of such field forces encountered to date.

A somewhat simpler but similar mechanism can be delineated for other more apparently "innate" competences. When, in animals, very discrete stimulations are performed in the core-brain (e.g., hypothalamus) part-movements related to feeding, drinking, etc., are obtained. Such part-movement loci appear to be relatively randomly distributed over a fairly large area. Lip smacking, for instance, may be produced from a point near another that produces arching of the back (Robinson, 1964). Even the genetic memory serving instinct appears to be distributed. When stronger stimulation or larger areas are excited, however, these part-movements become integrated into behavior patterns which serve one or another appetite or affect. Thus putting things into the mouth, chewing, and ingestion form the feeding pattern; crouching and turning away indicate incipient flight; the baring of claws and teeth, the arching of the back, and dilation of the pupils mark the agonistic pattern. The assumption is that this grosser electrical stimulation simulates what occurs ordinarily when appetitive and affective states are induced in these structures.

This assumption is borne out by a series of ingenious experiments performed by Elliot Valenstein which, however, raise additional problems. In these experiments with rats electrodes are implanted into the hypothalamic area from which eating, drinking, or gnawing can be elicited by electrical stimulation. When one of these behaviors was clearly observed to be stable, the environmental terrain was altered so that the initial achievement was no longer possible. A substitute terrain was made available for a whole night during which the electrical stimulation recurred at irregular intervals. The following morning identical stimulation (of the point originally excited) produced either the initial or an alternate behavior, depending on the terrain and when all possible alternatives were available, the newly trained achievement was often dominant. Valenstein reports:

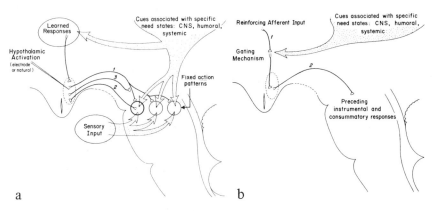

a   b

Fig. 14-8. (A) Reinforcement of motor patterns. Schema illustrates the relationships between the "reinforcing brain system" and the response system, as suggested by experimental results. (B) Role of sensory input. Schema illustrates the relationship between specific need states and the "immediate reinforcement" produced by sensory input. From Valenstein, 1970.

Following the standard tests confirming the presence of stimulus-bound behavior, the goal object to which the rat oriented was removed, and the animal was placed on a night schedule with the other two goal objects present. If, for example, the rat exhibited drinking during stimulation in the first series of tests, the water bottle was removed during the night, and only the food pellets and wood were left in the cage. The *stimulus parameters remained unchanged*. If the animal did not exhibit a new elicited behavior, it was placed a second, third, or even more times on the night schedule. In most cases, however, one night was sufficient time for a new behavior to emerge. After a new behavior emerged, the animals were given two standard tests with the initial goal object absent and a third standard test (*competition test*) with all three goal objects present. When the animal was not being stimulated, the three goal objects were always available; therefore, the animals had an opportunity to become satiated on food, water, and wood prior to testing. Eleven animals completed this sequence of testing, and these results constitute the first experiment . . . .

A second series of tests was administered after a variable amount of experience receiving stimulation in the absence of the goal object to which the animal first oriented . . . in most cases the second elicited behavior was exhibited as consistently as the first . . . . During the competition test, when all three goal objects were present, approximately equal amounts of the two elicited behaviors were displayed in most instances. Generally, one of the behaviors was elicited for three or four consecutive stimulus presentations and then the other behavior for an approximately equally long series. In most competition tests, the animals displayed more than one elicited behavior during several of the 20 stimulus presentations.

We were interested in determining whether the first behavior would reestablish its dominance if we gave a series of competition tests. Although a variety of patterns have emerged from this testing, we feel secure in concluding that once a second stimulus-bound behavior has been established, the initial behavior that was elicited by the stimulation is no longer the dominant response. In fact, several animals displayed a clear predominance of the second behavior during a series of competition tests. [Valenstein, Cox, and Kakolewski, 1969, pp. 247–49]

Valenstein has interpreted these results to mean that hypothalamic stimulation does not elicit any specific hunger, thirst, or other motivational state. On the basis of the interaction between the effects of the Olds type of self-stimulation and those stimulations which produce stimulus-bound behaviors such as eating, drinking, and gnawing, he comes to a conclusion similar to the one detailed in Chapter 10—that electrical excitation tunes the homeostatic mechanism, creates a bias which alters the response elicited:

An example may be helpful. Mendelson (1967) studied the behavior of animals displaying both self-stimulation and drinking in response to lateral hypothalamic stimulation. Mogenson and Stevenson (1967) have reported similar studies. Mendelson selected animals that would display stimulus-bound drinking at current levels below those which would support self-stimulation. At these low intensities the animals would not press the lever if water were not available, and when satiated they would not press the lever to receive water without hypothalamic stimulation. Mendelson concluded: "Thus if the rat is given the thirst it will press for water; if given the water it will press for the thirst." These results may be most important, but with respect to interpretation, the implication that the stimulation induced thirst does not seem justified. We would have to predict that these animals could be switched to displaying stimulus-bound eating, and the same phenomenon could then be demonstrated with food. It is now known from the recent work of Coons and Cruce (1968) that animals displaying stimulus-bound eating will self-stimulate at below "reward thresholds" if food is available.

Rather than evoking hunger and thirst, it would be much more parsimonious to postulate that the reinforcement produced by the execution of an elicited behavior summates with the reinforcement produced directly by that stimulation. It would follow that the summation of the reinforcement from executing the behavior and the subthreshold reinforcement from the brain stimulation may be sufficient to maintain the instrumental behavior. Indeed, Mendelson (1966) had demonstrated earlier that satiated animals which display stimulus-bound eating prefer the combination of food and brain stimulation to brain stimulation alone. [Valenstein, Cox, and Kakolewski, 1969, pp. 276–77]

But in his interpretation that the brain stimulation does not induce thirst, Valenstein may be throwing out the baby with the bath water. Warren Roberts (1969) points out that gross electrical stimulation does a disservice to the fine detail of the competent organization, the distributed loci of hypothalamic points from which part-movements can be reliably and invariably obtained. Roberts accuses Valenstein of taking a Lashleyan position on neural specificity which he argues is to be deplored because, as Peter Milner has pointed out (Roberts, 1969, pp. 17–19), it "discouraged many researchers from investigating functional specificity and localization for several decades." By contrast, Roberts suggests that the competent tissue consists of "overlapping but specific mechanisms."

The argument sounds familiar though the scene has changed. For almost a century the protagonists of localization vied with the protagonists of plasticity on the battlefields of the visual and the motor cortex. Now it is the hypothalamus.

The resolution of the conflict here lies, just as it did with perception and action, in the "third world," the junctional slow potential microstructure of the brain. Roberts recognizes the problem but can provide no neurological solution.

The high frequency of incomplete patterns gives . . . support to the conclusion that [localized] stimulation in the hypothalamus usually excites only a small fraction of the neurons in a given mechanism. It also indicates that there are relatively few if any [permanent] interconnections between the neurons controlling the different elements of these responses within the hypothalamus or in its efferent pathways. Thus, the tendency of these elements to occur together in normal behavior must result from some other mode of integration, such as a common humoral input, as may be the case with the thermoregulatory behaviors (Roberts, et al., 1969) or a common neuronal input from other central structures or peripheral receptors. [Roberts, 1969]

The common input, the integration, is, of course, furnished in
Valenstein's experiments by the combination of electrical brain
stimulation and reinforcement from the environmental terrain which,
according to the interpretation pursued in this book, make up arrival
patterns which compose a design of junctional slow potentials. This
slow potential microstructure, this momentary monitor state, now
guides behavior. These microstructures need not, of course, be
localized within the core brain tissue. The far-lateral hypothalamic
"go" mechanism is essentially a crossroad of fiber tracts carrying
signals that converge from many parts of the brain, including the
cerebral cortex.

Valenstein's results as well as the everyday experience that skills
are lasting once learned, demand, however, some more permanent
residue of experience than the momentary state of the junctional
microstructure. The substrate giving rise to terminal Images-of-
Achievement cannot be purely electrical. Some sort of enduring
modification, chemical or neuronal, must occur. We have returned to
the issues of Chapter 2. The next chapter reviews these issues and
pursues the modification of behavior in terms of the motivational
aspects of the memory process, the problem of reinforcement.

synopsis

The brain's motor mechanisms encode the environmental
contingencies that organize behavior. Thus the work of neurophysiologists and the efforts of behaviorists interested in behavior
modification (learning), in the process whereby environmental
contingencies guide behavior change, become mutually relevant. The
neural logic that controls behavior, just as the logic that constructs
percepts and feelings, is distributed in systems related to a broad
class of functions. This distributed logic forms a competent tissue
whose expressed function depends on the experience of the organism
with particular environmental contingencies. Expression depends on
a junctional mechanism akin to that which produces Images-of-
Achievements. Mere contiguity of contingencies does not modify
behavior; the contingencies must address the innate competences of
the organism or their modifications by prior experience (the
organism's expectancies).

reinforcement
and
commitment

reinforcement as induction

The claim made in Chapter 14 that the process of reinforcement induces changes in the competences of the brain needs closer scrutiny. Are there any similarities between the process of induction studied by embryologists and the process of reinforcement studied by behaviorists? Chapter 2 proposed induction as a model for memory storage. What neural mechanisms might be initiated during the reinforcing process that would allow induction to become operative in adult brain tissue?

The most controversial conception of reinforcement among behaviorists and psychoanalytically oriented psychotherapists is the drive reduction hypothesis. This conception is based on a two-factor theory of drive: physiological needs set up tension states in the organism which are manifested in increased general activity or neural activation; behavior which reduces such tensions is reinforcing. Some have argued (e.g., Sheffield, et al., 1955) that organisms seek tension increase—that behavior modification accompanies tension increase.

This argument eliminates the need for the second factor. Drive and reinforcement, however, are still considered covariant. Meanwhile, Estes (1959) has made a convincing case for a drive-stimulus rather than a drive-tension theory of drive, but his formulation leaves unanswered the question as to just what drive stimuli guide behavior. The answer resembles that given in the previous chapter: what constitutes a "stimulus" is not as simple as it seems. A drive stimulus, just as a sensory stimulus, results from the operation of a biased servomechanism, a homeostat. Homeostats are outfitted with receptors sensitive to excitation from the World-Within. Specialized areas sensitive to temperature, osmotic equilibrium, estrogen, glucose, and partial pressure of carbon dioxide are located around the midline ventricular system; these areas are connected to mechanisms which control the intake and output of the agent to which they are sensitive (Chaps. 9, 10).

In addition to these completely central mechanisms, other more peripheral sensitivities also play on the homeostatic process. The homeostat is often supplied with secondary mechanisms which aid in the more finely-calibered regulations of the agents in question. Stomach contractions in the hunger mechanism and mouth dryness in thirst are examples, as is the regulation of the circulation of blood in vessels of the finger tips to provide greater or lesser cooling. The blood-finger temperature differentially biases and is biased by the main hypothalamic thermostat.

Taking hunger as a model, we found that the core-brain homeostats with their central and peripheral sensitivities are constituted of two reciprocally active components. One component signals depletion and starts the regulatory process; the other component signals satiety and stops the process. We also saw that the "go" phase of the process is characterized by appetite and the "stop" phase generates affect. *Appetites and affects, feelings of interest, therefore turn out to be the motivational and emotional (as contrasted with perceptual) stimuli, the drives sought by the behaviorist.* In the language of this book appetites and affects are monitor Images, indicators of processes that track brain states and influence the temporal organization of behavior accordingly (Chap. 11).

How do the mechanisms that produce interest, appetite, and affect, modify behavior, reinforce the organism? By engaging the organism's memory mechanism. Chapter 2 proposed the hypothesis that enduring memory structures are "induced" in the brain much as tissue structures are induced during embryological development. The superficial similarity between induction as studied in embryological tissue and reinforcement as studied in conditioning situations is easily drawn: (a) Inductors evoke and organize the genetic potential of the organism. Reinforcers evoke and organize the behavioral capacities of organisms. (b) Inductors are relatively specific in the character they evoke but are generally nonspecific relative to individuals and tissue. Reinforcers are quite specific in the behaviors they condition but are generally nonspecific relative to individuals and tasks. (c) Inductors determine the broad outlines of the induced character; details are specified by the action of the substrate. Reinforcers determine the solution of the problem set; details of the behavioral repertoire used to achieve the solution are idiosyncratic to the organism. (d) Inductors do not just trigger development; they are more than just evanescent stimuli. Reinforcers do not just trigger behavior; they are a special class of stimuli. (e) Inductors must be in contact with their substrate in order to be effective. Contiguity is a demonstrated requirement for reinforcement to take place. (f) Mere contact, though necessary, is insufficient to produce an inductive effect; the induced tissue must be ready, must be competent to react. Mere contiguity, though necessary, is insufficient to produce reinforcement; shaping, deprivation, readiness, context, expectation, attention, hypothesis—these are only some of the terms used to describe the factors which comprise the competence of the organism without which reinforcement cannot become effective. (g) Induction usually proceeds by a two-way interaction— by way of a chemical conversation. Reinforcement is most effective in the operant situation where the consequences of the organism's own actions are immediately utilized as the guides to its subsequent behavior.

the neurochemistry of reinforcement

But when this much has been said, the question remains whether these descriptive similarities point to homologous mechanisms. My hypothesis states that they do. What evidence supports this? What neural processes become operative during induction?

What is required is an anatomical pathway that functions at multiple locations in the brain to release the reinforcing "inductor," the chemical that can induce the reciprocal tissue to differentiate. A provocative synthesis of recent neurochemical research has been suggested by Larry Stein (Figs. 15-1, 15-2):

All of the foregoing evidence is compatible with the idea that the reward mechanism contains a system of adrenergic synapses that are highly sensitive to pharmacological manipulation. Enhancement of noradrenergic trans-

a. Medial Forebrain Bundle
Reward

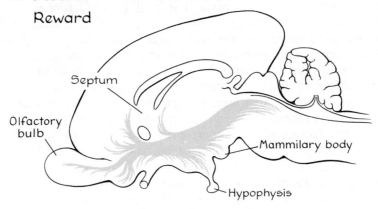

b. Periventricular System
Punishment

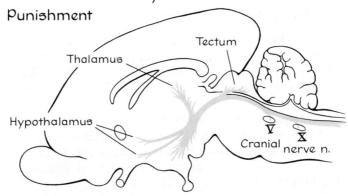

Fig. 15-1. Diagrams representing the medial forebrain bundle (upper figure—go system) and periventricular system of fibers (lower figure—stop system) in a generalized mammalian brain (sagittal plane). Redrawn after Stein, 1968, and Le Gros Clark, et al., 1938.

mission at these synapses facilitates behavior, and impairment of noradrenergic transmission suppresses behavior. In all probability, these synapses are the major site of action in the brain at which amphetamine and chlorpromazine exert their effects on goal-directed behavior . . . .

Where are these synapses located? If the medial forebrain bundle in fact constitutes the principal pathway of the reward system as suggested above, the adrenergic synapses in question evidently have already been described by a group at the Karolinska Institute (Fuxe, 1965; Hillarp, Fuxe, and Dahlstrom, 1966). Using a histochemical technique for visualizing cate-cholamines at the cellular level, these investigators report a system of norepinephrine-containing neurons whose cell bodies have their origin in [the mesencephalic core brain] and whose fibers ascend in the medial forebrain bundle and terminate in adrenergic synapses in the hypothalamus, limbic lobe, and neocortex . . . . Using a completely different technique, Heller, Seiden, and Moore (1966) independently confirmed the existence of this ascending fiber system. These workers lesioned the medial forebrain bundle on one side at the level of the lateral hypothalamus and then assayed different regions of the brain for changes in norepinephrine content. Because the axons in the medial forebrain bundle are largely uncrossed it was possible to compare norepinephrine levels on the lesioned and nonlesioned sides. Norepinephrine was extensively depleted by the lesion, but only in forebrain structures on the lesioned side; control lesions in the medial hypothalamus caused no important depletion of norepinephrine. These results confirm the presence of norepinephrine-containing fibers in the medial forebrain bundle; in addition, they validate the conclusion that these fibers comprise an ascending system, since decreases in norepinephrine levels occurred only in structures located above the lesion . . . . [Stein, 1968, p. 110]

Scheibel and Scheibel (1967; Figs. 15-3, 15-4) have also described this system of neurons which they suggest function as nonspecific afferents to the cerebral cortex. The axons of these cells are characteristically long and at their terminations produce climbing fibers which twine around the apical dendrites of pyramidal cells with a loose axodendritic coupling in contrast to the well defined synapses that characterize specific afferents. Taken together with the experiments by Fuxe, Hamburger, and Hokfelt (1968) noted by Stein, which show that the nonspecific couplings are largely aminergic (that the axons and the cells of origin contain norepine-phrene or noradrenaline) suggests that this system of neurons is responsible for instigating the induction process by stimulating the secretion of RNA and facilitating protein synthesis. The stimulating effect of noradrenaline on protein synthesis appears to be mediated by cyclic adenine monophosphate. [See *The Role of Cyclic AMP in the Nervous System,* Neurosciences Research Program Bulletin, July,

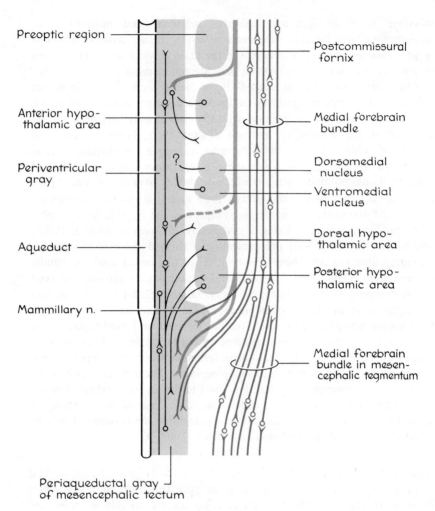

Preoptic region

Anterior hypo-
thalamic area

Periventricular
gray

Aqueduct

Mammillary n.

Postcommissural
fornix

Medial forebrain
bundle

Dorsomedial
nucleus

Ventromedial
nucleus

Dorsal hypo-
thalamic area

Posterior hypo-
thalamic area

Medial forebrain
bundle in mesen-
cephalic tegmentum

Periaqueductal gray
of mesencephalic tectum

Fig. 15-2. Diagrams of medial forebrain bundle (stippled) and periventricular system of fibers in horizontal plane. The scheme of organization shown here conceives of the hypothalamus as three longitudinally arranged columns—a periventricular stratum, a medial zone, and a lateral zone. Fiber bundles in the periventricular and lateral zones flank the medial zone which is devoid of major fiber bundles but does contain several prominent nuclei. Oblique lines denote the fornix system. AH: anterior hypothalamic area; DH: dorsal hypothalamic area; DM: dorsomedial nucleus; m: mammillary nuclei; PH: posterior hypothalamic area; PO: preoptic region; VM: ventromedial nucleus. Redrawn after Stein, 1968, and Sutin, 1966.

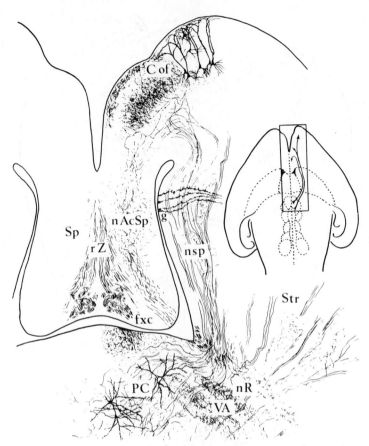

Fig. 15-3. Entire rostral projection of thalamic nonspecific system through inferior thalamic peduncle (part of medial forebrain bundle) upon cortex. Axons from anterior non-specific fields including paracentral (PC) and probably the medial portion of ventral anterior (VA) project rostrally via the inferior thalamic peduncle as the nonspecific projection (nsp), through the medial sector of the caudate division of corpus striatum (Str), to the base of orbitofrontal cortex (Cof). The axons branch widely in the subgriseal white matter and some continue into the nucleus accumbens septi (NAcSp). Other abbreviations include nucleus reticularis thalami (nR), columns of fornix (fxc), septum (Sp), and radiation of Zuckerkandl (rZ). Ependymal neuroglia (g) line the lateral ventricles. Modified rapid Golgi-stained section cut in horizon-tal oblique plane. 50-day-old partially demyelinated mouse. X 150; reduction in reproducing X 0.75. From Scheibel and Scheibel, 1967.

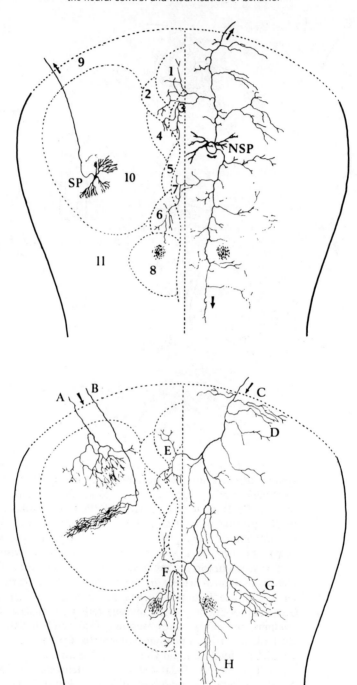

Fig. 15-4. Comparison between organization of axonal elements of the thalamic specific and nonspecific systems. Top: thalamofugal elements. A neuron of the ventrobasal complex (SP) projects a virtually uncollateralized axon (10), except for one small recurrent branch, toward cortex. A neuron of nonspecific system (NSP) generates an axon, which bifurcates into rostal and caudal running divisions, both of which are richly collateralized, ipsilaterally and contralaterally. Bottom: descending thalamopetal elements. A and B are axons from cortex to portions of the specific ventral nuclear complex. A is a characteristic tridimensional terminal pattern while B is a bidimensional discoid arbor. C is an axon descending from cortex to the nonspecific fields. The diffuse collateral system includes branches to area of nucleus reticularis and ventral anterior nucleus (D), contralateral nonspecific fields (E and F), the posterior nuclear complex (G), and meso-diencephalic junction (H). Other abbreviations include: 1, parataential; 2, anterior ventral; 3, interanteromedial; 4, anterior medial; 5, paracentral; 6, central lateral; 7, central medial; 8, centre median-parafascicular complex; and 9, n. reticularis. Drawing synthesized from a number of Golgi sections of rat and mouse. Scheibel and Scheibel, 1967.

1970, Vol. 8, #3.] Seymour Kety (personal communication) remarks that "it is interesting that the stimulation of protein kinase by cyclic adenine monophosphate can be markedly potentiated by magnesium or potassium ions and inhibited by calcium which suggests means whereby an effect of adrenergic stimulation could be differentially exerted on reasonably active and inactive synapses!"

I would add to this synthesis an emphasis on the neuronal matrix on which the aminergic reinforcing pathways exert their effect. This matrix, largely cholinergic, constitutes what Chapter 14 delineated as the competence of the brain's tissue. There is evidence (Fig. 15-5) that aminergic stimulation affects the cholinergic mechanism, at least in the "go" and "stop" mechanisms of the brain stem. Recall also that in Krech, Rosenzweig, and Bennett's experiments (Fig. 2-6) acetylcholine was shown involved in the effect of enriched environments on cortical growth. Could this more enduring cholinergic process be initiated by the aminergic reinforcement mechanism or does it function independently?

Glickman and Schiff (1967) solely on the basis of an extensive review of the results obtained in experiments exploring the effects of electrical brain stimulation on behavior provide a partial answer to this question. Their review emphasizes two types of innate response

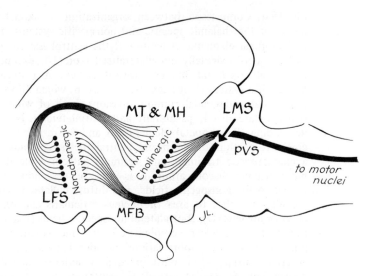

Fig. 15-5. Diagram representing hypothetical relationships between reward and punishment mechanisms inferred from chemical stimulation experiments of Margules and Stein (1967), Margules (in press), and Stein, et al. (1968). A rewarding stimulus releases (go) behavior from suppression (stop) by the periventricular system (PVS) in the following sequence of events: (1) Activation of medial forebrain bundle (MFB) by stimuli previously associated with reward (or the avoidance of punishment) causes release of norepinephrine into the amygdala and other forebrain suppressor areas (LFS). (2) Inhibitory action of norepinephrine suppresses activity of the LFS, thus reducing its cholinergically-mediated excitation of medial thalamus and hypothalamus (MT & MH). (3) Decreased cholinergic transmission at synapses in MT and MH lessens the activity in the periventricular system, thereby reducing its inhibitory influence on motor nuclei of the brain stem. Redrawn after Stein, 1968.

sequences, those involved in "approach" (go) and those in "withdrawal" (stop) from a stimulus object. They give the evidence for a relationship between electrical stimulation sites in the core brain stem that beget these types of behavior and the positive and negative rewarding effects of electrical self-stimulation (recall Figs. 5-1 and 5-2). They also sketch some possible mechanisms whereby cortical controls can regulate (inhibit and facilitate) the core-brain response mechanism. They fail, however, to come to grips with the problem of behavior *modification* by such cortical control. This inadequacy results from the fact that they had unavailable to them the data that indicate the distributed nature of the response mechanism (Chapter 14) and thus the necessity for a modifiable state with integrative properties. The delineation of a system of aminergic afferents originating in brain stem and reaching the apical dendrites of cortex now provides an anatomical base for such a modifiable integrating process.

The experimental evidence upon which the induction hypothesis is based comes necessarily almost exclusively from animal research. However, a recent survey of the locus of brain lesions in man that produce severe disorders in memory processes gave surprisingly confirmatory support for the existence of a mechanism such as the one outlined here. Localized lesions of cortex (including hippocampus) or of the basal ganglia failed to correlate with memory difficulties. When, however, core brain stem structures were involved the patients showed "an inability to form new memories, that is, antegrade amnesia (prolonged practice does not help)" despite the "preservation of an alert, attentive, wide awake state of mind" and "of normal capacity to think, solve problems, etc"; and where in the end stages of the disease intelligence test scores are "little if at all reduced from premorbid level despite gross memory defects." Anatomically "the nuclei that were devastated by the disease all lay in medial position, that is, within 2-3 mm. of the ependyma. In other words their position vis-a-vis the third ventricle [and aqueduct of Sylvius] appeared to be more important in determining their susceptibility than was any other attribute" (Adams, 1969, pp. 98–102).

Neurophysiologists have also contributed to the investigation of the mechanisms that allow induction to become operative in the human as well as the animal brain. A few years ago W. Grey Walter (Walter, et al., 1964; Walter, 1967) analyzed the slowly occurring changes in the brain's electrical activity in a variety of situations. He found a negative variation in electrical potential contingent on one stimulus alerting the organism to respond to a subsequent, expected stimulus. In my experience (Donchin, et al., 1971; Figs. 15-6, 15-7) such negative variations are induced by a variety of preparatory states of expectancy and the locus of occurrence of the potential change depends on the type of task in which the preparatory set is demanded: e.g., when a monkey or person waits without making an overt response, the CNV occurs maximally in the frontal cortex; when an anticipated motor response is demanded the negativity occurs first in the motor cortex and precedes the execution of the movement; when a continuing response such as a prolonged preparatory depression of a lever is necessary the negativity occurs maximally in the somatosensory cortex. When the expected second

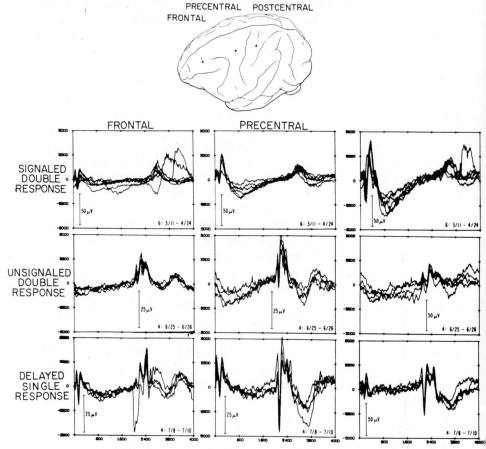

Fig. 15-6. Comparison of transcortical negative variation (TNV) at frontal, precentral, and postcentral recording sites in a rhesus monkey during various waiting tasks. In the signalled double response task, monkeys were required to press a lever within 400 msec. of the onset of a light stimulus, hold the lever down for two seconds, and release within 400 msec. of the onset of a tone. In the unsignalled task, monkeys were required to voluntarily initiate each trial by depressing the lever without a stimulus, holding for two seconds then releasing rapidly after tone onset. In the delay condition, the light and tone were presented, separated by a two second interval, but the monkey was required to withhold response until the tone came on. Each individual trace represents a computer average of 40-50 trials. Monkeys were reinforced with a small food pellet after each correct trial. Compare with Fig. 15-7. From Donchin, et al., 1971.

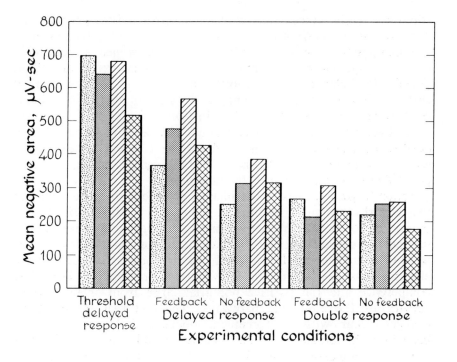

Electrode position

Frontal   Central
Motor   Posterior

Fig. 15-7. Comparison of CNV recorded at different scalp locations in humans in five experimental variations of a reaction time task. In all tasks, two visual stimuli separated by a 1.5 sec. interval were presented. Subjects were required to press a button with the dominant thumb after the second stimulus in conditions A-C. In conditions D and E subjects were required to press immediately after the onset of the first stimulus, hold the button down during the interstimulus interval, and release when the second stimulus appeared. Feedback consisted of a red or green light indicating correct or incorrect performance after each trial. Subjects were required to press within 350 msec. in tasks B-E. In this threshold condition, time to react was reduced so that subjects were making at least 25% errors. Negative area was calculated by integrating the sum of all negative points (relative to pretrial baseline) during a two-second epoch following the onset of the first stimulus. Electronegative brain waves were digitized, averaged, and integrated with a LINC-8 computer.

stimulus finally takes place a sharp positive deflection ends the negative variation. Another series of investigations has related these terminal positive electrical potentials to the occurrence of reinforcing events in operant conditioning situations (Clemente, et al., 1964; Grandstaff, 1969; Lindsley, 1969). Thus the CNV and its terminal sharp positivity signal expectancy and its fulfillment, the context-content process of stimulus determination discussed in Chapter 14.

A direct effect has also been produced by negative (cathodal) and positive (anodal) currents imposed on the cerebral cortex during learning (Stamm, 1961; Morrell, 1961). Negative currents impair, positive ones tend to enhance, learning rates.

Taken together, these experiments provide impressive evidence that electrical potential changes are induced in the brain prior to and during reinforcement. We know practically nothing, however, about the mechanisms that produce the electrical potential changes. Nor do we know much about the neurochemical processes induced by the electrical changes. Could the CNV reflect or mobilize cholinergic competence and the positive potentials arise from or give rise to activity of the aminergic pathways? The fact that the electrical changes occur with reinforcement opens a field of inquiry at behavioral, histological, and chemical levels which until a few years ago was completely closed. The conception of reinforcement as a process of induction provides a testable thesis for biological research into that enigma which has defied behaviorists for half a century.

registering reinforcement

Recall once more the habituation experiments (Chaps. 3, 11). By taking a set of physiological measures we can see that an organism is orienting to a novel stimulus. This reaction habituates when the stimulus is repeatedly presented. Recall also that after excision of the amygdala the physiological measures of orienting such as the galvanic skin response (GSR), heart rate, and respiratory changes no longer occur despite the fact that under other circumstances these physiological responses remain unaffected. Paradoxically, however, *behavioral* orienting not only remains intact but fails to habituate. I interpreted this to mean that amygdalecto-mized subjects do not register the effects of the orienting process in the way normal subjects do. In conditioning situations, also, these same indicators of registration fail to appear in the lesioned monkey (Bagshaw and Coppock, 1968; Fig. 15-8). Whereas in the normal animals there is a gradual incrementing of the number of phy-siological responses that occur at the time of stimulus presentation and a lengthening of the period during which anticipatory responses occur, in the operated subjects no such anticipatory—nor incrementation of—GSR is obtained. This result suggests that the amygdala is intimately involved in the temporal extension of a process set into operation in response to repetition of events—a process of serial registration of relevant events in memory. It is as if some sort of "internal rehearsal" were taking place in the normal organism, without which appropriate registration does not occur.

Behavioral evidence has supported the view that the amygdala allows experience to be registered appropriately (Douglas and Pribram, 1966). In simple discrimination tasks of a highly repetitive nature, this difficulty in registration is hardly perceptible. When, however, the reward contingency is shifted (Barrett, 1969) so that it

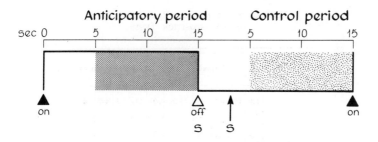

TRIALS	GRP	5-10 SEC ON	10-15 SEC ON	5-10 SEC OFF	10-15 SEC OFF
FIRST 40	NORM	3.7	7.0**	3.9	2.5
	AMX	3.2	3.3	3.9	2.0
SECOND 40	NORM	5.7**	8.8*	6.2	4.5
	AMX	2.7	4.8	3.5	4.3
All 80	NORM	9.3	14.5*	10.3	7.0
	AMX	5.8	8.2	7.3	6.3

* = p < .08
** = p < .05

Fig. 15-8. Mean number of GSR occurring in 10-sec period of light-on just preceding light offset (CS) in the first 40 and in the second 40 trials for each group. Note that the normal control monkeys learn to anticipate (rehearse) the offset of the stimulus and that amygdalectomized subjects fail to do this. From Bagshaw and Coppock, 1968.

reinforces the previously nonreinforced cue (discrimination reversal) or novelty is introduced, as in an experiment in which the monkeys must transpose what they have learned to another similar but not identical situation, amygdalectomy takes its toll (Schwartzbaum and Pribram, 1960; Fig. 15-9; Bagshaw and Pribram, 1965). In these tasks the monkeys who have suffered amygdalectomy appear to overreact to novelty (when compared to their controls) and this reaction continues long after normal subjects have become familiarized to the situation. The results, added to those obtained with psychophysiological measures, suggest that the amygdala ordinarily exerts control over the process of contrast enhancement, the neural mechanisms of lateral inhibition which takes place in the input channels (and whenever there are sheets of neuronal aggregates). The operation of the

NUMBER OF TRANSPOSED RESPONSES MADE
ON TRANSPOSITION TESTS

Day	Normals					Amygdalectomized				
	439	441	443	447	Mdn.	397	405	438	442	Mdn.
1	6	5	6	6		2	5	2	4	
2	5	5	5	6		3	6	2	2	
Total	11	10	11	12	11.0	5	11	4	6	5.5

Fig. 15-9. The effects of amygdalectomy on transfer of training to a new but related task (see Fig. 11-3 for description). Note that the amygdalectomized monkeys treat the task as completely novel whereas their normal controls transpose their responses on the basis of their earlier experience. From Schwartzbaum and Pribram, 1960.

neural system, of which the amygdaloid complex is a part, is conceived to provide a damping effect on the disequilibration produced in rapidly changing situations. These situations tend to create a shift from self-decrementing to lateral-inhibition in the ubiquitous reciprocal couplet which constitutes the neural inhibitory mechanism, the screen of the input systems (Fig. 15-10). In short, the presence of a normally functioning amygdala appears to initiate "internal rehearsal" leading to the registration of consonant, i.e., context-fitting events by damping the tendency of each novel occurrence to markedly disequilibrate the organism.

The evidence that registration takes place by some sort of

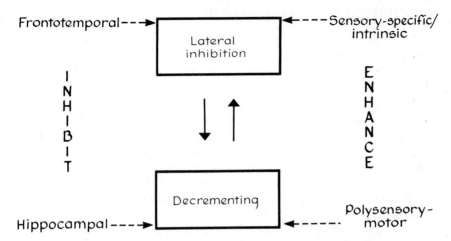

Fig. 15-10. Diagram of the model of cortical control over afferent decrementory and inhibitory processes (fronto-temporal system includes amygdala).

"internal rehearsal" which extends in time the effects on the brain of consonant occurrences immediately brings to mind the neuronal mechanism of induction. The operation of the amygdala system can be conceived to enhance the induction process by preventing interference (Pribram, Douglas, and Pribram, 1969), thus allowing adequate time for the "internal rehearsal" to run its course. Only when interference is controlled can enduring commitment occur and behavior become permanently modified.

Fig. 15-11. Graph of the results of changing the number of negative cues in a set of discrimination problems. From Douglas, et al., 1969.

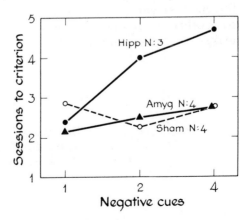

monitoring right and wrong

A supplementary mechanism, additional to registration has been identified as important to the lasting modification of behavior that we call commitment. Another more subtle process deals with what mathematical psychologists refer to as "negative instances." This process follows the earlier occurring registration phase and is characterized by the organism's beginning actively to ignore occurrences which had at one time been, but are now no longer, reinforced. There is good evidence that the hippocampal formation, part of the forebrain adjacent to the amygdala, is involved in this process. We have shown, for instance, that when the number or unreinforced (i.e., negative) cues is varied from one to four in a discrimination situation, the performance of normal subjects is hardly affected. Hippocampectomized monkeys, however, take considerably longer to learn the task when four nonreinforced cues are present, and their learning rate is proportional to the number of such nonreinforced cues (Douglas, et al., 1969; Fig. 15-11). Normal subjects have gone to the second phase of learning: they learn to ignore the now nonreinforced contingencies. In hippocampectomized monkeys the mechanism of the second phase is impaired; they are unable to evaluate their errors when these are made on the basis of nonreinforcement. This inability to evaluate errors .is especially manifest in situations that demand the extinction of previously learned behavior (Douglas, 1967; Kimble, 1969). But studies of extinction raise their own sets of problems which form the substance of the next chapter. Performance, rather than learning, is involved in the extinction paradigm.

The mechanism that allows active ignoring of errors undoubtedly operates over a wider range of conditions than those tested in the laboratory so far. In all such situations a rapid calculation of consonance among previous outcomes of behavior (previous reinforcements) must be accomplished. The structure of the hippocampal cortex, so similar to that of the cerebellum in many respects, makes it anatomically suited to this task (Fig. 15-12). A fast-time

Fig. 15-12. Drawings of the cytoarchitecture of the hippocampal gyrus: the denate gyrus and the hippocampus. Upper figure from Cajal, 1911; lower figure from Lorente de No, 1949.

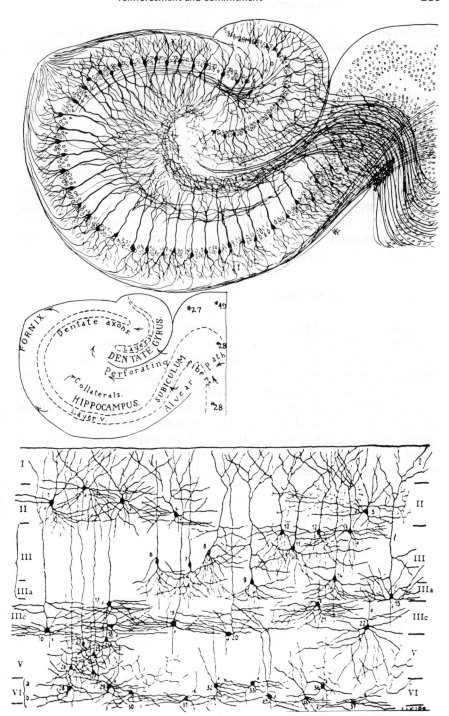

calculation of the probability of error or dissonance (based on estimations of momentary states of homeostatic processes and the effects on them of the outcomes of performance on the last or several last trials) can then serve as the context within which the consonant, the correct can be evaluated. Considered in this light, the hippocampus can be considered the cerebellum of the reinforcement and commitment mechanism.

Let us now turn to the third set of problems concerning the modification of behavior: modification during performance. Chapter 14 concerned the competence of the organism to learn. The present chapter detailed the neurology of the reinforcing process leading to commitment and outlined the brain mechanisms involved in maintaining that commitment. Yet commitment is not achievement. The next chapter must show how commitments become realized in the performance of Acts.

synopsis

Long lasting modifications of competences may be produced by a process similar to that which induces embryonic tissue to differentiate. The characteristics of embryological induction and those of behavioral reinforcement are remarkably similar. Evidence indicates that an aminergic chemical induction process stimulates the production of RNA and protein synthesis in the junctional mechanism of a distributed neural system. The induction mechanism must be protected from interferences for all of its steps to take effect. A number of brain processes ensure commitment to the continuation of a series of reinforcing occurrences after its initiation.

achievement

performance theory: valuing behavior

During the 1950s and 1960s an impasse developed in classical learning theory derived from animal experiments: response strength, i.e., the probability that a response should recur, ought, according to learning theory, to be proportional to the amount and immediacy of appropriate reward, and inversely related to the effort expended to obtain that reward. But in certain situations such is not the case:

Recently, there has accumulated a considerable body of experimental evidence suggesting that these common assumptions underlying learning theory fail to give an adequate description of changes in response strength. In fact, there is the suggestion that under some circumstances the variables of reward, temporal delay, and effort may have just the opposite effects from those predicted by the assumptions .... [Lawrence and Festinger, 1962, p. 6]

This paradox is not new to those working in physiological orientation. Lesions in the ventromedial region of the hypothalamus that

291

produce overeating do *not* induce the subject to work more for food; on the contrary, these animals work less than their controls under similar conditions of deprivation. After fully exploring the conditions that determine this dissociation a reasonable interpretation was made in terms of a go-stop, motivation-emotion distinction.

Situations calling for extinction of behavior epitomize the difficulty with learning theory. According to the theory, commitment should reflect the "strength" with which something has been learned. Learning rate as a measure of "strength" is directly proportional to the ease of task and to the number and immediacy of reinforcement. Therefore, once established, the strength of a commitment, as gauged by learning rate, should be reflected in the rapidity of extinction of behavior in a new situation. Just the opposite occurs. The more rapid the learning, the faster its extinction; learning rate is inversely related to ease of or resistance to extinction.

Experiments show that resistance to extinction is not merely dependent on a failure in new learning, a failure to make new discriminations, an insufficiency of information, or the development of competing responses. Various other interpretations have therefore been tried. For instance, Douglas Lawrence and Leon Festinger (1962) propose that information demanding several "competing," "incongruent," or "dissonant" sets of responses induce behavior to persist beyond the point expected if only one set were operative. Abram Amsel (1958) has focused on the frustration (affect) experienced by the organism in such incongruent situations. Most of the body of experiment and much of the spirit of the argument concerns the state aroused in such dissonance and frustration-producing situations. For instance, dissonance and frustration arise when the result of action does not lead to consequences which sufficiently "justify" it. If the information consequent to the action were available beforehand and choice were free, the action would not have been undertaken. That is, dissonance and frustration result when consequences do not match expectations, i.e., when the organism cannot handle the consequences of his behavior. Behavior thus becomes an expression of an emotional process rather than being motivationally guided by its outcomes. Is this the whole story?

Morphine addicts commonly know that often the strength of their commitment, their addiction is proportional to the amount of "hustling" required to obtain the drug. In fact, in most cases patients who go through withdrawal symptoms have an (understandable) aversion to the drug. Experiments with rhesus monkeys indicate a similar relationship between addiction and reinforcing schedules in animals (Clark and Polish, 1960; Clark, Schuster, and Brady, 1961).

Personality variables, of course, play a noticeable role: yet overall the realization of the hustling→addiction relationship has established the laws regulating morphine distribution in the British Isles; addicts obtain their drug by prescription and cause little behavioral disturbance. Because no underworld rackets can cater to hustling, the whole addiction problem is minimized for society. (Recently, unfortunately, the scene has changed somewhat because of the new youth drug culture and the influx of immigrants. Nonetheless the problem has not grown to United States proportions.)

The similarity to the frustration–dissonance-producing paradigm is unmistakable—thus I jokingly refer to dissonance as "addictionance." And the observation thus leaves us with the same unsettled and unsettling question: Is the fact that behavior comes under the control of emotional processes the only explanation for resistance to extinction? What other alternatives are possible?

Recourse to an information theoretic analysis supported by some intriguing experiments shows how organisms can become addicted or committed. In most situations a number of alternative responses are available to the organism. When an input decreases this number the input is said to have provided information. The amount of information measures the reduction of available alternatives, the amount of uncertainty which an organism might experience in making a choice. As we noted in Chapter 11, information measurement theory thus equates the measure of information with the measure of uncertainty. The term "information" is in a sense used prospectively (how much information can be obtained?) while the term "uncertainty" is used retrospectively (how much reduction in uncertainty has taken place?). When an organism performs a familiar task, "uncertainty" in this sense is no longer reduced by his actions. Nonetheless, behavior continues to be guided. This is, of course, the situation faced in most instances when the core homeostatic mechanism controls behavior. Organisms have been hungry, thirsty, and sexy on earlier occasions, their commitments are enduring and display a repetitive and cyclic appetitive-affective course. How then do these mechanisms exert controls on behavior?

The answer proposed is that actions are guided by the values placed on them. A change induced in the values of the variables that guide behavior is, in the ordinary sense of the word, of course, providing information. In the more restricted usage of information theory, however, the process is akin to biasing the servomechanism—setting the value around which the process stabilizes. Because this precise use of the word "value" is identical to its more usual use in the social disciplines (e.g., Zimbardos, 1969) the distinction between "information" and "value" is worth pursuing a bit further.

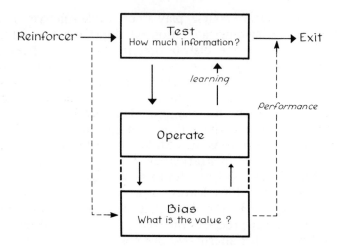

Fig. 16-1. Learning viewed as a feedback, performance as a feed forward process. TOTE notation.

Richard Whalen (1961) performed an experiment with rats which demonstrates this distinction between information and value. He showed that a male's choice between two alleys of a maze depends on the accomplishment of an intromission with a sexually receptive female, but that running speed in the maze continues to vary directly with the number of such occurrences despite the fact that no further information of her whereabouts is obtained after the first few trials. Spence (1956) has reported a similar result when pellets of food are used as reinforcers.

Whalen's and Spence's results show that, once performance is established, reinforcing occurrences display an interesting property: an increase in the number of reinforcements increases performance rate monotonically (over a range). Thus, reinforcers place a value on the behavior—in these situations the behavior is biased. Behavior therefore can generate consequences consonant with the bias, the commitment of the organism; or the behavioral consequences can be dissonant. This constitutes, therefore, a feedforward rather than a feedback process (Fig. 16-1).

the means — ends paradox

A clue to what determines whether behavior is controlled by a feedback or a feedforward process comes from an analysis of the means-ends relationship and its paradoxical reversal.

George Mace (1962) has pointed out that affluence engenders this means-ends reversal.

What happens when a man, or for that matter an animal, has no need to work for a living? . . . the simplest case is that of the domesticated cat—a paradigm of affluent living more extreme than that of the horse or the cow. All basic needs of a domesticated cat are provided for almost before they are expressed. It is protected against danger and inclement weather. Its food is there before it is hungry or thirsty. What then does it do? How does it pass its time?

We might expect that having taken its food in a perfunctory way it would curl up on its cushion and sleep until faint internal stimulation gave some information of the need for another perfunctory meal. But no, it does not just sleep. It prowls the garden and the woods killing young birds and mice. It *enjoys* life in its own way. The fact that life can be enjoyed, and is most enjoyed, by many living beings in the state of affluence (as defined) draws attention to the dramatic change that occurs in the working of the organic machinery at a certain stage of the evolutionary process. *This is the reversal of the means-end relation in behaviour.* In the state of nature the cat must kill to live. In the state of affluence it lives to kill. This happens with men. When men have no need to work for a living there are broadly only two things left to them to do. They can "play" and they can cultivate the arts. These are their two ways of enjoying life. It is true that many men work because they enjoy it, but in this case "work" has changed its meaning. It has become a form of "play." "Play" is characteristically an activity which is engaged in for its own sake—without concern for utility or any further end. "Work" is characteristically an activity in which effort is directed to the production of some utility in the simplest and easiest way. Hence the importance of ergonomics and work study—the objective of which is to reduce difficulty and save time. In play the activity is often directed to attaining a pointless objective in a difficult way, as when a golfer, using curious instruments, guides a small ball into a not much larger hole from remote distances and in the face of obstructions deliberately designed to make the operation as difficult as may be. This involves the reversal of the means-end relation. The "end"—getting the ball into the hole—is set up as a *means* to the new end, the real end, the enjoyment of difficult activity for its own sake. [Mace, 1962, pp. 10–11]

Some of the conditions under which the means-end reversal takes place have been discovered. David Premack (1959) performed the experiments in an operant conditioning situation. He measured the rate of a response in a situation relevant to the organism (e.g., the rate of eating), then compared this rate with a second independently obtained rate (e.g., the rate of lever pressing). His results suggest that

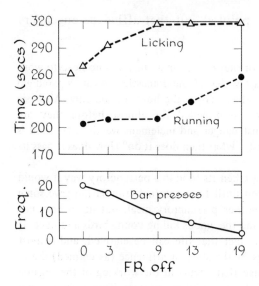

Fig. 16-2. Shown as a function of the number of licks required to turn off the wheel (FR OFF) are (1) average bar presses per session, (2) average duration of licking per session, and (3) average duration of running per session. The point to the left of the lick curve gives the base duration of licking. Redrawn after Premack, 1965.

reinforcement occurs whenever the response with the lower independent rate (lever pressing) coincides, within temporal limits, with the stimuli that govern the occurrence of the response with the higher independent rate (eating). An ingenious set of experiments supports this view, one of which is especially interesting:

> Parameters were identified for the rat which both made drinking more probable than running and running more probable than drinking. In the same subjects, depending upon which parameters were used, running reinforced drinking and drinking reinforced running. This relationship suggests that a "reward" is simply any response that is independently more probable than another response. [Premack, 1962, p. 255; Fig. 16-2]

Specifically, the experiment employed an activity wheel equipped with a brake and a retractable drinkometer:

> Drinking contingent upon running was arranged by retracting the drinkometer, freeing the wheel and making availability of the drinkometer contingent upon running. Conversely, running contingent upon drinking was arranged by locking the wheel, moving in the drinkometer, and making release of the wheel contingent upon drinking. [Premack, 1962, p. 255]

Unfortunately, Premack discusses only the relation between responses. He fails to define fully the immediate operations that define response. Response, in an operant situation, indicates that the organism has acted in and on the situation. Action (as spelled out in Chapter 13) is premised not on the patterned muscular contraction (movement) of the organism but on the environmental consequences of that movement. In fact, the operant "response," the indicator of the action, is one of these consequences. The "response rates" studied by Premack therefore refer not so much to the rapidity of the organism's movements, but to the rapidity with which some reliably observed consequences of these movements can be recorded. For instance, one set of experiments used a Cebus monkey. The monkey might well have been smacking his lips, circling in the cage, or turning somersaults—all irrelevant movements which should not be recorded in the situation as responses, since manipulation of lever, door, and bin were the actions under study. Even the particular movements involved in these actions are pretty much irrelevant to these experiments—the monkey could use his right or left hand, his feet, or even his head to accomplish the response.

Stated succinctly, an operant response is in reality a consequence, a part of an action. Premack's contribution is therefore that the occurrence rate of the consequences of action determines the means-end relationship. Affluence can thus be defined in terms of the *density of consonant consequences* generated in a situation, although rate is probably not the only variable involved. At the moment we can at least state that, other things being equal, the organism tends to organize his actions not just to reduce dissonance but to actively produce consonance. The production of consonance is no haphazard affair—behavior is generated in such a manner that consequences will accrue hierarchically—the more densely consonant within the framework of the less densely consonant. Essentially this hierarchical arrangement of Acts constructs a Plan or program. The importance of Plans to the organization of behavior has already been discussed fully in Miller, Galanter, and Pribram (1960). Here I will pursue only one aspect—the one relevant to the means-end problem and performance theory in general.

meaning and the formation of plans

Plans and the Structure of Behavior (Miller, Galanter, and Pribram, 1960) discussed two aspects of motivation: Plan and Value. Plan clearly directs behavior, i.e., Plans program choices. Value plays some other, less specified, role in the initiation and the "seeing through" of Plans. When Value is stated to be a bias on performance, a commitment, the conception of Value becomes clearer. Thus as reinforcers, the outcomes, the consequences of actions, display two properties. They can provide information, that is, reduce uncertainty for the organism, or they can bias behavior, place a value on it (Fig. 16-1). Let us examine these two properties of the reinforcing consequences of action more closely.

Part II showed that sensory excitations initiated temporary or long lasting changes in ongoing central nervous system activity. This constellation of neural happenings can be described as the processing of sensory input. When that input addresses the competences of the system it becomes perceived information. The amount of information can thus be defined as the amount of match between input and competence. This definition derives from information measurement theory: the amount of perceived information corresponds to the amount of information transmitted by a channel whose capacity corresponds to the neural competence.

Chapter 14, however, noted that the mobilization of an organism's competences depends on some flexible, modifiable mechanism which Chapter 15 showed to be the process of reinforcement which leads to commitment. The necessity for commitment arose because the neural substrate (in mammals at least) does not contain localized mechanisms that lead to the achievement of an Act. Instead mechanisms that invoke part-activities are distributed over a range of tissue, and these part-activities must become integrated, organized for achievement. This distribution of part functions is apparently ubiquitous in the nervous system, and Chapters 6, 7, and 8 considered the consequences of this neurological fact for the organization of sensory processing in perception (thus the need for flexible integrative processes such as the holographic transformation, etc.). I want now to add an important corollary: sensory processing, because it is reinforcing, generates Meaning. An old adage states that all of the problems of psychology ultimately reduce to two: the nature of similarity and the nature of reinforcement. But note that really these are not two problems at all: similarity and reinforcement are one and the same—though looked at from the vantage of stimulus language in one case (similarity) and from the vantage of response language in the other (reinforcement). The process of reinforcement progressively increases discriminability and decreases similarity; the process of discrimination, the perceiving of Meaning, is reinforcing.

The neural machinery involved in this view of the learning mechanism is stated succinctly in the following quotation:

> But perhaps the model has its greatest power in the description of what constitutes reinforcement for the organism. The neural mechanism, because of the hierarchical nature of its selective control over its own modification, allows a change in the representation to occur over successions of trials. Whenever the input perceived is such that complete match between representation and input is not achieved the representation is modified to include this information, and trials continue. Thus an organism can, given a relatively

unchanging or slowly changing environment, search that environment for the additional information that is needed to reduce the uncertainty. The neural model would thus account for search by an information-hungry organism until corrective change of the representation no longer occurs—i.e., stability is achieved. [Pribram, 1960b, p. 8]

Looking, sniffing, listening, touching, and the like are in and of themselves rewarding activities once the organism has become committed to a task. Monkeys, when mastering a problem, will discard the food rewards given them for their responses because their cheek pouches are filled and they cannot hold any more in their hands and feet, and still they will continue testing avidly. Also, a monkey will put a peanut reward obtained on a correctly performed trial in his cheek pouch only to retrieve and eat it when he makes his next error. The guiding of performance has shifted from a food to an information appetitive process. But in order for input to become guiding, i.e., meaningful to the organism, he must process the input in successions of information generating steps in terms of his competences and commitments, much as the digestive system processes ingested substances before they become nourishing. Thus, Meaning is formed by the hierarchical nature of the information processing mechanism.

Chapters 12 and 13 detailed parallels between the sensory and motor mechanisms of the brain. What corresponds in the motor mechanism to the engenderment of Meaning when information is processed by the sensory mechanism? The ready answer is that a hierarchical process similar to that which characterizes the sensory systems occurs in the motor mechanism. The Image-of-Achievement is not informed by "objects" or "interests" but by the play of forces produced by the behaving organism. From these forces must come the commitments which bias the motor competences toward achievement. Furthermore, because of the cerebellar fast-time circuit, the Image-of-Achievement is predictive. Given (1) that the neural mechanism "because of its selective control over its own modification, allows a change in representation to occur over successions of trials," and (2) that whenever "complete match between representation and input is not achieved the representation is modified to include this information and trials continue . . . until corrective change of the representation no longer occurs," then any succession of *predictive* representations in essence constitutes a program or Plan.

In review, achievements are organized performances and steps toward an achievement theory of performance have been taken. These steps account for the differences in function of reinforcers during learning (when they provide information) and during performance (when they value, bias behavior). At least one class of variables, response rate, has been shown to play a major part in determining the contingencies under which an organism no longer learns yet continues to perform—the means-end reversal. Performances achieve because of the hierarchical nature of the reinforcing (in stimulus language, the discriminative) process: Meanings are derived when information is hierarchically processed in sensory systems, and Plans, programs, are constructed by hierarchical processing in the predictive motor mechanism. Part IV continues detailing the neurology of the processes which engender Meaning and Planning by describing the interactions of the brain's receptive and motor mechanisms with each other and with those of other brains.

summation

Before proceeding let us look over the journey thus far. Part I delineates a two-process coding mechanism of brain function consisting of a state and operations on that state. The state part of the mechanism encodes in a microstructure composed by the slow potentials that are generated at the junctions between neurons. Recoding operations are performed by nerve impulses initiated by disturbances of the state; they continue until the disturbance has been equilibrated. The modifications of the junctional microstructure (memory) occur in three categories: enduring, temporary, and evanescent.

Part II relates the two-process mechanism of brain function to subjective experience. In addition to feature detectors (innate) and feature analytic mechanism (modifiable) a flexible organization distributes information within a neural system. This property derives from the junctional microstructure and is functionally similar to optical information processing devices called holograms.

In addition, Part II addresses the manner in which external "reality" becomes constructed by bilaterally symmetrical sensory stimulation, and how specific feelings such as hunger and thirst, alertness and sleepiness, assertiveness and depression stem from the core brain's neural and chemical mechanisms. Each core-brain mechanism is made up of a "go" and a "stop" part, the "go" part involved in "appetitive," motivational feelings and the "stop" part in "affective," emotional feelings. However, these appetitive and affective feelings, feelings of interest, have a far wider neurological base than the core-brain mechanisms; involved is a considerable amount of cortical control over brain processes including those in the core brain and sensory input systems. An organizational, "cybernetic" theory of motivation and emotion based on the two-process mechanism of brain function is evolved.

Part III analyzes the neural regulation of behavior. It distinguishes between movement and action. Movement, patterned muscular contraction, is controlled by a two-process logic similar to that controlling sensory processes. The similarity is caused by the presence, in the reflex organization, of a system of efferent fibers that relay signals from the central nervous system to receptors embedded in muscle tissue. This system of fibers makes the reflex a servomechanism—a TOTE process—not a stimulus-response arc. Controls on muscular contraction must therefore involve signals not only to contractile muscle but to these receptors; if they fail to be informed, the shortened muscle produces a "silent period" in receptor excitation which interferes with smooth performance. In fact, movement can be controlled entirely by changes in the settings made on the spontaneous discharge of the muscle receptors, much as the heating plant in a house is controlled by setting the bias on the thermostat.

The significance of this type of control for the performance of Acts is considered. Acts are defined as the environmental consequences of movement. Puzzles created by experimental results concerning the role of the cerebral motor cortex are resolved by evidence that it is actually a sensory cortex for action—that the motor representation (state part of the two-process mechanism) deals with the field of forces exciting muscle receptors and not with some final common residue of brain function controlling the specifics of contraction of this or that muscle fiber. This representation is holographic-like in nature and not altogether different from other sensory representations. One important difference, however, is due to an input from the cerebellar hemispheres which compute, in fast-time, the predicted next step if the action were to continue its current course. Thus, achievements rather than percepts or feelings become encoded by the motor mechanism.

The neural basis for the modification of behavior is discussed in terms of achievement. Temporary modifiability depends on the fact that the elements making up the motor representation, the competences of the organism to perform one or another Act, are distributed in the neural substrate just as are the elements (bits of information) in the sensory representation. Flexible combinations come about when the elements are combined, integrated into a particular pattern. The process of reinforcement makes this integration more lasting. The hypothesis is proposed that reinforcement "induces" permanent changes in neuronal connectivity. However, these changes can lead to consistent behavior modification only when the organism's induced commitments are protected from destruction through

distraction. Two such protective brain mechanisms exist: one registers reinforcement—the occurrence of outcomes of behavior consonant with the commitment. This is accomplished by a mechanism
that allows internal rehearsal to take place free from interference by
successions of novel occurrences. The other mechanism evaluates
outcomes that are no longer reinforcing. These neural mechanisms
insure that the organized state consequent to reinforcement lasts
sufficiently for learning to occur.

Thus behavior persists (and yet remains modifiable by reinforcers)
under some circumstances when performance does not yield any
novelty, any information. An achievement theory of performance
develops from this distinction between the effects of reinforcers
during learning and during performance. The theory is backed by
behavioral data on the means-ends reversal (such as results of experimental extinction), by observations on addiction and on the influence of response rate on the relationship between behaviors. These
data lead directly to a consideration of the manner in which the
brain makes Meaning and of the neurological construction of Plans,
two processes that critically depend on achievement.

We have thus come to a point where the focus of interest must
shift from the modifications of the behavior of organisms by their
environments to the modifications of environments by the consistent
behaviors, the performances and achievements, of organisms. One
essential difference separates perception and feeling from action.
Perception without intervening action tends to merely assimilate (in
the Piagetian sense of the word) the environment into the organism;
feeling, even when expressed, tends to merely project (in the
Freudian sense) an organism onto his environment. Action, more
realistic, achieves accommodation (Piagetian) between the organism's
perceptions and his feelings.

Action has a further consequence. It achieves accommodation
between organisms. To this communicative property of action the
fourth part of this book is addressed. In this realm man's actualization in his achievements really set him apart. Let us, therefore, take a
look at the neural mechanisms responsible for communicative
achievement in order to discern just what makes man Homo Sapiens.

synopsis

Commitment entails two phases: (1) a continuation of the learning
process that modifies the competences of the organism, and (2) the
pursuit of performance toward achievement. An achievement theory
of performance is formulated from the results of experiments on
extinction, on addiction, and on response rate determinants of the
means-end relationship in reinforcement.

part 4

the structure
of the
communicative process

"The limits of my language mean the limits of my world."
                                    Wittgenstein, 1922

seventeen

signs

Man's most impressive achievements have issued from behaviors that form his communicative actions. Part IV examines the structure of primate communication from the vantage of the two-process mechanism of brain function, the neurological organization of perceptions and feelings, and the neural regulation of behavior. Chapter 16 indicated that communication involves a hierarchical interdigitation of receptive (sensory and core-brain) processes with motor mechanisms; the succeeding chapters will examine this interdigitation in detail. Two classes of communicative Acts can be distinguished on the basis of whether the meaning of the Act depends on the context in which it occurs. Context-free communicative Acts are labeled "signs" and their neurological organization is pursued in the present chapter. Context dependent communicative Acts are labeled "symbols" and the brain mechanisms responsible for their construction are detailed in Chapter 18. To some considerable extent the parts of the brain involved in constructing "signs" are different from those involved in constructing "symbols." In man, however, a higher order relationship develops. Linguistic signs are used symbol-

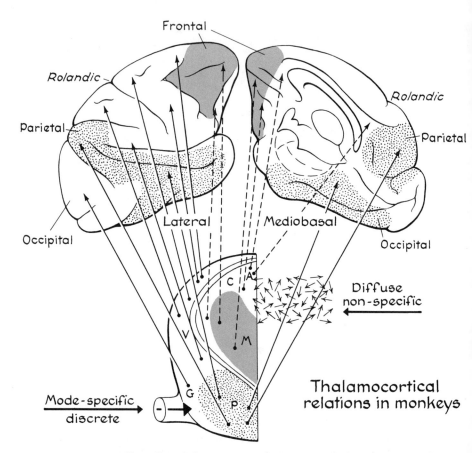

Fig. 17-1. Schematic representation of the projections from
the dorsal thalamus to the cerebral cortex in the monkey. The
lower half of the figure diagrams the thalamus, the straight
edge representing the midline; the upper half of the figure
shows a lateral and mediobasal view of the cerebral hemispheres. The broad black band in the thalamic diagram
indicates the division between an internal core which receives a
nonspecific, diffuse input and an external portion which
receives the modality-specific, discrete projection tracts. The
stippled and cross-hatched portions represent the "association" systems: the medial nucleus of the internal core and its
projections to the anterofrontal cortex; the posterior nuclear
group of the external portion of the thalamus and its
projections to the parieto-temporo-occipital cortex. See Fig.
17-2 for details. Redrawn after Pribram, 1958.

Electro-physiology | Comparative histomorphology | Retrograde thalamic degeneration after cortical removals | Cytoarchitecture & Strychnine neuronography

External Portion

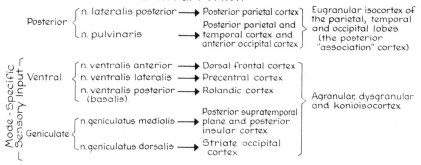

Internal Core

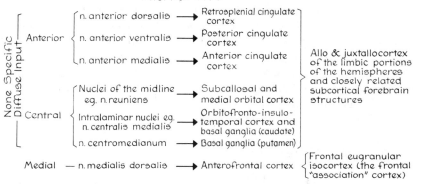

Fig. 17-2. Diagram of the distinctions between an internal core and an external portion of the forebrain. Particular studies used in making the classification are as follows: Electrophysiology: Magoun, 1950; Starzl, et al., 1951; Silver stain: Morin, et al., 1951; Comparative histomorphology: Kappers, et al., 1936; Rose and Woolsey, 1949; Retrograde thalamic degeneration after cortical removals, Monkey: Walker, 1938; Chow, 1950; Chow and Pribram, 1956; Pribram, et al., 1953; Cytoarchitecture and Strychnine neuronography: von Bonin and Bailey, 1947; Bailey, et al., 1950; MacLean and Pribram, 1953; Pribram and MacLean, 1953. Redrawn after Pribram, 1958.

ically in propositional language and linguistic symbols are used significantly in thinking. Thus Chapter 19 poses the problem: "How do the two parts of the brain (the sign and symbol parts) get together in talk and thought?"

The key concept throughout these chapters is context dependency. In essence, signs are conceived to be context-free constructions derived from the action of the association cortex (Figs. 17-1, 17-2) on the input systems. A rose is a rose is a rose regardless of whether it appears in a garden, on a dinner table, or in the garbage pail.

A symbol, on the other hand, derives its meaning from the context in which it appears. Thus the current widely used symbol for peace has stood in other contexts for victory, for a greeting, etc. There is a special affinity between symbols and other context dependent behaviors, such as those that guide interpersonal interactions, because the parts of the brain involved in symbolic behavior (the fronto-limbic forebrain, which includes the frontal cortex (Figs. 17-1, 17-2) and the by now familiar amygdala and hippocampus) are those that are involved in monitoring feelings—appetitive and affective interests and the realization of right and wrong.

The usage in these chapters of the terms *sign* and *symbol* is specific and defined. This use departs from that commonly held in philosophy (e.g., Ayer, 1946; Morris, 1946; Langer, 1951) and in linguistics (e.g., Jakobson, 1956) in one important aspect. Most usages, since they are concerned with an analysis of human language, regard linguistic symbols as a class superordinate to linguistic signs or vice-versa. Neurological considerations make me distinguish signs and symbols as independent classes to be brought together only in propositional language and thought.

what a sign can be

When I began to test monkeys, I customarily used shelled peanuts to reward the animal for making correct choices leading to problem solution. A considerable amount of time was spent shelling peanuts in preparation for a test session. I suddenly realized that there was no reason why the monkeys shouldn't shell their own peanuts—and, in fact, it turned out that they usually did this without delaying the experimental procedure. Being interested in discrimination learning, I conceived that the learning to respond appropriately to a peanut shell was in a sense a more primitive form of the discrimination being taught; that the shell was a consistent indicator, a sign, of the goodies within just as the plus sign painted on the cover of the box containing the peanut. The painted sign was, of course, a more remote, abstracted (and arbitrarily chosen rather than naturally occurring) representation consistently signaling the edible nut and the behavior which would generate its appearance, but the commonality with the peanut's shell was there nonetheless.

These early experiences convinced me that discrimination learning is an exploration of the organism's ability to handle signs. But this formulation lacked the operational rigor one likes to apply to the results of one's experiments—a sign, because of its consistent reference, its freedom from contextual influence, is something *I* can attribute to a situation and *you* can learn this attribution, but can animals really use signs? Isn't human language a prerequisite to the use of signs? When pursued to its origin, my uneasiness stemmed from the fact that in all my experiments I made up the sign and asked the monkey to respond simply by a press of a panel or lever, the displacement of a lid, or the like. Signs are communicative Acts and I had obviously made such Acts but had asked the monkey to reply in a manner which might or might not mean communication to him. So the ambiguity developed.

This ambiguity was resolved in one sweep by an exciting result obtained by Robert and Beatrice Gardner (1969) working with a young female chimpanzee named Washoe. Because of previous failures to enable chimpanzees to talk they decided to try to teach her to communicate by using her hands rather than the vocal cords. American Sign Language devised for the deaf and dumb was chosen as the ideal vehicle since it is easy to learn because of its iconicity; the hand and fingers are maneuverable to resemble, to some considerable degree, the object or action described by the sign. Washoe, about three and one-half years old at the time of this writing, has learned over 150 signs of the American Sign Language System (Fig. 17-3). The Gardners and Washoe readily communicate with each other using this method. Washoe has, in fact, *invented* several new signs which are now in common use by humans being taught the system.

We will return to the far-reaching importance of the Washoe experiment several times in the next three chapters. Here we need to discuss only the accomplishment—primates *can* construct and communicate by signs, context-free, consistent attributes of a situation which are discriminated and recognized. And a great deal is known about the brain mechanisms involved in discrimination learning and recognition.

discrimination learning and recognition

The Imaging aspects of pattern recognition were discussed in Chapters 6, 7, and 8. The involvement of a memory mechanism was handled in terms of the formation of a neural screen,

Signs	Description	Context
Come-gimme	Beckoning motion, with wrist or knuckles as pivot.	Sign made to persons or animals, also for objects out of reach. Often combined: "come tickle," "gimme sweet," etc.
More	Fingertips are brought together, usually overhead. (Correct ASL form: tips of the tapered hand touch repeatedly.)	When asking for continuation or repetition of activities such as swinging or tickling, for second helpings of food, etc. Also used to ask for repetition of some performance, such as a somersault.
Up	Arm extends upward, and index finger may also point up.	Wants a lift to reach objects such as grapes on vine, or leaves; or wants to be placed on someone's shoulders; or wants to leave potty-chair.
Sweet	Index or index and second fingers touch tip of wagging tongue. (Correct ASL form: index and second fingers extended side by side.)	For dessert; used spontaneously at end of meal. Also, when asking for candy.
Open	Flat hands are placed side by side, palms down, then drawn apart while rotated to palms up.	At door of house, room, car, refrigerator, or cupboard; on containers such as jars; and on faucets.
Tickle	The index finger of one hand is drawn across the back of the other hand. (Related to ASL "touch.")	For tickling or for chasing games.
Go	Opposite of "come-gimme."	While walking hand-in-hand or riding on someone's shoulders. Washoe usually indicates the direction desired.
Out	Curved hand grasps tapered hand; then tapered hand is withdrawn upward.	When passing through doorways; until recently, used for both "in" and "out." Also, when asking to be taken outdoors.
Hurry	Open hand is shaken at the wrist. (Correct ASL form: index and second fingers extended side by side.)	Often follows signs such as "come-gimme," "out," "open," and "go," particularly if there is a delay before Washoe is obeyed. Also, used while watching her meal being prepared.
Hear-listen	Index finger touches ear.	For loud or strange sounds: bells, car horns, sonic booms, etc. Also, for asking someone to hold a watch to her ear.
Toothbrush	Index finger is used as brush, to rub front teeth.	When Washoe has finished her meal, or at other times when shown a toothbrush.
Drink	Thumb is extended from fisted hand and touches mouth.	For water, formula, soda pop, etc. For soda pop, often combined with "sweet."
Hurt	Extended index fingers are jabbed toward each other. Can be used to indicate location of pain.	To indicate cuts and bruises on herself or on others. Can be elicited by red stains on a person's skin or by tears in clothing.
Sorry	Fisted hand clasps and unclasps at shoulder. (Correct ASL form: fisted hand is rubbed over heart with circular motion.)	After biting someone, or when someone has been hurt in another way (not necessarily by Washoe). When told to apologize for mischief.
Funny	Tip of index finger presses nose, and Washoe snorts. (Correct ASL form: index and second fingers used; no snort.)	When soliciting interaction play, and during games. Occasionally, when being pursued after mischief.
Please	Open hand is drawn across chest. (Correct ASL form: fingertips used, and circular motion.)	When asking for objects and activities. Frequently combined: "Please go," "Out, please," "Please drink."

Signs	Description	Context
Food-eat	Several fingers of one hand are placed in mouth. (Correct ASL form: fingertips of tapered hand touch mouth repeatedly.)	During meals and preparation of meals.
Flower	Tip of index finger touches one or both nostrils. (Correct ASL form: tips of tapered hand touch first one nostril, then the other.)	For flowers.
Cover-blanket	Draws one hand toward self over the back of the other.	At bedtime or naptime, and, on cold days, when Washoe wants to be taken out.
Dog	Repeated slapping on thigh.	For dogs and for barking.
You	Index finger points at a person's chest.	Indicates successive turns in games. Also used in response to questions such as "Who tickle?" "Who brush?"
Napkin-bib	Fingertips wipe the mouth region.	For bib, for washcloth, and for Kleenex.
In	Opposite of "out."	Wants to go indoors, or wants someone to join her indoors.
Brush	The fisted hand rubs the back of the open hand several times. (Adapted from ASL "polish.")	For hairbrush, and when asking for brushing.
Hat	Palm pats top of head.	For hats and caps.
I-me	Index finger points at, or touches, chest.	Indicates Washoe's turn, when she and a companion share food, drink, etc. Also used in phrases, such as "I drink," and in reply to questions such as "Who tickle?" (Washoe: "you"); "Who I tickle?" (Washoe: "Me.")
Shoes	The fisted hands are held side by side and strike down on shoes or floor. (Correct ASL form: the sides of the fisted hands strike against each other.)	For shoes and boots.
Smell	Palm is held before nose and moved slightly upward several times.	For scented objects: tobacco, perfume, sage, etc.
Pants	Palms of the flat hands are drawn up against the body toward waist.	For diapers, rubber pants, trousers.
Clothes	Fingertips brush down the chest.	For Washoe's jacket, nightgown, and shirts; also for our clothing.
Cat	Thumb and index finger grasp cheek hair near side of mouth and are drawn outward (representing cat's whiskers).	For cats.
Key	Palm of one hand is repeatedly touched with the index finger of the other. (Correct ASL form: crooked index finger is rotated against palm.)	Used for keys and locks and to ask us to unlock a door.
Baby	One forearm is placed in the crook of the other, as if cradling a baby.	For dolls, including animal dolls such as a toy horse and duck.
Clean	The open palm of one hand is passed over the open palm of the other.	Used when Washoe is washing, or being washed, or when a companion is washing hands or some other object. Also used for "soap."

Fig. 17-3. Signs used reliably by chimpanzee Washoe within 22 months of the beginning of training. The signs are listed in the order of their original appearance in her repetoire. From Gardner and Gardner, 1969. *Science*, 165: 664-72, 15 August, 1969. Copyright 1969 by the AAAS.

a set of feature filters and holographic microstructures, through which and onto which input is projected to construct an Image. This chapter will detail some of the factors which influence this screen during learning and recognition.

In Chapters 6, 7, and 8, the Imaging process was discussed as a relatively passive mechanism thrown into operation by input. However, some of the active aspects of the process were dealt with even earlier. For instance, Chapter 5 showed the necessity for a feed-forward, a corollary discharge, without which stability and constancy of the Image would be impossible. By Chapter 16 it became obvious that the entire perceptual mechanism was involved in the generation of meaning—a very active process indeed. The Image as we have come to know it is holistic and holographic. However, when we actually look out upon the world, or listen to it, we *select* one or another aspect—we attend, choose, limit our view in some fashion—especially if we are actively engaged in the looking, listening, etc.

Sign learning and recognition involves, therefore, more than just Imaging. Attentive choice, selection becomes involved, much as in the prosecution of a motor skill. Evidence shows, in fact, that control over Imaging involves pathways through brain structures usually considered to be motor in function. This should not come as a great shock to the reader since he has already found that motor function, i.e., behavior, is effected largely through control over peripheral receptors.

The thesis of this chapter is that signs are constructed when actions operate on perceptual Images. A sign is an Act representing a perceptual Image. Discrimination learning, pattern recognition, selective attention, all involve neural choice mechanisms, choices that beget actions which in turn modify what is Imaged.

This thesis is derived from a series of experiments on monkeys—a series which has turned topsy-turvy the ideas on how the so-called association areas of the primate brain work. Theodore Meynert (1867–1868) and Paul Flechsig (1896) in the latter part of the nineteenth century attributed an associative function to all those parts of the brain cortex which do not connect relatively directly with peripheral receptors and effectors. They were guided by both fact and theory—the fact that all parts of the cortex are highly interconnected, and the theory from the then prevailing empiricist doctrine of the association of ideas. This associationistic view of brain function is still important when the language and thought of man are scrutinized. But as far as discrimination learning, pattern recognition, and the like, the early empiricist approach to brain function which states that the association cortex merely "associates," integrates inputs from a variety of primary sensory receiving areas, has proved wanting.

Specifically, many experiments done with monkeys have shown that discrimination learning and pattern recognition is still possible after removal of large expanses of cortex surrounding the primary projection areas (Pribram, Spinelli, and Reitz, 1969; Fig. 17-4). Yet

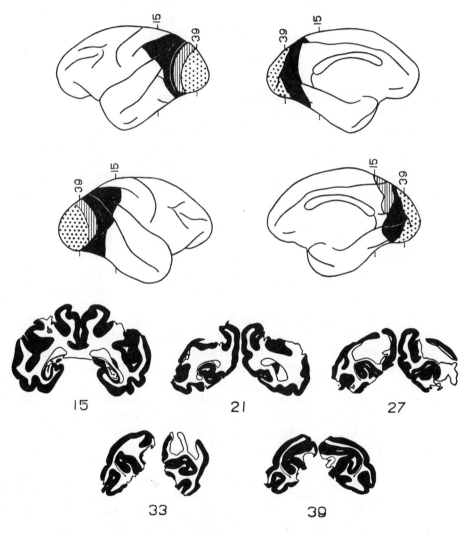

Fig. 17-4. Reconstruction of bilateral prestriate lesions after which monkey could still perform a visual discrimination (the numerals 3 vs. 8). From Pribram, Spinelli, and Reitz, 1969.

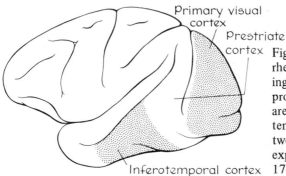

Fig. 17-5. Schematic view of rhesus monkey brain, showing location of the primary projection and "association" areas in the cortical visual system. Note the area in between which was removed in experiment illustrated in Fig. 17-4.

much more restricted removals made at some distance from the primary cortex produce severe deficiencies in both sign learning and recognition (Mishkin and Pribram, 1954; Fig. 17-5). Simply disconnecting the intracortical pathways which join these areas with the primary has no effect. On the other hand, cutting the pathways which connect the cortex with subcortical structures produces as severe a disturbance as does removal of the cortical tissue itself (Pribram, Blehert, and Spinelli, 1966; Fig. 17-6).

For the associationistic view these results pose another of those paradoxes which have been so stimulating to research in the neurobehavioral sciences during the past century and a half. How can a sector of the brain cortex "associate" the effects of inputs to other more primary parts of the brain when disconnection from those parts has no effect?

The puzzle was compounded by the finding that the impairments were not all-of-a-piece. Localization of function on the basis of sense modality was found within the so-called association cortex. A sector in the parietal lobe affects somesthetic discrimination, and no other; a sector in the anterior portion of the temporal lobe concerns only taste (gustation); a mid-temporal sector is selectively involved with audition; and a sector in the inferior part of the temporal lobe serves vision (Fig. 17-7). Further, no intersensory association defects are produced by lesions in this so-called association cortex (reviewed by Pribram, 1969a).

The problem thus becomes the identification of the functions of these sensory specific regions. Most of the experimental work attempting to solve this problem has been performed in the visual sphere and therefore concerns the cortex of the inferior part of the temporal lobe. Enough has been done with auditory and somatosensory procedures, however, to know that the results obtained in vision research are applicable to the other parts of the "association cortex" serving other sensory modalities.

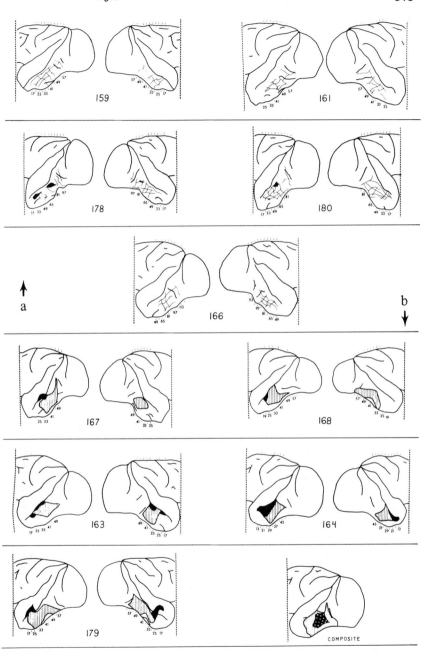

Fig. 17-6. (A) Reconstructions of the crosshatch lesions (fine lines). (B) Reconstructions of the undercut lesions (black indicates superficial cortical damage; stripes indicate the deep lesion). From Pribram, Blehert, and Spinelli, 1966.

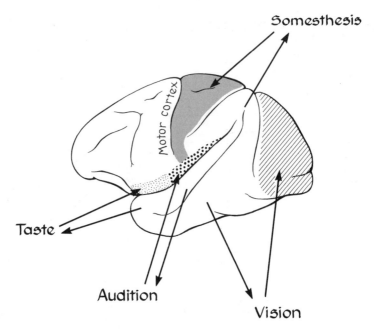

Fig. 17-7. View of lateral surface of monkey brain showing modality specific primary sensory areas and the sensory specific subdivisions of "association" cortex.

Initially the question arose as to whether resections of the inferior temporal cortex of monkeys would impair all forms of visual performance. It was quickly established that the tracking of a visual object, such as a flying gnat, remained undisturbed by the lesion. This finding was later confirmed with the use of an eye camera, photographing the reflections of the cornea of objects looked at (Bagshaw, Mackworth, and Pribram, 1970).

Only when choices, discriminations, were undertaken by the brain-injured monkeys did deficits show up. Impaired performance was recorded on a great variety of visual choice procedures: color, form, pattern, brightness were all affected (Mishkin and Pribram, 1954). The only common denominators in these tasks were that they were visual, that choices were involved, and that the degree of behavioral impairment was proportional to the difficulty experienced by normal monkeys in learning the tasks.

These results immediately led the investigators to ask whether the difficulty shown by the brain-injured monkeys centered on their inability to learn (and remember) the problem rather than their inability to perceive the cues which guide problem solution. In order to test this hypothesis, comparisons were made on a variety of different visual performances of monkeys with resections of the inferior temporal cortex and of others with partial removals of the primary visual area. On the whole, the hypothesis that learning and perceiving could be separated by making lesions in different parts of the cortex was supported by the evidence. Perceptual problems, such as being able to pull in a peanut attached to a string which crosses several other unbaited strings, were adversely affected by lesions in the primary visual area but not by those in the inferior temporal cortex; the reverse picture was obtained when learning tasks were used (Wilson and Mishkin, 1959; Fig. 17-8).

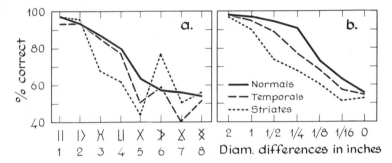

Fig. 17-8. (A) Mean performance of three groups of monkeys (*a*: controls; *b*: lesioned in primary; and *c*: lesioned in inferotemporal visual cortex) on Patterned Strings tests. Problems are shown in order of their difficulty for the normal group. (B) Mean performance of the three groups on Size-Discrimination Thresholds. From Wilson and Mishkin, 1959.

Note the qualifying statement "on the whole," however. The dissociation between effects on perception and learning of the two types of lesions was neither complete nor unambiguous. Some slowing of the learning process resulted from the primary cortex lesion—as might be expected if the monkeys were adjusting to impaired acuity and large scotomata in their visual field. More puzzling was the finding that some acuity loss (e.g., size, Mishkin and Hall, 1955; flicker fusion, Mishkin and Weiskrantz, 1959) was recorded for the monkeys with inferior temporal cortex lesions. Since acuity had to be ascertained by the use of discrimination techniques, the ready explanation to the puzzle was that choices were involved and therefore so were learning and remembering. Checks on human subjects who had suffered a loss of temporal lobe for one reason or another, however, made this explanation suspect (Goldman, et al., 1968). Changes in the threshold of flicker fusion were obtained even when a verbal report of fusion (method of limits, ascending and descending series) was used.

Again the reader should not be completely surprised by these results—nor should we, the investigators, have been. Pattern recognition, sign discrimination, involves both Imaging and memory. The familiar face has become familiar through learning but is perceived holistically and with immediacy.

how the brain controls its input

What led us into quandary was that we could not initially conceive of a mechanism that would partially—but not wholly—separate perception and learning. In the classical view of cortical function, an input is perceived by means of the primary cortex; what is learned is then added, as it were, by the association of other inputs and the storage of those associations, in the "association" cortex. In fact, Wilder Penfield (1969) has, on occasion, called the temporal lobe cortex the memory cortex because electrical stimulation of this part of the brain of epileptic patients produces sequences of mnemic experiences. This classical view, however, does not fit with the paradoxical findings of the disconnection experiments.

As indicated in the introduction to this chapter, the paradox in all of its facets is resolved if one seriously considers the hypothesis that the inferior temporal cortex influences visual processes not so much because it *receives* visual information *from* the primary cortex, but because it *operates* through corticofugal connections *on* visual processes occurring *in* subcortical structures. What evidence makes it likely that such cortical control over subcortical visual mechanisms exists and that it functions as we might expect from the knowledge derived from the neurobehavioral data?

Recall that undercutting the inferior temporal cortex and thus severing the connections between this area and subcortical stations produces the same impairment seen as does resection of the area. Where do these connections lead?

Fibers have been traced by anatomical (Whitlock and Nauta, 1954), and physiological (Reitz and Pribram, 1969; Fig. 17-9) techniques from the inferior temporal cortex. Some of these fibers reach the thalamus from which the afferent connections to the temporal cortex are derived. But a much larger number of fibers reach subcortical structures ordinarily thought of as motor in function—basal ganglia such as the amygdala and the putamen; visuomotor structures such as the superior colliculi of the upper brain stem (see Fig. 17-10).

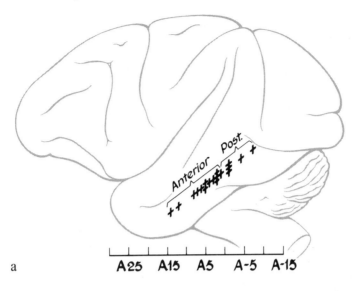

a   A25   A15   A5   A-5   A-15

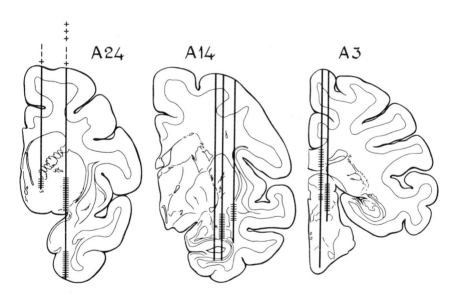

b   Anterior stimulus   Posterior stimulus

Fig. 17-9. (A) Side view of the brain showing stimulation sites
in experiment that traced the subcortical connections of the
inferotemporal cortex. (B) Selected cross sections showing
sites (≠) where response was evoked by inferotemporal cortex
stimulation. Note especially the responses in putamen and
superior colliculus. Redrawn after Reitz and Pribram, 1969.

Further, the effects of electrical stimulation of the inferior temporal cortex can be recorded at a variety of stations along the input pathways. Changes in the electrical activity evoked by flashes of light are produced by the temporal cortex stimulation. These changes have been recorded at the primary cortex, at the lateral geniculate nucleus of the thalamus, and even in the optic nerve. The connections from basal ganglia and colliculus to the thalamic and

Projections of Cerebral Cortex Onto Basal Ganglia

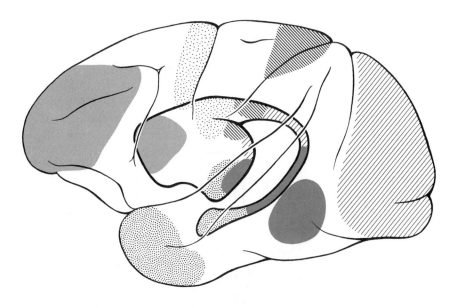

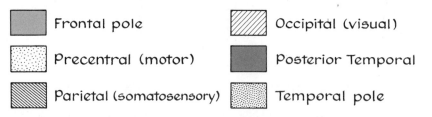

☐ Frontal pole   ▨ Occipital (visual)

☐ Precentral (motor)   ☐ Posterior Temporal

▨ Parietal (somatosensory) ☐ Temporal pole

Fig. 17-10. A brain inside the brain: diagram of the projections of cerebral cortex onto the caudate nucleus and putamen. There is considerable overlap not shown in diagram. Based on data reported by Kemp and Powell, 1970.

retinal locations have not been fully worked out but enough has been done to know of the existence of such connections, albeit, with regard to the brain's control over retinal (and therefore optic nerve) events, the evidence is as yet only electrophysiological (Spinelli and Pribram, 1966, 1967; see Fig. 18-9) and not histological.

In the auditory system the pathways from the temporal cortex to the periphery have been delineated more completely. Here again the colliculi (this time the auditory colliculi) are an important site of connections; from them the pathway descends to the cochlear nuclei (either directly, by way of the superior olive, or by both routes, Nobel and Dewson, 1966).

There is thus no longer any question that the connections exist whereby the so-called association cortex can exert control over input. That this control intimately involves motor mechanisms fits with the neurobehavioral evidence that the temporal cortex plays a role when *active* choices have to be made. But how do such choices effect the classification of input, the construction of signs, and of attribution of significance?

attention

One of the most striking aspects of Images is their richness. As a rule, this richness cannot be apprehended all at once but must be sampled piecemeal, attribute by attribute. Now color, now shape, now texture, now content are selected for emphasis. This limitation of the attentive process does not, however, diminish the immediacy or the kaleidoscopic nature of Imaging—if anything, both are enhanced by proper attending. How?

The answer lies, of course, in the continuous interaction between Imaging and attending. The neurological mechanism for achieving this is available. As we have seen, processes originating in the so-called association areas have access to the functions of the input systems. Evidence suggests that this access utilizes the subcortical and perhaps the cortical filters or screens within the input systems to control what is attended.

The evidence accrued from experiments using techniques of estimating the rapidity with which excitability recovers within the input channels (recall Figs. 11-6, 11-7). When responses are evoked in a sensory system by some fairly abrupt event in the environment, say a flash of light or a click of sound, the response of the system takes a finite period. Should a second flash or click occur before the system has "recovered" from its reaction to the initial event, the response to the later event will be affected by the earlier one. The length of time of the reaction to excitation is therefore important in determining the manner in which input becomes processed. In our experiments we were able to show that electrical stimulation (or even ablation) of the so-called association cortex could alter this length of time.

The sites where such influence is most likely to be exerted are, of course, the neuronal inhibitory interactions which occur in the input channels, the interactions which, when grouped as logic elements, compose the screens through which and onto which input is transmitted. By increasing lateral inhibition, for instance, sensory contrast can be enhanced and the recovery of the system slowed (since lateral inhibition is assumed to reciprocally influence decrementing; recall Fig. 3-10).

Slowing of recovery in the primary visual system is in fact observed when the inferior temporal cortex is electrically stimulated (Spinelli and Pribram, 1966; Fig. 11-7). This result was especially welcome because it indicated the neurological mechanism by which the so-called association cortex exerts its control over the primary input systems. We wanted to explore this mechanism further, but, as so often happens at the laboratory bench, we found we had incomplete knowledge of the variables involved in the phenomenon under observation. When we tried to replicate we could not obtain the effect reliably. Because the problem was so important, we persisted and found a way to gauge the conditions necessary to obtain the effect.

Needing a more stable indicator of excitability, we abandoned, for the moment, the multiple flash presentations. We reasoned that the retina was the site of instability and that electrically stimulating a more central location in the visual system by means of an implanted probe would produce more reliable results. However, the cost of achieving stability might be that we would no longer be able to influence the excitability of the sytem. Indeed, electrical stimulation of the inferior temporal cortex failed to influence excitability as tested with the cortical probe.

Lauren Gerbrandt, a postdoctoral fellow, extracted us from this dilemma with a simple observation. He showed that the amplitude of the responses evoked by electrical probe stimulations within the visual system were a function of the attentiveness of the monkey during the experiment. When the monkey was enclosed in a box, the response was small. When the box was opened and the monkey was looking around, the response was large, Further, inferior temporal cortex stimulation could make the small response obtained in the closed box into a large response, but had no influence on the large response. Finally, using the size of this probe-evoked response as a monitor, he could predict in the closed box situation whether

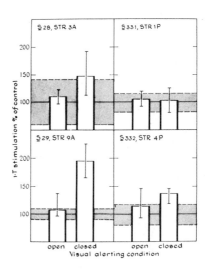

Fig. 17-11. Effect of IT stimulation on size of response evoked in striate cortex by stimulation of the lateral geniculate nucleus. Note that only in the closed box situation does the effect (in three of the four monkeys) transcend the variance (shaded band) of the unstimulated condition. From Gerbrandt, Spinelli, and Pribram, 1970.

inferior temporal cortex stimulation would or would not affect the recovery function of the visual system.

Whenever the monkey was attentive, the effects we had earlier obtained were not observed. When, however, the monkey became "bored," tended to nod into sleep, etc., the effect on the recovery function was clear-cut. In our initial experiments we had performed a long routine of daily procedures: paired flashes, paired clicks, click-flash and flash-click combinations, patterned flashes, etc., were presented in regular order, day-in, day-out, week-in, week-out. Not only the monkeys, but also Spinelli and I, who were performing the experiments, became disenchanted with the routine. Spinelli and I took turns keeping watch on the other two to see to it that sleep would not intervene. We watched the monkey through a peephole; when he nodded, we tapped the enclosure gently. A small displacement of the stool of the nodding investigator accomplished the same end. In short, we got our results because the monkeys were not attentive. Subsequent teams testing monkeys only on the recovery cycle phenomenon, working with monkeys fresh to the situation and apparently interested in the goings-on of the experiment, obtained different results. Only when, through repetition, the situation became boring to us and to the monkey did the recovery-cycle effects again emerge (Gerbrandt, Spinelli, and Pribram, 1970; Fig. 17-11).

Taken together, these experiments show that the effects of electrical stimulation of the inferior temporal cortex and those produced when a monkey is "attending" are similar, and that the two processes show a considerable amount of convergence onto some final common mechanism. It becomes reasonable, therefore, to suggest that the process of attention involves the influence exerted by inferior temporal "association" cortex on the input mechanism. Through this influence attention is able to alter the time course of inhibitory interactions in screens and thus the characteristics of the Image initiated by any particular input.

The influence of the temporal lobe areas on the input system is thus the specification of a particular operation and the production of a setting in which certain operations are enhanced. How then does the mechanism affect discrimination, the recognition process?

feature filters and mechanisms of identification

Much work has shown that pattern recognition involves the identification of the features that distinguish objects. Machine simulations of the process have relied heavily on identification in their programs. The discovery of neural units that are sensitive to features, i.e., capable of responding selectively to lines at different slants, movement, color, and the like, has therefore been heralded as the answer to the recognition problem. Without detracting from the importance of the discovery, earlier chapters pointed out that all the problems in perception could not be handled by a feature detection mechanism. Let me pursue the point by suggesting that the problem of pattern recognition, which depends on memory, also fails to be met if only detection is considered. I shall therefore distinguish between feature detection and feature indentification. Feature detectors are, of necessity, built into the neural apparatus and, of necessity, they cannot be radically modified by experience if they are to do the job of detection. Feature detectors are therefore stable, "wired-in," native elements of the input systems which preprocess signals before further operations on them are performed. On the other hand, the mechanism of identification. Feature detectors are, of necessity, built into the and modifiable by experience. Because of the immediacy of recognition, however, identification must, at any given moment, share preprocessing with detectors. It is this sharing which has led to confusion about the two mechanisms and to the feeling that feature detectors do the whole job.

Feature detectors play a somewhat limited role. Along with other mechanisms, they are thought to provide the essential reference, the backdrop against which other more labile configurations of neural events transpire. They are the wired-in parts of the screen, the warp across which the woof of experientially sensitive neural microstructure is woven. At any given moment the fabric of the screen processes the neural events impinging on it—preprocesses them on the way to subsequent cell stations. The warp of the screen is unaffected by the processing, but a residue is left on the woof, another thread has been woven into the fabric.

Some of the various mechanisms whereby experience can affect the nervous system have been detailed in Chapters 2 and 14. In terms of the screen these mechanisms could be thought to tune, to change the bias of the logic elements which compose the screen. Small changes in the time course of recovery of excitability, such as those produced by stimulation of the inferior temporal cortex, could, were they to become permanent, alter the response characteristics of a logic element until it "resonated" rather specifically to one configuration of the neural microstructure and not to others. Spinelli (1970; recall Fig. 7-8) has simulated in a computer program such a system which he calls Occam. The program can "recognize" a wave form after it has been exposed to it on several occasions and can identify this pattern even if given only a part of it. Further, the program can discriminate among dozens of wave forms.

The neural mechanism by which identification is achieved might be thought of as operating something like this. Ordinarily, the logic elements of the screen, the columns of cortical cells, are more or less connected to each other by their directionally sensitive elements. Recall that Chapter 7 suggested that the directional sensitivity of the receptive fields of cortical cells provided pointers to adjacent cells thus making of a cortical column a data structure, a list. Lateral inhibition, by separating logic elements from one another, structures the list. Each logic module, each list, can be thought of as a dipole which becomes polarized by the input signals. A good case can be made for the existence of electrical dipoles in the cortex (see Elul, 1964; Barrett, 1969). The electrical dipole could become constituted of the changes in molecular conformation discussed in Chapters 2 and 8. Conformational modifications can be measured by nuclear magnetic resonance spectroscopy and X-ray diffraction studies since each distinct conformation resonates at a different natural frequency. Large molecules, such as the lypoproteins and glucoids which make up the synaptic and dendritic membranes in the brain's microstructure, are known to be liable to conformational change.

Whenever a neural signal traverses such a membrane, conformational changes would tend to become stabilized, aligning molecular structures for the duration of the signal and for some limited time after. These temporarily stabilized conformations, if sufficiently extensive, would, in effect, produce electrical polarization of the microstructure. This polarization would be enhanced when the influence of each dipole on its neighbor was minimized through lateral inhibition. Without such inhibitory interactions, the alignment of dipoles would tend to weaken much as like poles of magnets aligned in parallel tend to disturb the alignment. The alignment of dipoles by input is therefore enhanced by the effects of temporal cortex stimulation on lateral inhibition (recall Fig. 15-10), an enhancement which provides constancy to the relationship between input and logic elements. This constancy also cuts the cortical system into smaller functioning units, allowing readier adaptation of each unit to its input. As Ross Ashby has pointed out (1960; Fig. 17-12), a completely interconnected system is ultrastable and therefore difficult to adapt. Only by "cutting the system to pieces" through constancy can modification occur.

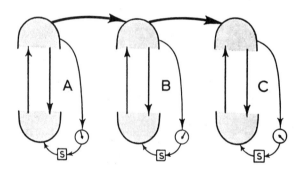

Fig. 17-12. Ashby's diagram of the development of constancies in his homeostat. Top hemispheres indicate stimulus variables, lower hemispheres neural response variables. S is a selector switch and ↗ a monitor. Note similarities to TOTE. From Ashby, 1960.

Such a system of logic dipoles, neural list structures, is advantageous because it is a parallel processing content-addressable mechanism. The logic elements are addressed simultaneously and not searched sequentially; storage location becomes unimportant. Preprocessing and modifications based on experiences occur side-by-side at practically the same time. In short, some parts of the preprocessor are changed by the processing. The neural mechanism is self-organizing.

To summarize: In real life the perceptual process of Imaging and the cognitive process of recognition cannot easily be separated. We identify, objectify what we sense to be significant almost the moment it is sensed. But, for purposes of scientific analysis—especially if the interest is in mechanism—it becomes worthwhile to tease apart, as we have done in these chapters, the various sub-processes involved. Since we find that the neural mechanisms of the subprocesses are so interwoven in actuality, we come to understand more thoroughly how the unity of the psychological process comes about. When this unity is expressed, a sign is identified or actualized, but the actualization (as all Acts) must be achieved sequentially. Any momentary signing is therefore incomplete—it stands for, derives meaning only from the totality of the image intended for expression.

significance

A final question must be discussed: How do some aspects of Images take on meaning, become significant? In the monkey discrimination experiments, a painted pattern takes on meaning, becomes a sign, as a consequence of the monkey's behavior. Making the discriminative choice utilizes the neural apparatus necessary to action. The fact that the pathways from the inferior temporal cortex which affect visual attention lead through motor structures provides the structural basis for the interaction of motor and sensory processes, the influence of those screens giving rise to Images-of-Achievement on the screens from which perceptual Images are constructed. Signs are therefore achieved through action. It is this active aspect of signing that generates meaning: perceptual learning through reinforcement. The meaningfulness of signs turns out to depend on a mechanism that calls attention to, reinforces, alternatives, (see Fig. 17-13). Monkeys deprived of inferior temporal cortex select from a restricted range of alternatives (display less uncertainty) when making visual choices, whether the alternatives are clearly separated in the form of dime store junk objects (Pribram, 1960b; see Figs. 19-11, 19-12) or are the features that distinguish patterns from each other (Butter, 1968; Fig. 17-14). A slowing of recovery of the input systems occurs when the organism is generally attentive or when the inferior temporal cortex is electrically stimulated (recall Figs. 11-5, 11-6). Such slowing of recovery reduces the redundancy of the input channels; at any moment in time fewer channels are carrying identical signals. Thus smaller pieces of neural hologram become constituted by any particular set of signals. When small pieces of physical hologram are used to reconstruct Images, depth of field increases and more of the Image is in focus, although at the cost of some slight loss in detail. The mechanism works much like shortening a zoom lens—more comes into focused view and, in fact, direct evidence for such a zoom mechanism has been obtained in man. Measurements of the receptive fields of single units in the

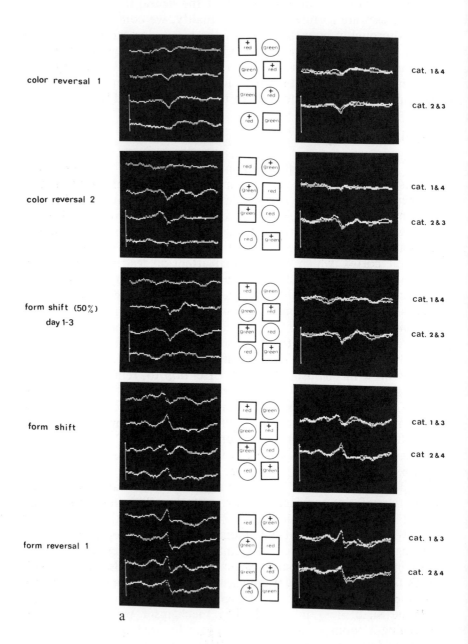

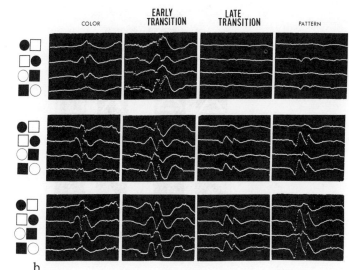

b

Fig. 17-13. Results of an experiment demonstrating the functions of the inferotemporal cortex by behavioral electrophysiological techniques. The experiment is similar to the one described by Figs. 7-3 and 7-4. A monkey initiates a flashed stimulus display and responds by pressing either the right or left half of the display panel to receive a reward while electrical brain recordings are made on line with a small general purpose computer (PDP-8). In this experiment the flashed stimulus consisted of colored (red and green) stripes and circles. Reinforcing contingencies determined whether the monkeys were to attend and respond to the pattern (circle *vs* stripes) or color (red *vs* green) dimension of the stimulus. As in the earlier experiment stimulus, response, and reinforcement variables were found to be encoded in the primary visual cortex. In addition, this experiment showed that the association between stimulus dimension (pattern or color) and response occurs first in the inferotemporal cortex. This is presented in panel t h r e e of B where the electrophysiological data averaged from the time of response (forward for 250 msec and backward 250 msec from center of record) show clear differences in waveform depending on whether pattern or color is being reinforced. Note that this difference occurs despite the fact that the retinal image formed by the flashed stimulus is identical in the pattern and color problems. Once the monkeys have been overtrained this reinforcement produced attentional association between a stimulus dimension and response also becomes encoded in the primary visual cortex as is shown in a. From Rothblat, and Pribram, in preparation.

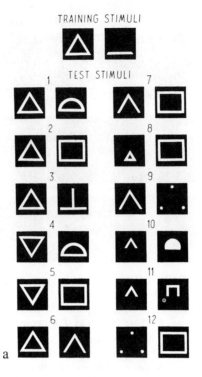

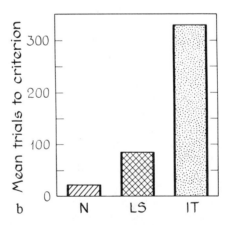

Fig. 17-14. Experiment performed to investigate whether IT lesioned monkeys attend to specific features of the training triangle (top figure) as well as do unoperated controls. (A) cues used; (B) results. N: normal; LS: lateral striate (primary visual cortex); IT: inferotemporal cortex. From Butter, 1968.

human visual cortex show that size constancy is achieved by a process which maintains a constant angle relating to a fixation point at the geometric center of the receptive field (Marg and Adams,1970). Thus, when I intend to focus on a large segment of a scene I shorten the zoom. Paradoxically, when I then selectively attend to one or another aspect of the scene, the meaning of that aspect becomes context consistent—i.e., free from variation in interpretation. When, on the other hand, I intend to focus on a limited segment of a scene to the exclusion of the rest, I lengthen the zoom. The segment in focus thus becomes severed from the context in which it originally occurs with the consequence that it can take on a variety of meanings depending on the bias or set of the viewer.

But this context sensitive narrowing of focus is another aspect of the problem of meaning. Chapter 18 deals with this aspect, meaning derived from communication by symbolic processes. Symbols as well as signs engender meaning.

synopsis

Man's achievements derive largely from his unique communicative capacities. These develop when the brain's motor mechanisms become engaged in perception and feeling. The resulting coding operations construct signs and symbols. Signs are made and recognized when motor mechanisms operate on the junctional patterns initiated by input; symbols, when motor mechanisms operate on junctional core-brain receptive processes. The neural organization of significant and symbolic processes differs: signs become communicative Acts that remain invariant over a large variety of contexts; symbol communications almost completely depend on the context in which the symbols occur. The sign's freedom from context derives from the function of pathways from the association cortex of the brain that influence via motor stations, the junctional mechanism of the logic structures of the sensory input mechanism discussed in Chapters 7 and 8. This corticofugal control on input is coordinate with the process of selective attention.

symbols

tokens

Symbols are tokens. Tokens derive meaning from their past use and from the current state of the organism using them. They are thus different from signs: Symbols, as representations, are biased by the context in which they occur. The sign 🌹 is a rose, is a rose. The symbol 卍 has a different meaning for the Jew than it has for the Hindu.

This chapter aims to show that symbols are constructed when actions operate on feelings, on interests. The evidence concerns the functions of the primate frontal cortex, the part of the brain which was, for a decade or so during the 1940s and 1950s, isolated by lobotomy (leukotomy) in an effort to restore psychiatric patients to sanity. Though the therapeutic efficacy of this procedure remains questionable, its advent generated a large amount of neurobehavioral reasearch which is only now beginning to form an interpretable body of knowledge.

the delayed reaction experiment

The story begins shortly after World War I in the psychological laboratories of the University of Chicago. The then new functionalism in psychology raised many procedural questions. One of these was asked by Walter Hunter (1913), a graduate student at the time: Was it possible that children and animals really had "ideas"? And would it be possible to prove that they did? He devised a test during which, in full view of the child, a tidbit such as a piece of chocolate was hidden in different locations on successive occasions (trials). In each trial either the child was relocated or a screen was interposed between him and the hiding place. Some minutes (or even hours) later, the child was exposed to the hiding place which over successive trials had shifted and so, contrary to what occurs in sign discrimination, had lost any consistent distinctiveness. If he finds the tidbit he must have carried the "idea" of the hidden tidbit and its location in his head during the delay between hiding and finding. Children and a host of animals were shown to be proficient at this task which became an indicator of their ability to recall.

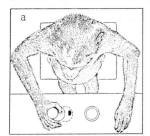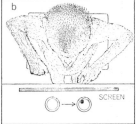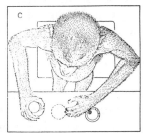

Fig. 18-1. Drawing of alternation task which requires a monkey to remember which cup he lifted last in order to lift the correct one on his next trial and be rewarded with a peanut. He is rewarded if he remembers to lift cups in a simple alternating sequence: left, right, left, and so on. After each trial a screen comes between him and the cups and remains there for periods that can be varied from seconds to many minutes. In part *c* of this sequence the monkey has forgotten to alternate his response. Experiments demonstrate that frontal and limbic brain lesions interfere with a monkey's ability to perform this particular task. Changing the task only slightly (see Fig. 18-6), however, allows the brain-lesioned monkeys to perform as well as unoperated controls. From Pribram, 1969d. "The Neurophysiology of Remembering," Copyright © 1969 by Scientific American, Inc. All rights reserved.

During the 1930s Carlysle Jacobsen at Yale became interested in devising a procedure to test for the impairment produced in nonhuman primates when the frontal cortex of the brain is damaged. Clinical studies and laboratory observations of monkeys had suggested that frontal injury destroyed some sort of thought processes. It seemed reasonable to Jacobsen, therefore, to use the test which had become the scientists' indicator of recall to study the effects of frontal brain damage.

By this time several versions of the test had become standardized. The first involved the hiding of a tidbit in one of two identical boxes within view of the animal, closing the lids, interposing a screen between subject and boxes for a few seconds (usually 5–15), raising the screen, and allowing the subject to choose between the boxes. Sometimes the screen was transparent, sometimes opaque. Only the opaque trials constituted the true test—the "delayed reaction task." In one modification of this test—the "indirect method"—a cue such as a colored object temporarily shown over the actual hiding place of the tidbit indicated which box would, after the delay, contain the reinforcement. After the delay the animal was allowed to choose between hiding places that now were indistinguishable. Another modification, the "delayed alternation" procedure, did not signal the hiding place at all. The location of the reinforcer was simply alternated from one box to the other from trial to trial (Fig. 18-1).

Jacobsen's approach (1928, 1936) to the study of the frontal cortex was successful: resection of the frontal pole of the brain interfered with adequate performance of all versions of the delayed reaction task. Therefore the frontal lobes must in some way be responsible for an organism's ability to recall recent occurrences.

The indirect form of the delayed reaction task is of special interest here. The indirectness of the method signaling the hiding place led some of Jacobsen's colleagues to devise other tasks to explore the ability to use tokens. The most famous of these is the Chimpomat. Chips such as those used in poker are provided by a slot machine, and the entire "game" is played with the chips which only later and in a remote location can be "turned in" for peanuts. Normal chimpanzees readily use these chips, these tokens, but chimpanzees whose frontal lobes have been resectioned fail entirely to take the steps that lead from token to reinforcement (Jacobsen, Wolfe, and Jackson, 1935; Fig. 18-2).

This method of training has been enhanced recently in another experimental effort to teach a chimpanzee to communicate. Chapter 17 described Washoe's ability to use signs. David Premack (1970) at the University of California in Santa Barbara has trained his

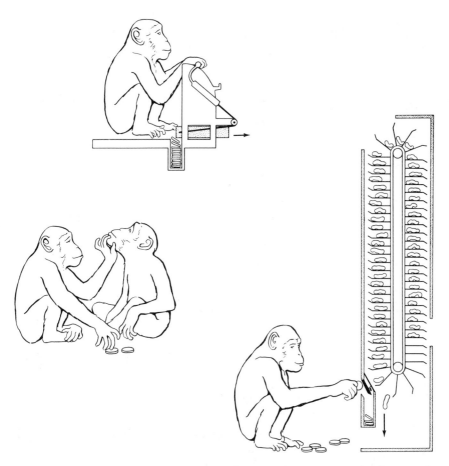

Fig. 18-2. Illustration showing chimpanzee trained to work for poker chips (upper left) and inserting earned tokens into an automatic vender for bananas and peanuts (lower right). Chimpanzees work, save, and hoard poker chips in a miniature economic system—even steal chips from each other (lower left).

chimpanzee, Sarah, very differently from the manner used by the Gardners with Washoe. Premack applied operant conditioning methods to determine just how complex a system of tokens can be used to guide Sarah's behavior. The Chimpomat had already shown that chimpanzees would work for tokens. Premack's chimpanzee has demonstrated that behavior dependent on tokens is not only possible, but that serial organizations of tokens can be responded to appropriately (Fig. 18-3).

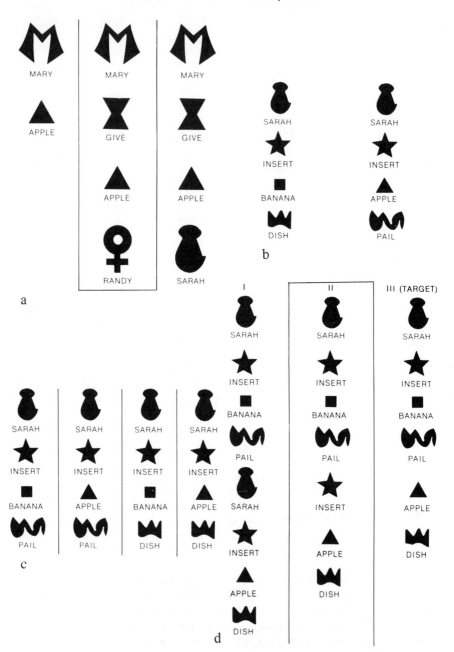

Fig. 18-3. Some examples of the sequences of symbols used by Sarah to communicate with her experimenter. From Premack, 1970.

In all of these experiments the crux of the problem is that the token does not call forth a uniform response. Depending on the situation (the context in which the token appears), the token must be apprehended, carried to another location, inserted into a machine or given to someone, traded for another token or traded in for a reward. Or, as in the original delayed response situation, the token stands for a reward which is to appear in one location at one time, in another location at another time.

I shall use the term symbols to describe these context-dependent tokens. (This distinction is consonant with that made by Noam Chomsky, 1963 and is used here to indicate that the primordia of the rules that govern human language are rooted in what are here called "significant" and "symbolic" processes.) As reviewed in Chapter 17, there is now a large body of evidence demonstrating that the cortex lying between the classical sensory projection areas in the posterior part of the brain is involved in discriminating context-free signs. The evidence which shows that the frontal cortex lying anterior to the motor areas is involved in context dependent symbolic processes follows.

Jacobsen believed that the processes tested by these procedures had to do with memory (short-term recall) and that these processes were attributable exclusively to frontal lobe function. Later studies have shown that, with two exceptions, his belief was justified. One exception is that lesions of the caudate nucleus of the basal ganglia, a part of the motor system of the brain, also disrupt performance in the delayed reaction task. Here again we have evidence of the involvement of the motor mechanisms which produce action in a higher order brain process. The other exception concerns performance in the delayed alternation task, which, though it does not use tokens, is disrupted by frontal lesions. Performance of this task is also impaired by ablations of all parts of the limbic system (Pribram, Wilson, and Connors, 1962).

There are thus behavioral as well as anatomical reasons for grouping the frontal pole of the brain with the limbic formations (Pribram, 1958; recall Figs. 17-1, 17-2). Removals of tissue in these systems does not impair sign discrimination but does impair performance on such tasks as delayed alternation (Pribram, et al., 1952; Pribram, et al., 1966; Pribram, Wilson, and Connors, 1962), discrimination reversal (Pribram, Douglas, and Pribram, 1969) and approach-avoidance (commonly called "passive" avoidance; Mc-Cleary, 1961). In all of these tasks some conflict in response tendencies, conflict among sets is at issue. The appropriate response is context (i.e., state) dependent and the context is varied as part of the problem presented to the organism. Thus a set of contexts must become internalized (i.e., become brain states) before the appropriate response can be made. Constructing sets of contexts depends on a memory mechanism that embodies self referral, rehearsal, or, technically speaking, the operation of sets of recursive functions. (The formal properties of memory systems of this type have been described fully by Quillian, 1967). The closed loop connectivity of the limbic systems has always been its anatomical hallmark and thus makes an ideal candidate as a mechanism for context dependency (Pribram, 1961; Pribram and Kruger, 1954).

As an aside, it is worth noting that much social-emotional behavior is to a very great extent context dependent. This suggests that the importance of the limbic formations in emotional behavior stems not only from anatomical connectivity with hypothalamic and mesencephalic structures but also from its closed loop, self referring circuitry. It remains to be shown (although some preliminary evidence is at hand: Fox, et al., 1967; Pribram, 1967b) that the anterior frontal cortex functions in a corticofugal relation to limbic system signals much as the posterior cortex functions to preprocess sensory signals.

Thus the relationship of frontal cortex with motor mechanisms on the one hand and with limbic formations on the other, suggests the existence of a frontal lobe process by which action and interest (appetitive and affective feelings) interact. The organism's ability to use tokens or symbols, generally so dependent on the frontal cortex, appears therefore to be derived from this interaction.

emotion and memory

Support for this suggestion comes from a variety of sources. Perhaps the most persuasive source is another set of neurobehavioral paradoxes. As indicated at the outset of this chapter, lobotomy or leukotomy in man was devised and used as a psychotherapeutic procedure. The development of the procedure of frontal lobotomy on man is directly attributable to the experiments on monkeys and chimpanzees already described—despite their disabilities in performing the delay tasks, the animals appeared to be undisturbed by their inadequacy. What could be simpler than to amputate the organ responsible for disturbance in patients? (See Fig. 18-4.)

The procedure worked to a certain extent. The paradox came, however, with the discovery that to all intents and purposes the problem solving abilities of lobotomized patients remained unim-

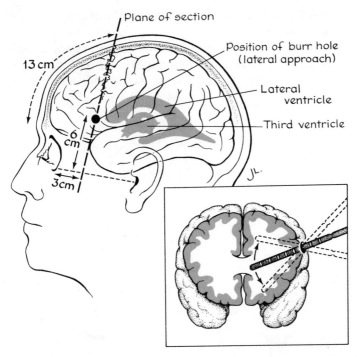

Fig. 18-4. Diagrams of frontal lobotomy procedure showing point of entry of leukotome in lateral and frontal views.

paired. In an attempt to analyze this paradox, I performed tests which showed that lobotomized monkeys (and chimpanzees, as well as man) really did become disturbed when frustrated, but the disturbance was of briefer duration than in control subjects (Pribram and Fulton, 1954). The experiment consisted of training the subject to perform 100 percent correctly in a discrimination and then, on test trials interspersed among the discrimination trials, withholding the reward from the subject. The resulting disturbed behavior interfered with performance on subsequent trials paced at regular intertrial intervals. The time taken to resume criterion (100 percent correct) performance was measured. Though the disturbed behavior was every bit as disruptive after frontal surgery as before it, the disruption did not last as long. This experimental result suggested that the frontal cortex ordinarily enhances the persistence of the disruptive effect, a suggestion compatible with the interpretation of subhuman primate frontal lobe function in terms of recent memory. Meanwhile, however, ordinary tests of recent memory in man, such as the recall of recently read telephone numbers (the digit span), failed to reveal anything abnormal although suffering was relieved and neurosis alleviated.

But the paradox did not end. To cure certain types of epilepsy, neurosurgeons began to invade the temporal lobe of man's brain as well. The results of animal experiments would indicate that feelings

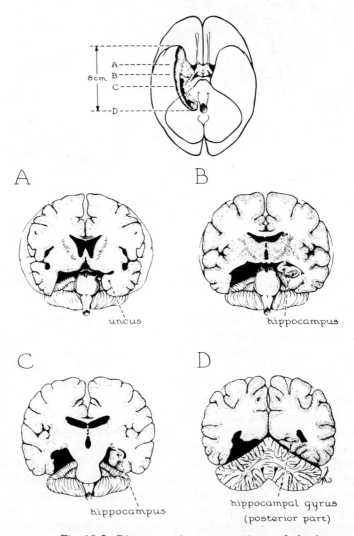

Fig. 18-5. Diagrammatic cross sections of the human brain, showing the extent of bilateral medial temporal-lobe resections which include amygdala and hippocampus and which lead to marked disturbances of memory processes. From Milner, 1959.

and emotions would be radically changed when the limbic structures of the temporal lobe fell under the surgeon's scalpel. Nothing obvious of this sort occurred. Instead, a peculiar kind of severe memory disturbance followed the resections. Immediate memory as tested by digit span remained intact. Also, the patient could recall in considerable detail his experiences before brain surgery and maintained the perceptual and motor skills he had acquired. What seemed awry, however, was his ability to register current experience in long term memory. Should a testing session be interrupted and resumed some minutes or hours later, the patient not only could not recall answers given but was also unaware that he had been asked questions or that he had participated in the test situation (Milner, 1958; Fig. 18-5).

Were it not for this doubling of the paradox it might be easy to dismiss the discrepant effects of frontal and temporal lobe surgery on memory and emotion on the basis of species differences. Such differences are, of course, the obvious factor; but why this curious juxtaposition of memory functions and emotions? Could it be that the impairment of function is basically the same in subhuman primates and in man, but that whatever makes man different, his linguistic ability for instance, also results in the species difference? Could the frontal lobe defect be expressed during problem solving in monkeys but only in highly nonverbal social interactions in man? Could the reverse be true of limbic deficits?

As far as the frontal lobes are concerned, these questions can be answered affirmatively. The patient's intact verbal facility allows the problem solving in delay situations to be apparently normal. Tasks only slightly more complicated than the simple delayed reaction and which monkeys were shown to fail are also failed by patients after lobotomy (even ten years after surgery) when these tasks were presented without the use of verbal instructions (Poppen, Pribram, and Robinson, 1965). Also, patients who have been given the delay task report that they verbally code the location of the hidden tidbit—and thus they can recall after surgery, even when the surgery intervenes between the hiding and the seeking.

The paradox is not so easily resolved for limbic lesions. For one thing, we do not clearly know that only limbic damage has been done in the temporal lobe resections made on man. The profound memory loss seen in patients can to some extent be mimicked in monkeys when the lesion is extended to the inferior lateral surface of the temporal lobe, the part which the previous chapter showed to be involved in identification and recognition of signs (Weiskrantz, 1967). Such monkeys fail to learn discriminations—possibly only because of destruction of the association cortex of the temporal lobe. In monkeys, at least, discrimination learning is not impaired when resection is limited to the medial part of the temporal lobe where the limbic structures (amygdala and hippocampus) are located (Pribram, Douglas, and Pribram, 1969).

short-term memory—
a context sensitive coding mechanism

Keeping in mind that the true story may be otherwise, let us explore the thesis that there is indeed a single brain function basic to both the emotional and the memory processes affected by limbic and frontal lesions. We have already seen that frontal damage does not reduce the occurrence of emotional behavior but only its duration in a frustrating situation. The delayed reaction task also demands a durational response. Could it be simply that frontal (and limbic) resection hastens the fading of memory traces? I tested this hypothesis in the following experiment (Pribram and Tubbs, 1967; Fig. 18 -6). Ordinarily trials are separated by equal intervals (right box, five seconds—left box, five seconds—right box, five seconds—left box, five seconds, etc.) in the delayed alternation task. Instead, I formed couplets: right box, five seconds—left box, 15 seconds—right box, five seconds-left box, 15 seconds, etc. Almost immediately the frontally lesioned monkeys began to perform properly despite the insertion of the long (15 seconds) interval. Thus the hypothesis of a more rapid fading of memory traces was disconfirmed.

The idea for doing the experiment came from a pet example used by Warren McCulloch to demonstrate the power of coding. When words are run together as in the song "Mairsey Dotes and Doesey Dotes" or in the phrases:

INMUDEELSARE
INCLAYNONEARE
INPINETARIS
INOAKNONEIS

it's difficult, if not impossible, to find meaning. But when the proper stops are put in, coding the string of letters into separate chunks, words can immediately be discerned: Mares eat oats; in mud eels are; etc. To the frontally lesioned monkey the alternation task may appear all run together, one response interfering with the next and the one past. Imposing the grouping resolves the difficulty. Orga-

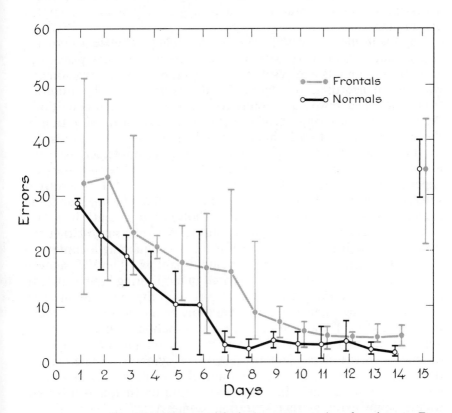

Fig. 18-6. The modified alternation task referred to in Fig. 18-1 which could be mastered readily by monkeys with part of their frontal cortex removed. The brain-damaged monkeys had been unable to solve the standard left-right alternation task even when the interval between trials was only 5 seconds. The task was then modified so that the intervals between trials described the pattern *R* 5 sec. *L* 15 sec. *R* 5 sec. *L* 15 sec. *R* 5 sec. *L* 15 sec. When this change was made, brain-damaged monkeys performed about as well as normal monkeys, as shown here. Performance curves of frontal (upper) and control (lower) groups. Errors are the number made each day before a monkey achieved 40 successful trials. Bars indicate the range of errors made by different monkeys. Data for the 15th day show the result when all the trials were again separated by equal intervals of 5 seconds. From Pribram and Tubbs, 1967.

nizing events into groups is a simple way to provide the context necessary to fundamental forms of coding as well as more complex programing.

Perhaps in man, this propensity to group and organize, to provide and maintain a context within which experience takes place, can grow out-of-bounds and result in disturbances such as obsession and compulsion neuroses. A diminution of this propensity by a limited frontal lobotomy would account for its success in such conditions. Perhaps also the change produced by lobotomy in the duration of the frustration reaction in monkeys and the duration of pain is due to this same change in the ability to impose on experience and maintain some context (see Ornstein, 1969). The post-surgical experience becomes short lived and at the mercy of the current situation. In the clinic the expression *stimulus-bound* has been coined to describe this aspect of the lobotomized patient's behavior.

These observations and experimental results thus suggest that the frontal cortex is involved in providing and maintaining a context, a temporary organization of brain events. Chapters 10 and 15 showed that the limbic formations participated in monitoring brain states. In a sense, the operation of the frontal cortex on the limbic monitoring of states can be likened to the operation of the posterior "association" cortex on the sensory specific functions. Organization is imposed—in the case of the frontal lobe, on monitor-Images to produce context dependent organizations—symbols; in the case of the posterior cortex, on a continuum of perceptual Images to produce context-free signs. In both cases action on Images is involved. Unless some external representation, some Act, is attempted, the operation does not come off.

However, the neural structures involved in the organization of signs are different from those which are involved in symbolic processes. Perceptual and motor *skills* remain intact in spite of frontal and limbic system damage. By contrast, the coding operation taking place in the grouping or chunking of events necessary to solution of the delayed alternation problem depends on just these systems. What then are the neural mechanisms involved?

the self-corrective regulation of behavior

The answer to this question can by no means be final at this time. But some indication of mechanism comes from the interrelation between frontal cortex and limbic systems and from an analysis of what is involved in performing the delayed alternation and delayed reaction tasks. The cue for correct performance on an alternation trial (which is administered with a correction procedure—i.e., the trial is repeated until a correct response has been made) comes from the just completed trial. The monkey must develop a simple strategy that takes into consideration the context established by the immediately preceding experience. In this case a "shift-response" strategy serves him well. Note, however, that the appropriate behavior at any moment depends not on the events occurring in the environment at that moment, but on the context established by the (short-term) memory of the behaving subject. In Chapter 15 we learned that the amygdala and hippocampus of the limbic systems register and value behavior. It is not surprising, therefore, that when these structures are damaged, the organism fails a task in which the correctness of a response depends on having registered (and evaluated) the prior one. In order to develop a context sensitive strategy, a context must at least be established and maintained.

The defective performance of alternation which follows frontal resection must, however, be explained differently. Context becomes established, but the organism doesn't seem to know how to use it. We faced a similar problem in explaining the effects of removal of the posterior "association" cortex. In that case (Bagshaw, Mackworth, and Pribram, 1970b) an eye camera showed that the monkeys normally scanned a figure and could apparently see sensory presentations perfectly well but could not operate on what they sensed.

Patients clearly show this inability to regulate behavior when meaning is sensitive to the context in which the behavior occurs. Clinical observation is replete with stories of inappropriate behavior (e.g., sexual advances made in embarrassing situations—to the expressed discomfort of the patient as well as the other person). Perhaps the most illustrative observation is that of one of Hans-Lukas Teuber's patients (1964) who regularly visisted the laboratory on Thursdays. One Thanksgiving afternoon he set out for the usual visit, saying to himself every step of the way: "Today is Thanksgiving, I should not go to the laboratory, no one is there." The special context of Thanksgiving day, though verbalized, had no effect on his behavior. Only when he reached the laboratory and found no one there did he return home—no wiser than he had been at the outset of his journey.

So much for the alternation task. The frontal deficit which shows up in the classical direct and indirect forms of the delayed reaction task tell us a bit more about the relationship between context sensitivity and short-term memory. In this case, correct performance on a trial depends not on the context set by some prior Act, but on

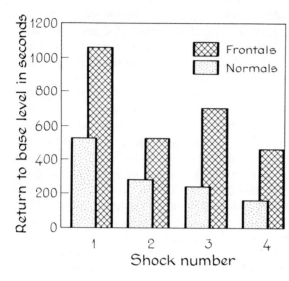

Fig. 18-7. Graph showing time for skin resistance to return to pre-shock level, expressed as group mean return time. From Grueninger, et al., 1965.

the temporary appearance of a discriminative cue which initiates the trial. A great number of experiments have shown that registering this evanescent cue properly, i.e., internalizing it by making some reaction to it, is critical to correct performance (Pribram, 1969c). Of what does proper registration consist? Neurophysiologically, unless some perturbation of the brain's electrical activity is evidenced, an error is made. Just this sort of perturbation indicated orienting and formed the basis for subsequent habituation. And, in fact, the orienting reaction is grossly altered by frontal lesions in both man and monkey (Luria, Pribram, and Homskaya, 1964).

By now we are well acquainted with the fact that there are a number of indicators of the orienting reaction as defined by Sokolov. These include behavioral turning towards the stimulating event; a change in heart and respiratory rate; a GSR; a shift in blood flow from peripheral to central structures (as gauged by finger and temple artery plethysmography); and activation of the EEG. After frontal resection (Fig. 18-7), as after amygdalectomy, only the behavioral and the EEG indicators remain (though the duration of EEG activation is shortened). At the same time, repetition of the event fails to habituate the behavioral response. This, as already detailed, has led to the suggestion that orienting consists of at least two separate processes: an alerting, searching, and sampling component, and a registration in awareness and memory of the events sampled. The frontal cortex and the amygdala influence this process of registration. When registration is impaired, the organism not only fails to recall events, but is much more subject to retroactive and pro-active interference among closely juxtaposed events. Patients and

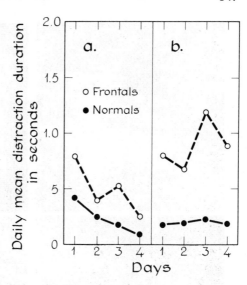

Fig 18-8. Graph showing daily mean distraction duration (mean distraction trial latency minus median latency) for (a) Condition 1–stimulus varied, location constant; (b) Condition 2–location varied, stimulus constant. From Grueninger and Pribram, 1969.

monkeys with frontal lesions show this susceptibility to interference in their short-term memory processes (Grueninger and Pribram, 1969; Fig. 18-8).

Electrophysiological evidence suggests that the frontal cortex normally controls interference through a corticofugal effect on input channels. Electrical stimulation of the frontal cortex produces results opposite to those obtained by stimulation of the posterior "association" cortex (Fig. 18-9). Frontal excitation enhances channel redundancy (recall Figs. 11-6, 11-7); the channel tends to operate, at any moment, all of a piece. Thus, the possibility of interference between successive inputs diminishes. In the experiments performed, the time course of change produced was in milliseconds; retro- and proactive interference in behavioral situations takes a considerably longer time course. Nonetheless, the direction of the electrophysiological effect is suggestive: presumably in behavioral situations in which interference effects are observed, the frontal cortex is "turned on" for a longer period than we were able to do electrophysiologically.

Taken together, these analyses of the delayed alternation and reaction tasks suggest that frontal lobe damage impairs those brain processes in which coding of perturbations of states is an essential element. These processes occur in the operations of short-term memory that involve context-sensitive decisions, rather than in well established context-free operations, and are reflected in both problem solving and in emotional behavior. Viewed prospectively, the defect shows in problem solving: the organism is not able to regulate his behavior on the basis of the perturbing events that signal changes in

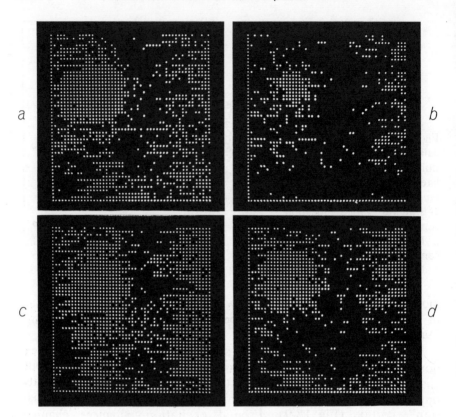

Fig. 18-9. Visual-receptive field maps show how information flowing through the primary visual pathway is altered by stimulation elsewhere in the brain. Map *a* is the normal response of a cell in the geniculate nucleus when a light source is moved through a raster-like pattern. Map *b* shows how the field is contracted by stimulation of the inferior temporal cortex. Map *c* shows the expansion produced by stimulation of the frontal cortex. Map *d* is a final control taken 55 minutes after recording *a*. From Spinelli and Pribram, 1967.

context. Viewed restrospectively, the defect shows in emotional expression: the organism has failed to monitor, register, and evaluate perturbations that continuously complicate context and so add to the troubling present. In the temporal domain this loss of context-sensitive operations is reflected in the fact that the stream of happenings is not segmented and so runs together in a present which is forever, without past or future. The organism becomes completely a monitor at the mercy of his momentary states, instead of an actor on them.

recall and the symbolic process

What remains is the relationship between short-term memory and symbolic processes. Take memory first. The neurological process of memory storage is ordinarily thought to run something like this: an event occurs and is registered in short-term memory where it circulates for a time as a trace in neural loops from which it is finally transferred into a longer term molecular store. The transfer process is called the consolidation of the memory trace. If one is concerned solely with the memory storage process, this picture is not altogether inadequate. We have already noted that habituation probably depends on a feedback loop which decrements neural activity. A number of such loops might well constitute a buffer storage mechanism within the sensory systems. We have also noted that reinforcement may prolong certain neural activities so that chemical changes and even glial and neural growth are induced. Variations on these basic mechanisms would readily account for the evidence obtained in experiments testing the consolidation hypothesis.

But this "storage oriented" way of looking at the memory process does not account for all of the facts of remembering—for recognition and recall. Recognition entails the juxtaposition of input to long-term storage. The juxtaposition can, in many instances, occur immediately without the intervention of short-term memory—which suggests that recognition occurs by a parallel processing, content addressable memory mechanism which can reconstruct the recognized Image even from inputs which only partially replicate those which initially resulted in storage. Recognition is, however, not always so immediate; in more complexly patterned situations, identification may take some time and depend on some slower process of aligning cortical dipoles or the like. This type of recognition resembles most the classical neurophysiological view of the memory process.

But in recall the situation is different still (Fig. 18-10). The stimulating event triggers a short-term memory mechanism which searches memory for a best fit. In the case of recognition there was no real search; a best fit was immediately or very quickly attained through cross-correlation among simultaneously occurring and interfering wave fronts. Recognition is therefore iconic to the stimulating event and not dependent on the context in which it occurs. In recall, on the other hand, the fit engages some arbitrary "associative" contextual relationship: According to the model detailed in Chapter 17, frontal stimulation enhances decrementing and therefore increases the join between memory modules. Large segments of the

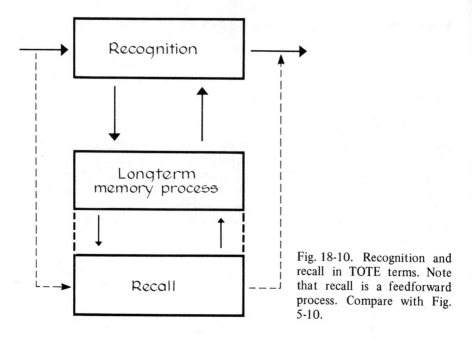

Fig. 18-10. Recognition and recall in TOTE terms. Note that recall is a feedforward process. Compare with Fig. 5-10.

holographic mechanism become involved, the zoom is extended so that attention is focused on one or another detail; attention is concentrated. The extent and location of this increased connectivity among memory modules depends on the past history of those modules, how their alignment has been tuned by the immediately prior (as well as by longer range) experience. The setting of the alignment of dipoles might provide the holographic reference which, when activated by a nonspecific input, initiates, via a feedforward process (Fig. 18-10), the reconstruction of a "ghost" Image previously associated with that reference. Here perhaps we have the key to understanding the role of the frontal cortex in recall and its relationship to symbolic processes.

caring

Chapter 17 suggested that the control over input exerted by the posterior "association" cortex via motor structures provides a mechanism for making Images meaningful. In the current chapter we have reviewed the evidence that this mechanism is shared by the frontolimbic forebrain which often acts reciprocally to the posterior cortex. Thus signs and symbols "intend," make meaning, differently. Signs derive meaning by selective attention to aspects of the Images they signify. Symbols derive meaning by establishing a context within which interests, feelings become organized. Signs intend some part of the World-Out-There; signs signify attributes of that domain. Symbols refer to occurrences in the domain of the organism's World-Within. Symbols express what the organism has registered from his experience and his valuation of that experience— what he is interested in, what he cares about. Caring largely consists of being sensitive and responsive to changes occurring in the communicative context. Caring for someone is not so much doing something, as doing it at the right time in the right place, when needs are felt and communicated. Caring is context-sensitive and, when executed skillfully, leads to gracious communication, to behaving with style. The major effect of frontal lobe surgery is that it makes the patient care less.

So much for the difference between signs and symbols; we turn now to the relationship between them. This relationship concerns human language, the fascinating topic of the next chapter.

synopsis

Symbolic processes appear to be derived from the interaction of motor mechanisms with the brain's frontal cortex and limbic formations. These parts of the cerebrum are characterized by a multiplicity of interconnections, an organization which in computer programing leads to context-sensitive communications. Context-dependent behavior is necessary to the solution of certain problems that involve short-term memory (recall), such as delayed reaction and alternation, and also to a variety of appropriate communicative interpersonal responses usually described as motivational/emotional. The involvement of frontal cortex and limbic formations in both intellectual and emotional communication is therefore attributed to their function in context-dependent processes.

talk and thought

communication and talking

I recently attended a meeting of psychologists who addressed the problem of human learning. Animal psychologists, S-R psychologists, social psychologists, educational psychologists, mathematical psychologists, cognitive psychologists, psycholinguists, and psychophysiologists all had their say. As I was to summarize the contents of the conference, I listened carefully for commonalities among the welter of presented material. A restricted number of problem areas was being explored, but a rich diversity of terms confused and blocked communication among the separate factions of psychologists and resulted in profusion of tongues. Each language system had been developed through experimentation and observation in response to a felt need to explore the psychological universe. The variety of linguistic subcultures resulted more from the variety in the actions taken to resolve the problems, than from variety in problems per se. Thus the conference on human learning proved a microcosm of human learning, a study of how an elite of talking animals uses the linguistic tool.

These observations confirmed some views about language that I had gradually been developing from research in primate behavior and studies of language disabilities in brain injured man. Although these views are far from being finalized, I can now voice and therefore test explicit expressions of the disturbing problems. These problems are among the most critical in science, for on their resolution depends our understanding of how man's humanity has developed and of what it is constituted: man has always, and correctly, felt that "in the beginning was the word."

the paradox of broca's aphasia

　　　　Initially, one of those recurrent paradoxes aroused my interest. I was attempting to make sense of the variety of disturbances of language that result from brain injury. Classifications had been proposed, but these differed from one another not only in the names assigned to the disturbances but in the very basis upon which the classification was made. Further, in clinical practice, some of the most fundamental types of disturbance, agreed to by most of the classifiers, proved to be so rare as to make me question their existence.

The major issue devolved on the occurrence of motor aphasia.

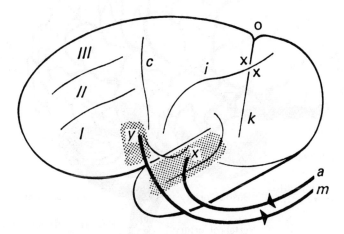

Fig. 19-1. Wernicke's (1880) schema of the cortical mechanism of speech. *c* central sulcus; *i* interparietal fissure; *o* parietal-occipital fissure; *k* anterior occipital fissure; *I-III* first to third frontal convolutions; *xx* transitional gyri; *x* sensory speech centre; *y* motor speech centre; *xy* association tract between the two speech centres; *ax* auditory tract; *ym* tract to the speech muscles. From Freud, 1953.

Early in the history of neurology (i.e., a hundred years ago) disturbances of language that were related to the input of signals to the brain were distinguished from those that were related to output. Input disturbances were called "sensory," "receptive," or "Wernicke's aphasia"; output disturbances of speech were called "motor," "expressive," or "Broca's aphasia." Carl Wernicke (1886) located the lesion producing receptive aphasia in the posterior superior part of the temporal lobe of the brain; Pierre-Paul Broca (1861) placed the lesion producing expressive aphasia in the posterior inferior part of the frontal cortex (Fig. 19-1). During the past century accumulated evidence has shown that damage in the posterior superior temporal cortex produces language disturbances ranging from an inability to name objects to severe disabilities which disrupt the entire linguistic process. During this same century, the support of Broca's localization, and indeed of even the occurrence of Broca's aphasia has been equivocal.

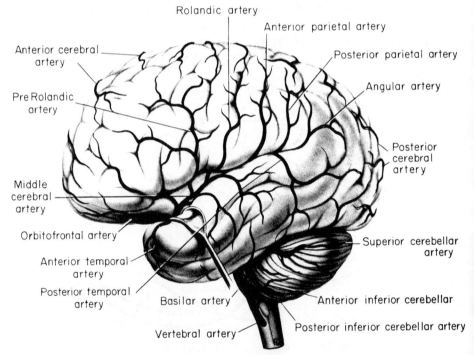

Fig. 19-2. Principal arteries on the lateral surface of the cerebrum and cerebellum. Note placement of middle cerebral artery within Sylvian fissure and the extent of its branchings. From Truex and Carpenter, *Human Neuroanatomy,* 6 ed. © 1969. The Williams & Wilkins Co., Baltimore, Md.

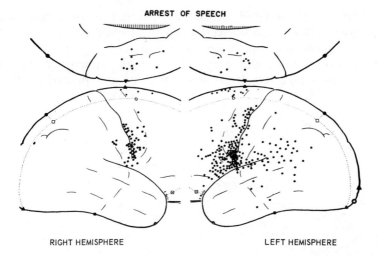

ARREST OF SPEECH

RIGHT HEMISPHERE   LEFT HEMISPHERE

Fig. 19-3. Arrest, hesitation, slurring, distortion, and repetition of speech was obtained with stimulation in the lower Rolandic motor cortex extending forward to Broca's area of the left hemisphere and to the supplementary motor areas on medial surface of both hemispheres; such responses are also obtained from stimulation of the posterior temporo-parietal region of the left hemisphere. From Roberts, 1961.

Patients who had articulatory disturbances associated with posterior inferior frontal lesions were easily identified. Some could write what they could not speak; others could neither speak nor write; and occasionally a patient could not write (agraphia) but could talk readily. Often these motor disturbances would be associated with a more profound language disability, but more often they were associated with a general mental deterioration shown by confusions of orientation in space and time.

I wondered therefore, as had others before me, just what constellation of disabilities Broca had encountered in his early localization attempt. His original descriptions convinced me that he had, in fact, observed language impairments—not just articulatory disturbances. What also came clear, however, was that his reference to the posterior inferior frontal cortex was largely accidental. Broca's patients had suffered strokes which involved the middle cerebral artery, which supplies the territory around the Sylvian fissure of the brain (Fig. 19-2). Broca had been taught that language was a function of the frontal lobes: his teachers derived their doctrine from the phrenologists who had reasoned that man's high forehead and his linguistic ability were two of his most distinguishing features; ergo they might well be related. Broca reasoned that the only place where his aphasic patient's lesion overlapped the frontal cortex was in the posterior inferior portion. Hence Broca's area.

Support for Broca's reasoning came from experiments on monkeys and men in which electrical excitation of the posterior inferior

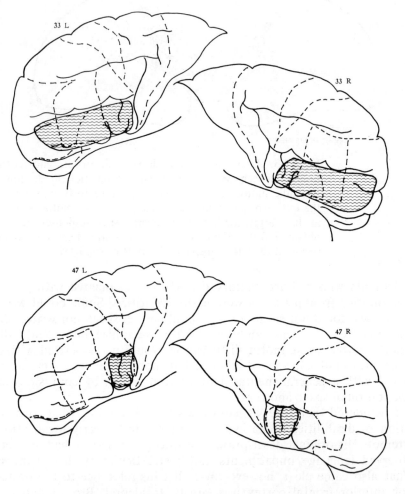

Fig. 19-4. Diagrams of frontal cortex of two patients showing bilateral removal of the inferior frontal convolution which contains (on the left) removal of Broca's area. No marked disturbances of speech resulted. One resection extends forward to include entire inferior frontal gyrus. Compare with Fig. 18-4 which shows that site of entry of leukotome in classical lobotomy procedure traversed Broca's area. From Pool, et al., 1949.

frontal cortex produced tongue movement and, in man, the arrest of ongoing speech (Fig. 19-3). Such support, though indirect, hindered the appreciation of other, contradictory evidence.

Evidence against Broca's claim is simply that excision of Broca's area in man's brain, and damage to this area, has been inflicted without causing any severe linguistic disturbance. The story begins with the psychosurgical procedure of frontal lobotomy, or leuko-tomy as it was called in Europe. Well over 10,000 lobotomies were performed during the 1940s and 1950s, most of them according to a technique popularized by Freeman and Watts (recall Fig. 18-4). Mettler and Rowland (1948) wanted to know precisely what part of the brain was isolated by the procedure, and so in a carefully performed series of studies they marked the skulls and brains of a hundred cadavers used in anatomical laboratories for the teaching of medical students. The markings were made according to the directions given by Freeman and Watts. The markings fell directly over the posterior inferior frontal cortex which, on the left side of the brain, is Broca's area. Presumably therefore all of the lobotomies performed for psychosurgical reasons injured Broca's area to some extent. Yet not a single report of aphasia due to lobotomy occurred.

Mettler was encouraged by his finding to plan, as part of an experimental psychosurgical project, the selective removal (topec-tomy) of Broca's area and its mate in the opposite hemisphere in catatonic patients who had not talked for more than twenty years. Two such patients were operated upon, and, apart from some tran-sient articulatory disturbance (dysarthria), these patients began to talk and continued for years to talk fluently (Fig. 19-4).

The results of these studies proved that an intact Broca's area, the base of the third frontal convolution in man, is not necessary for normal speech. It is still possible, however, that a malfunctioning, damaged Broca's area can disrupt normal speech—the next section pursues the evidence that this could be so.

language disruptions by brain damage

Aphasics have more recently been examined with quantitative psychological testing techniques. Such tests can generate profiles of the disturbances and this innovation has renewed the effort to describe the variety of aphasic disabilities. Despite the refinement of techniques, however, the students of aphasia continue to polarize into those who claim a unitary deficit due to a lesion in the posterior part of the temporal lobe, and those who suspect that the lesions responsible are as various as the disturbances, and extend over the reach of the brain's lateral surface.

I was exposed to the evidence for the multiple determination of language disabilities at the Moscow neurosurgical hospital in the clinic of Alexander Romanovitch Luria (1964). I examined patients who had difficulty in naming objects but who showed no other language disability; other patients had difficulty with sentence structure but could name readily; still other patients mixed up the syllables within words, though they made grammatically correct sentences and indicated the names of objects reasonably well. Obviously, all aphasics were not alike.

I continued to puzzle over this dilemma between the unitary and the multiple views of language disturbances caused by brain injury, called conferences on the subject, visited clinics, and talked in depth with the proponents of each position. My conclusion has been that the facts are not as disparate as are the descriptions and systems that have been built on the facts. What seems to divide the interpretations is a definition of what constitutes language and the uses language is believed to serve.

The proponents of the unitary view base their interpretation on the communicative aspects of language—language is a system of signs and symbols by which the organism can communicate his conception of the world and his feelings about himself. The proponents of the multiple view, on the other hand, are interested not only in the communicative use of language but also in linguistic structure and the *varieties* of uses to which language is put (see Fig. 19-5). The examiner of the unitary view tries, as a rule, to find out how well the patient understands what is going on around him and whether the examiner understands what the patient is trying to tell him. The examiner with the multiple view approaches the patient to find out whether the *form* of linguistic use is disturbed, not whether the disturbed form is still useful.

Given this insight into the differences in approaches and biases of the investigators, the facts they had gathered come in clearer perspective. All investigators agree that damage to the posterior superior temporal cortex of the dominant hemisphere results in a communicative disability in the use of language. When the lesion extends anteriorly from this locus, the disability tends to be more expressive; when the lesion extends posteriorly, the disability is more profound, i.e., the patient appears not only to have difficulty in expressing himself but also appears to be confused as to what is to be expressed. Further differences in sensory and motor modality depend on the direction of extension of the lesion. A posterior inferior extension will likely damage the visual mode to produce reading difficulties (alexia); a posterior superior extension into the parietal cortex will

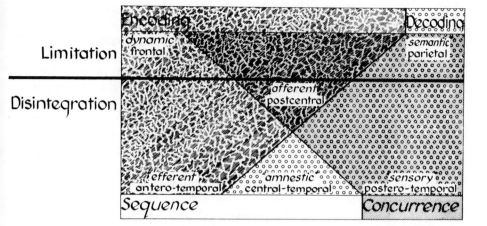

Fig. 19-5. The linguistic dimensions underlying six forms of aphasia. This diagram resulted from extensive discussions between Roman Jakobson, Alexander Romanovitch Luria, and myself. Two major linguistic axes were distinguished: one extending posterior-frontally in the brain which serves a decoding-encoding dimension; the other extending dorso-lateral-mediobasally in the brain which serves a simultaneity (concurrence)-successivity (sequence) dimension. In addition two forms of language disturbance lying beyond the confines of cortex surrounding the Sylvian fissure were identified: frontal lesions result in the loss of verbal control over behavior and posterior parietal lesions result in semantic disturbance akin to the agnosias. From Jakobson, 1964.

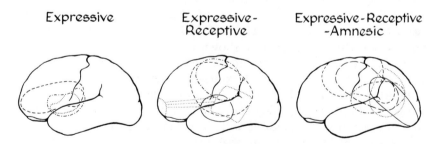

Fig. 19-6. Cranial defects in 12 cases with marked aphasia. All lesions are in the left hemisphere. The complexity of aphasic disorders tends to be greater with lesions involving posterior portions of the dominant hemisphere. From Teuber, 1964.

likely impair semantic relationships in language, especially those which involve the somatic mode such as pointing, touching, pushing, and pulling. An anterior superior lesion will likely result in agraphia because of involvement of the hand representation of the motor cortex; an anterior inferior lesion will likely result in dysarthria because of involvement of the tongue representation. But the important consideration is that this "language field" of the brain is a fairly large area of cortex, fed by the middle cerebral artery, in which the representations of the ear, throat, tongue, and mouth overlap. Within this cortical field a great deal of the machinery of human verbal communication becomes represented, and therefore malfunction resulting from partial damage produces disability in such communication (Fig. 19-6).

But there is more to the problem of language. As we saw in the previous two chapters, nonhuman primates can communicate about the world around them and about their world within by primitive signs and symbols. But linguistic structure remains undeveloped in nonhuman primates. Therefore the question arises: what changes have taken place that make man's brain human, i.e., that make possible language systems as we know them? A corollary question asks why the human use of language is such a powerful tool in the adaptation and advancement of mankind. The next sections examine these questions.

against association by cortico-cortical connections

The common answer to the question of what makes man's brain "human" is that its cortex establishes associations more readily than does nonhuman cortex. This answer stems from an empiricist tradition and the tracing of large bundles of nerve fibers which interconnect various areas of the brain. Three facts stand against this common view. The first derives from the experiments on nonhuman primates that have shown the primary functional connections of the cerebral cortex to be subcortical rather than cortico-cortical. This result may, of course, be limited to the brains of nonhuman primates—if cortico-cortical connections *are* found to be critical to human psychological processes, the major change in brain that makes humanity possible will have been identified.

The road of inquiry will probably not prove that straightforward, however. Other arguments speak against the association fiber hypothesis of brain function and the disconnection hypothesis of dysfunction. I have made a case throughout this book for the existence of holographic transformations as one way by which the nervous system codes and recodes its signals. One of the attributes of holograms is

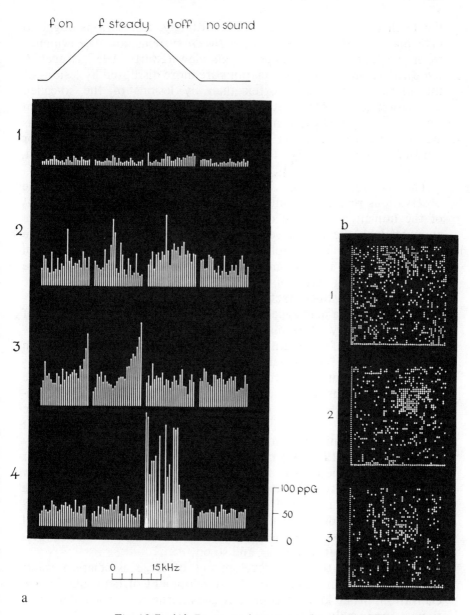

f on   f steady   f off   no sound

1

2

3

4

100 ppG
50
0

0   15 kHz

a

b

1

2

3

Fig. 19-7. (A) Response histograms from four different units in *visual* cortex sensitive to modulated *auditory* frequencies. Increased firing rates can be seen to specific aspects of the stimulus in units 2, 3, and 4. (B) The visual receptive fields of units 2, 3, and 4 of (A). X-axis and y-axis are equal to 25° of visual angle. The visual axis falls approximately at the center of the display. From Spinelli, Starr, and Barrett, 1968.

the facility in associative recall. Accordingly, associations ought to take place *within* a system, not *between* systems, and the evidence from monkeys at least supports this view (Evarts, 1952; Wegener, 1968). Even intermodal associations are more disrupted by lesions of the primary projection cortex than by lesions of the so-called association areas. Also, neurophysiological evidence obtained from single neurons shows that many units in the primary projection areas are sensitive to excitation in a modality different from the major sensory mode served by that system (Spinelli, Starr, and Barrett, 1968; Fig. 19-7).

The second, and more direct line of evidence comes from the observations regarding hemispheric specificity in man. The two sides of the human brain serve different functions even though they are connected by the largest set of associative fibers in the brain, the corpus callosum. This cerebral commissure is considerably larger in man than it is in nonhuman primates. Sperry and his colleagues have performed a long series of experiments designed to investigate the functions of this fiber tract by cutting it, thus severing the connections between the hemispheres, which then operate independently of each other (Sperry, Gazzaniga, and Bogen, 1969; Figs. 19-8, 19-9).

Prior evidence from brain damaged patients had established that in most people one hemisphere governs language, the other regulates nonverbal perceptual performances (Milner, 1954). Usually the language functions are managed by the left hemisphere which controls the right side of the body. Since the majority of people are right-handed, the left hemisphere is, in them, called the dominant hemisphere. Monkeys and apes also show some rudimentary dominances, but these are not generalized to as many situations nor to as many functions as in man. Left-handed persons may also show divided dominances—despite their left-handedness, their language abilities may be regulated by the left hemisphere. Even in right-handed people, dominance may be dissociated; writing and ball pitching may best be done with different hands, right-handedness may accompany left-eyedness, and so on.

It seems odd that the development of large association tracts should go hand in hand with the development of hemispheric specialization. What kind of connectivity is it that rends asunder functions it supposedly associates?

This question has not been asked until now. My own answer is that perhaps the connections, rather than functioning to associate, tend to separate through suppression the various parts of cerebral mantle. Clinical documentation shows that during simultaneous excitation of two points on receptor surfaces, one point dominates,

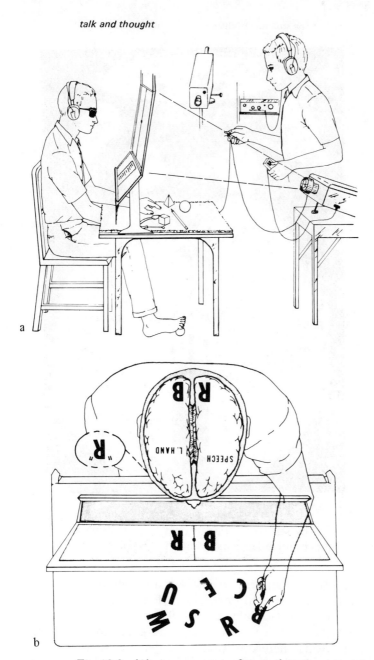

Fig. 19-8. (A) Arrangement of general testing apparatus used in demonstrating commissurotomy symptoms. (B) Manual identification of stimuli in left visual field is successful with left hand although subject is unable to name the object. From Sperry, 1970.

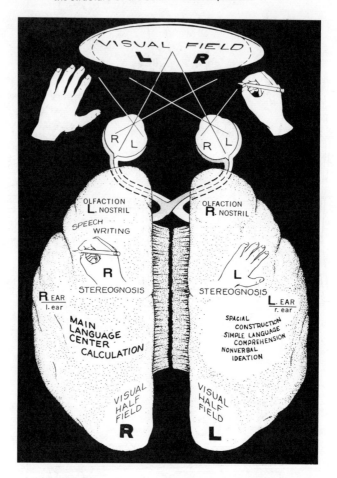

Fig. 19-9. Scheme of functional lateralization demonstrated by separate testing of right and left hemispheres after section of forebrain commissures. From Sperry, 1970.

while the other is suppressed (Teuber and Bender; 1951). Also, the behavioral deficits that follow lesions of some parts of the brain, e.g., the frontal eye fields (Kennard, 1939) or the visual cortex (Sprague, 1966), disappear when additional lesions are made in appropriate sites. It is clear, therefore, that an imbalance of function has been caused by the initial insult to the brain, an imbalance that results in the suppression of a function. Inhibitory processes are most likely responsible, though little is known of how the mechanism actually works. The hypothesis that is suggested states that cortical dominance is due to a similar inhibitory suppressive mechanism.

Although many of the results of the split brain experiments are readily explained by a mechanism of simple transfer of memory traces across the corpus callosum, other more complicated results demand a more sophisticated explanation. Perhaps the suppression hypothesis will be able to serve usefully in bringing these puzzling exceptions into line when sufficient data are available. In any case, the proponents of cortico-cortical association via fiber tracts must explain the paradox that greater connectivity and greater specialization arise together. That this should be so makes sense; how it can be accomplished is not so easy to detail.

The third line of evidence that makes me suspect the association-by-fiber-tracts view of the language mechanism comes from studies in verbal learning. Several investigators in this area, independent of physiological evidence, have come to view storage of an event not so much as the result of making a bond or strengthening that bond, as the production of a distribution of representations of that event and thus an increase in the probability that it will be selected over other coded representations (e.g., see Voss, 1969, p. 99; and Tulving, 1970). Fiber tracts may well help to distribute representations, though they may not be essential to the reduplicating process. But conceiving fiber tracts as mechanisms of distribution is not the same as conceiving them to make associative bonds, even though associations may be enhanced by virtue of the distribution.

the linguistic act

What alternative, then, can account for the immense difference in the languages of nonhuman primates and those of man? I believe a clue to such an alternative comes from the aphasia studies. In man, the mechanisms whereby signs and symbols are produced somehow merge into one linguistic device, but this is not necessarily the result of associating sign and symbol with each other. Rather a new mechanism is evolved which allows signs to function as linguistic symbols and symbols as linguistic signs.

Let me review briefly the distinction between sign and symbol as set forth in the earlier chapters. Signs are representations that refer to the consistent attributes of the world of the senses. Signs are thus context-free constructions that take meaning through action on that world, classifying, categorizing, and even naming its existences. On the other hand, symbols are representations that refer to the world within the organism. The symbols are produced, just as are signs, through action, but it is the remembrance of the effect of the action that produces the symbol. Symbols thus are context-sensitive constructions that take meaning from the history of their use and the current state of the organism using them.

Signs and symbols are thus Acts, environmental representations produced by the organism. Any increase in the capacity to act would therefore be reflected in an increase in significant and symbolic behavior. I believe that sign and symbol come together in man as a corollary of his demonstrated increased capabilities for action. But, as we have seen, these capabilities are so intertwined with the capabilities to image (especially to construct Images-of-Achievement) that it is probably better to formulate the issue in terms of greater capacity to make any sort of coded representations. Stated in this way the problem becomes a tautology: man's capacity for language is due to the capacity of man's brain for making coded representations, i.e., language.

Tautologies are often good starting points for inquiry. Let us examine the structure of man's language to see what it requires of the structure of man's brain.

Man's languages have two primary characteristics: they provide a prolongation of reference (Bronowski, 1967) and they are productive (Jakobson, 1964, 1966). Both characteristics appear in primordial form in the signs and symbols of nonhuman primates, but the extent to which they are developed in man is hardly foreshadowed by these rudiments. Even a retarded child will spin sentences before he is a few years old that are so far beyond the nonhuman level that he can be easily identified as a member of the genus homo by this action alone.

A child begins communicating, just as does the nonhuman primate, with what are called holophrases—single utterances signifying something or symbolizing some state. Although linguists have not classified holophrases in this fashion, my own observations show that holophrases are of two kinds: more or less continuous grunts, coos, and explicatives which refer to the baby's internal state, and shorter repetitive syllable-like sounds often accompanied by directive gestures that indicate something about the world the baby sees, hears, touches, or tastes.

Around the age of two years the holophrases become more precise and their referent more readily distinguishable until couplings of holophrases occur. Such couplings—and later strings—are also observed in chimpanzee utterances. But the child quickly goes on to make propositions, which, at the time this book is written, has not been observed in ape communication.

Propositions or sentences develop around a function called *pre-*

dication by linguists. Predication implies another function, that of nominalization or noun formation. The line of development from signs as they were described in Chapter 17 to nouns (or deictic signs) as found in human utterances seems to be straightforward. Verbs, such as "run," "catch," "flow," and other parts of speech, such as adjectives and adverbs, give somewhat more trouble until one realizes that they also describe existences and occurrences and are therefore forms of nominalization. In a sense such verbs are names for actions rather than things; the adjectives and adverbs are names for attributes—and the difference lies in the number of transformations over which things, attributes, and actions remain invariant.

Predication is, however, premised on more than existence and occurrence. Predication makes a statement about beliefs, the truth or falsity of ongoings which take the form of propositions, the rules which proclaim the is-so and the is-not of such beliefs. "Black-sand-water" is a string of holophrastic-like utterances which a chimpanzee might make pointing to a beach in Hawaii. I would understand him. A child would say: "Look, the sand *is* black *next to* the water." He expresses an assurance, a belief. He would be very upset if you explained to him that he is subject to an illusion caused by heating of the air over the asphalt landing strip. But it would be foolhardy to try to communicate the difference between propositions "the sand is black next to the water" and "the illusion of water is produced on asphalt by heat" to a chimpanzee.

In other words, predication is premised on what in Chapter 18 I called symbolization. Predication is an expression by the human organism that to him, at this time, in these circumstances, this is the way it is (or is not). According to this view, predication derives from a productive context-sensitive process, a logical operation that groups beliefs in terms of equilibrations and disequilibrations of the monitor functions of the brain. Some groupings are right (yes), other wrong (no). And sometimes the grouping becomes rather complicated before it feels right.

Nominalization derived from signing provides the extended context-free referent in human language: "purple," "people," "eaters" for example. Predication derived from symbolizing (and utilizing nominalization) gives human language its productivity: the variations of groupings (eaters of purple people or purple people who are eaters?) that can feel right could be almost infinite.

The brain mechanisms that participate in the production of both signs and symbols are, as we have seen, the action systems. Here is the alternative to cortico-cortical associations through fiber connec-

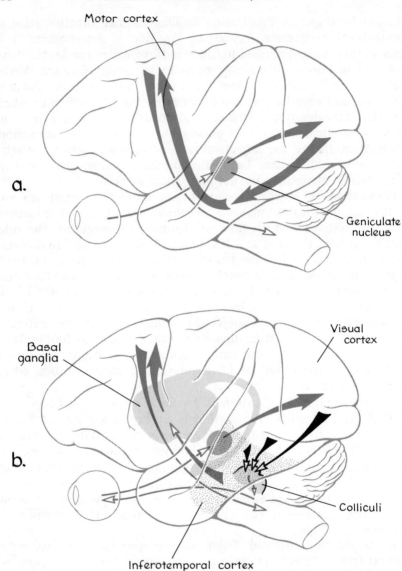

Fig. 19-10. Comparison of classical (upper figure) and proposed (lower figure) mechanism by which "association" cortex
functions. Classical view emphasizes transcortical connections
leading from primary sensory areas through association areas
to motor cortex. Proposed mechanism emphasizes cortico-
subcortical connections of "association" areas with basal
ganglia and other *sub*cortical motor structures.

tions. In fact, here the motor mechanisms of the brain may well be responsible—especially that part of the sensory-motor cortex where the representations of Images-of-Achievement of the vocal apparatus are engendered, since this cortex overlaps so extensively the apparatus in which auditory images are formed. The increase in the size of the posterior superior temporal cortex (and adjacent angular gyrus) in man can also be attributed as readily to an enhancement of their subcortical motor connections as to any augmentation of associative processes (recall Fig. 17-10). This central-motor interpretation would, of course, fit the data obtained for nonhuman primates; the associative interpretation would not. But considerably more research on man's brain, now ethically possible with implanted electrodes in selected clinical situations, is necessary before definitive answers to these alternatives will be available (Fig. 19-10).

A final word, however, about this central-motor theory of the origins of human language. If indeed it is only through action, an effect on environment (in this case other brains), that the significant and symbolic processes of language are brought together, an explanation is at hand for both the multiplicity of the forms of languages and for the fact that an infant in isolation does not give form to any language. Only by action on other like brains can the human potential be realized. Communicative action thus considered becomes the root rather than the fruit of language.

What then is the fruit of man's language? As noted, powerful communication is possible with holophrases and by nonverbal, gestural means. And communicative action is necessary for human languages to develop. But the example of the conference given at the outset of this chapter reminds us that communication is as often blocked by the development of language systems as it is enhanced—yet man goes right on talking. If not communication, what has been the evident adaptive function of this productivity achieved through predication, of this extension in referent achieved through nominalization?

the linguistic and holographic aspects of thinking

Man uses language as a tool to accomplish his purposes. Often his purpose is to merely express his existence. At other times he uses language in an effort to obtain information from or to achieve control over his environment. On still other occasions he uses language to explore and achieve control over his World-Within.

Whenever language is used in this last, internal fashion, it becomes thought. Thinking is not, however, solely a linguistic enterprise. Thinking derives from prolongations of states of active uncertainty which can be resolved only when the Images involved are reconciled. Sometimes these imaginal resolutions are overt, as in Kekule's discovery of the hexagonal structure of the benzene ring, a musician's twists of tonal phrases, or a painter's play with colors. More often, however, the nonlinguistic aspects of thought are implicit, partly because verbal communication can be much more explicit.

My hypothesis is that *all* thinking has, in addition to sign and symbol manipulation, a holographic component. Holographic representations are excellent associative mechanisms; they powerfully and instantaneously perform cross-correlations. These are the very properties that have been attributed to thought in the problem solving process—the difficulty has been to make explicit the neural mechanism involved. Both this difficulty and the ubiquitous use by the brain of holographic transformations stem from another attribute: holograms are composed by transformations which, when they are simply repeated, essentially reconstruct the original from which the holographic representation was composed. Holograms are the "catalysts of thought." Though they remain unchanged, they enter into and facilitate the thought process.

According to this view, thought is a search through the distributed holographic memory for resolution of uncertainty, i.e., for acquisition of relevant information. This formulation is inadequate, however, unless the term *relevant information* includes appropriate configurations as well as items or bits in the information-theoretic sense. More often than not, when problems generate thought, contextual and configurational matchings are sought, not just specific items of information. These matchings, I believe, can occur best while the coding operation is in its holographic mode. Perhaps the power of thought in problem solving resides in the repeated return to the configurational form of representation that serves a rehearsal function and allows the occurrence of additional distributions in memory. Some of these distributions will, because of correlations with brain states different from the initial one, become imbedded in new representations. They thus become available, when properly triggered, as new possibilities in problem solving.

We are now faced with the two-part question of how problems become actively engaged, and how their resolution is recognized or abandoned. Investigating this question, I experimented to learn something about the neural mechanisms of thought. Brain operated monkeys were placed in a problem solving situation (Pribram, 1959; Figs. 19-11, 19-12). The monkeys had to develop two strategies in

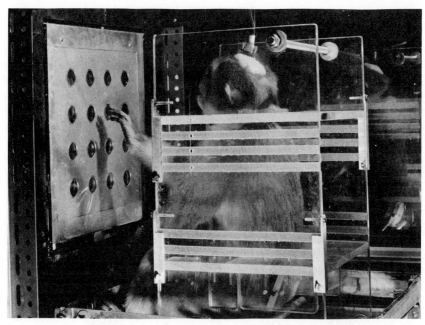

Fig. 19-11. Photograph of monkey performing in Discrimination Apparatus for Discrete Trial Analysis (DADTA). The control and data analysis portion of DADTA system, a general purpose computer (PDP-8) programs stimulus presentation, records behavioral and electrophysiological results on magnetic tape, and provides typed or oscilloscope display readouts. Simple collations of data are performed on-line. More complex analyses are performed on taped data-store.

order to meet the test specification, i.e., to pick out its invariant properties. One strategy involved searching the situation until a peanut was found; the other strategy involved sticking to the choice which had brought the reward. Monkeys with posterior cortex lesions were unable to search successfully; monkeys with frontal lesions failed to stick to their choices. Two aspects of thinking were thus delineated: one concerns the recognition of, the other the tolerance for a problem. The distinction resembles the one made in decision theoretical formulations between signal detection and response bias, between input related and criterion effects. Thought, as search, is initiated (by the posterior mechanism of the brain) when a mismatch between input and memory is not resolved through action. Thought is maintained (by the frontolimbic mechanism) until a more or less preset criterion for what is considered a match is met.

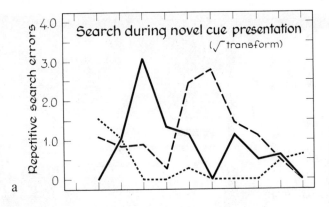

a

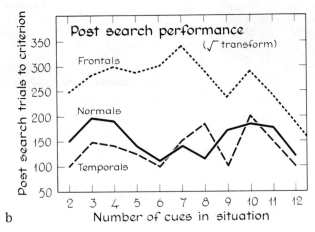

b

Fig. 19-12. (A) Graph of the average of the number of repetitive errors made in the multiple choice experiment during the search trials when the novel cue is presented. Search trials are those anteceding the first "correct" response in a succession of trials, i.e., those anteceding the movement of the object (cue) under which a peanut has been placed. Note that although records of the control and inferotemporal groups show peaks that indicate confusion between novel and familiar cues, the monkeys with frontal lesions are not confused. (B) Graph of the average of the number of trials to criterion taken in the multiple object experiment by each of the groups in each of the situations after search was completed, i.e., after the first correct response. Note the difference between the curves for controls and for the frontally operated group. From Pribram, 1967.

thought, interest, and reason

This description of the thought process recalls the descriptions given of interest in Chapter 11. Recognition of a "problem" is comparable to the recognition of any other feeling state. Thought, like interest, is defined as the recourse to internal mechanisms to achieve control over that state. What then is the difference between thought and interest?

Interest demands for its maintenance some sensory receptor excitation consonant with the emotional/motivational aroused state—something or someone in the World-Out-There in which or in whom to be interested. Thought, by contrast, becomes self contained, part of the World-Within. A common distinction is made between communication guided by interest and that guided by thought. When interest is manifest the resulting communication has the feeling of immediacy; when thought through, the communication becomes reasoned. This distinction is often interpreted to mean that thought is determined by rules but that motivational/emotional interest, the appetites and affects are not. Clinical experience, codified initially by Sigmund Freud (1954), has shown, however, that emotional and motivational interests are as lawfully determined as is reasoned thought. Further, reasoned thinking can be dysrational, i.e., deluded, inappropriate, unproductively repetitive, etc., whereas a direct approach to a situation, especially a complex situation, can often show a greater creative yield than does problem solution through reasoning (perhaps because the direct approach has more opportunity for Imaged correlation among fundamental attributes of the problem).

This is not to be taken as pejorative of reasoned thought, however. It is, of course, in reasoned thought that language plays such an important role. This role is caused in part by the ease of communicability of language, in part by its precision. But perhaps most important is the fantastic flexibility which arises when symbols are used linguistically to signify and when signs become linguistically symbolic. In essence, the symbolic use of signs is speech; the significant use of symbols constitutes thought. Through thoughtful reasoned speech man begins to regulate his affairs—and achieves a new level of communication. Through the operation of the means-ends reversal this new level not only leads a life of its own but replicates. The cultural, sociobiological laws of reproduction may well resemble those operating in the reproduction of individuals. We have already encountered a parallel between those processes governing induction and those governing reinforcement. Others have talked of social homeostasis (Cannon, 1941) and of societal life as a cognitive process (Lorenz, 1969). Will biological laws of such compass really be found ubiquitous? Before we can seek laws, however, we have to examine the assumptions upon which the search will be conducted. The final chapter explores these assumptions.

synopsis

Man's brain brings sign and symbol together in propositional language. Evidence from language disturbances produced by brain lesions and stimulation suggests that linguistic Acts derive from the operations of a multifaceted cortico-subcortical system in which junctional patterns derived from sensory input have unusually ready access, through an overlap of connections, to those involved in motor mechanisms. The existence of this brain system makes possible propositions: communications about the truth, the symbolic rightness or wrongness, of significant perceptions. The accrual of such propositional communications constitutes a human language.

the regulation of
human affairs

culture as language

Some years ago in the Hamilton station of the laboratories at Bar Harbor, Maine, John Calhoun (1956) performed an interesting experiment on the development of a culture. His subjects were two separate inbred biological strains of mice. One strain inhabited terraced apartments constructed of earth and herbaceous debris. Socially dominant mice maintained penthouses, the hoi polloi lived below. The second strain of Calhoun's mice was nomadic. They dug small burrows to come in from the rain and cold, moved on when these became soiled or otherwise unusable. Calhoun asked the question: Is apartment construction and habitation an inborn trait, or is this complex social organization culturally transmitted? To answer the question he took newborn infants from each strain and cross-fostered them by the mother of the opposite strain. Exchanging newborns between strains was not in itself sufficient, however, to answer the question. Sets of cross-fostered infants had to be separated from parental influence at weaning and raised so that communication would occur only with unacculturated cross-fostered

375

others. Colonies of offspring of these cross-fostered strains were thus founded, with the strains kept carefully separated. Biology took its course and many generations of offspring mice were observed.

The result of the experiment dramatically demonstrated the nature-nurture relationship. Cross-fostered mice of the apartment dwelling strain did not immediately build apartments. The first and even the second generation social interactions were hardly distinguishable from the apparently unstructured relationships of the cross-fostered nomads. Calhoun noted one small difference, however. Nomadic mice distributed the dirt of their digging helter skelter. Apartment mice made neat piles of such diggings. In fact, over successive generations, the piles became somewhat taller and provided small hills for dominance play and struggle.

To make a long story short, after some 15–20 generations the apartment mice had completely reestablished the apartment culture; nomads remained levellers both architecturally and socially. The genetic primordium for the apartment culture consisted of hillock construction from diggings. The full blown complexity of the culture became actualized only after generations of transmitted cultural achievement.

In Chapter 3 we discussed the problem of constructing codes, the transformations involved, and the power gained by alternative representations of occurrences. We also detailed how the more complex codes are based on the simpler ones, how programing languages are gradually achieved once rudimentary codes (assemblers and compilers) are available.

Cultures can be thought of as nonverbal languages. They have significant and symbolic aspects, and human cultures display grammatical constructions. The rudiments of cultural languages just as of verbal languages are Acts achieved by the brain. This book has been concerned with the psychological functions that beget achievement and the communicative processes that nourish them until they truly become languages.

The brain is the instrument that accomplishes all this and so one is tempted to identify the cultural-linguistic accomplishment with the brain. In a sense such identity is admissible. Calhoun's apartments devolved from the structure of DNA in a strain of mice; without their special brains these mice would not develop the apartment culture. The accomplishment is, in a sense, already contained in the mouse brain and in his DNA.

Yet this simple identity statement leaves one vaguely dissatisfied. In fact, most statements of the nature-nurture issue, what we are now talking about, leave too much unsaid. The brain, because of its capacity for recording and remembering experience, is the obvious bridge—but another problem is immediately encountered. Man's language allows him to talk about himself, and the talk is often phrased in terms of man's "mind." What then is the relationship between language, brain, and mind? In this final chapter, let us explore this fascinating problem upon which man's view of man is ultimately based.

the languages of brain, behavior, and mind

Modern views of the mind-body problem stem from the time of Descartes. Essentially two views are held, and each has several modifications. These views are (1) the identity position already alluded to and its derivative, the pluralistic view espoused in its most sophisticated form by critical philosophers; and (2) the dualistic position sponsored by Descartes. Each position is logically defensible and sheds some light on the mind-body problem. I will maintain, however, that each is incomplete, and will propose an alternative, different in its content and aim. I will call this alternative the Biologist view of the problem. But first let us briefly review some of the arguments made by the classical theories.

Identity theory regards mental phenomena and brain events as identical. As already noted, an extension of this view identifies mind with the genetic potential inherent in cytoplasm. Many philosophers immersed in the Anglo-American tradition for the most part espouse this position, pointing out that the language we use to describe events may be derived from physiological or behavioral observations or from social communication about introspective evidence. Each language, however, deals with the same basic "event-structure" but approaches it from its own aspect. A plurality of aspects can thus portray the basic identity. Although some philosophers who espouse this view would never directly admit it, the identity referred to by these aspects must be either "real" or "ideal" in the Platonic sense. If "real," experiments and observations should disclose the commonalities indicated by the aspects. This is, in fact, what we as scientists try to do. However, as we have found out from the brain studies detailed in these chapters, what is "real" has to be constructed by the brain's control over the sensory process. "Reality" as a construction is thus not altogether different from another construction which we might call "ideal" just because of the level of abstraction attained. But Willard v.O. Quine (1960) has shown clearly, constructions are languages and languages are to some extent mutually untranslatable. The dilemma of the identity theorist is therefore that he can never reach that which is assumed identical without construction which entails an additional language, an additional aspect which, though it may subsume others, can never become itself identical with them. The identity theorist thus ends up as a pluralist, and identity remains an unachieved goal. Identity theory is not totally wrong; it just cannot satisfy except as a *belief* that a monistic explanation is worth striving for.

the world of languages

Dualistic theory does not fare much better. Since Descartes, an emphasis has been placed on the distinction between the phenomenon subjectively experienced and the objective world which can be instrumentally validated. Dualism points up an important distinction. There is a difference between the subjective and the objective constructions we experience, a difference between the "phenomenal" and the "real" world. The difference lies in how each is validated. Empiricists have emphasized that we perceive the world through our senses. Empirical studies augment these perceptions through instrumentation that refines the senses. We construct the physical, the "real" world from detailed descriptions fed to our senses, from information about the world. The phenomenal "ideal" world, on the other hand, is a world of ideas. We validate experience in this world through social communication, through enactment, through communicative acts. In science this distinction between real and phenomenal becomes externalized in a distinction between descriptive and normative, between more or less certain facts and those which are completely dependent on convention. A systems approach such as the one taken in this book provides an understanding for the way in which the distinction has come about and its usefulness. On another occasion I discussed this topic as follows:

I believe that... the behavioral, biological-social scientist interested in the mind-body problem finds his universe to be a mirror image of the universe constructed by the physical scientist who deals with the same problem. And it should not come as a surprise when each of these isomers, the one produced by the physicist and the one produced by the behavioral scientist, on occasion displays properties that differ considerably from one another, much as do optical isomers in organic chemistry.

I believe these images are mirrors because of differences in the direction generally pursued from each investigator's effective starting point, his own observations. The physical scientist for the most part, constructs his universe by ever more refined analysis of input variables, that is, sensory stimuli to which he reacts. The form of the reaction (cathode-ray tube, solid-state device, chromatography, or galvanometer) is unimportant, except that it provides a sufficiently broad communicative base. Constancies are gradually retrieved from manipulations and observations of these input variables under a variety of conditions. As these constants achieve stability, the 'correctness' of the views that produced them is asserted: the physical universe is properly described.

In the social disciplines the direction pursued is often just the reverse. Analysis is made of *action* systems (Parsons and Bales, 1953). The exact nature of the input to the actor (including the observing scientist) is of little consequence, provided it has sufficient communicative base; the effect of action on the system is the subject of analysis. It matters little (perhaps because the cause is usually multiple and/or indeterminable) if a currency is deflated because of fear of inflation, depression, personal whim, or misguided economic theory. The effects of deflation can be studied, are knowable. And once known, the action becomes corrective; the resulting stabilization, constancy, is interpreted as evidence for the 'correctness' of the action that produced the correction. Appropriate norms for the social universe become established.

One striking difference between the two images thus formed is immediately apparent. The physicist's macroscopic universe is the more stable, predictable one: "It does not hurt the moon to look at it" (Eddington, 1958, p. 227). For the most part, it is as he moves to ever more microscopic worlds that uncertainties are asserted. The scientist concerned with social matters finds it just the other way round: it seemingly does little harm to the man to look at him; but seriously look at his family, his friendships, or his political-economic systems and what you had started out to look at changes with the looking. Here indeterminacy comes to plague the macrostructure; it is in the stabilities of micro-analysis that the mirage of safety appears . . . .

The problem can be grasped . . . if it is dealt with in terms of isomeric forms of the same event universe—isomers differing in that their *structures* mirror each other. Put another way, the problem resolves itself into a meshing of the descriptive and the normative sciences. The suggestion is that structure in descriptive science ordinarily emerges from the analysis of the relations between systems and their subsystems; that in the normative sciences, it is largely the other way round: structure emerges when the relation between a system and its 'supersystem' is studied.

If this view is correct, we should find normative statements about the nature of the physical world when these are constructed from the examination of relations between a set of systems and a higher order system. Is not relativity just this sort of statement? This is not a social scientist speaking about the 'criterion problem':

The modest observer . . . [is] faced with the task of choosing between a number of frames of space with nothing to guide his choice. They are different in the sense that they frame the material objects of the world, including the observer himself, differently; but they are indistinguishable in the sense that the world as framed in one space conducts itself according to precisely the same laws as the world framed in another space. Owing to the accident of having been born on a particular planet our observer has hitherto unthinkingly adopted one of the frames; but he realizes that this is no ground for obstinately asserting that it must be the right frame. Which is the right frame?

At this juncture Einstein comes forward with a suggestion—

"You are seeking a frame of space which you call the *right* frame. In what does its *rightness* consist?"

You are standing with a label in your hand before a row of packages all precisely similar. You are worried because there is nothing to help you to decide which of the packages it should be attached to. Look at the label and see what is written on it. Nothing.

"Right" as applied to frames of space is a blank label. It implies that there is something distinguishing a right frame from a wrong frame; but when we ask what is the distinguishing property, the only answer we receive is "Rightness," which does not make the meaning clearer or convince us that there is a meaning (Eddington, 1958, p. 20).

Obversely, we should find descriptive statements about the nature of the social world when these derive from a study of the relations between a system and its subsystems. Doesn't the following passage fit this requirement?

Role behavior depends first of all on the role positions that society establishes; that is certain ways of behaving toward others are defined by different positions (Hilgard, 1962, p. 482).

Aren't statements about roles unambiguously descriptive? [Pribram, 1965, pp. 447–49]

The problem with dualism arises not when separate "mirror images" of the world are considered but when the question is asked: How do these worlds interact? It is the same question asked of the identity position: How can two or several linguistic constructions influence each other, how can they be translated into some common view?

The ordinary answer to this question is that the mental construction intervenes in the construction of the real world. Immanuel Kant (1963) especially emphasized the role of understanding, that is of cognitive activity in the construction of all experience—even that of reality. Recently Roger Sperry (1969) has suggested that *intervention*

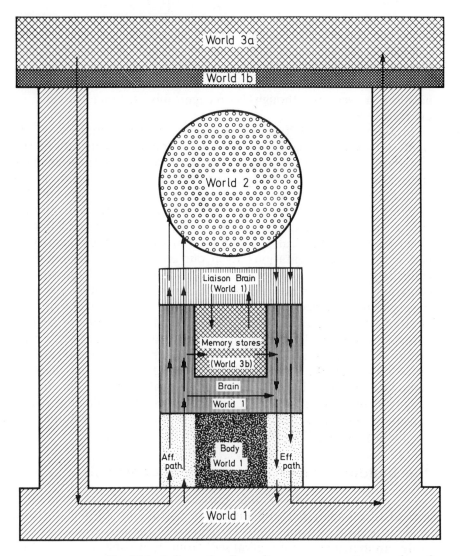

Fig. 20-1. Information-flow diagram representing modes of interaction between the three Worlds as shown by the pathways represented by arrows. Except for the liaison between the brain and World 2, all of information occurs in the matter-energy system of World 1. For example, in the reading of a book, communication between the book and the receptor mechanisms of the eye is subserved by radiation in the band of visual wavelengths. Any individual can at will range widely in his relationship to World 3. From Eccles, 1970.

is not really what occurs—he prefers the term *supervention* to describe the superordinate aspect of the phenomenal, the mental. He emphasizes the separateness of mind as a construction of the operations of the brain. The fact, however, that these constructions can feed back into the brain through the senses, makes the supervention position a variant, though a recognizably distinct variant, of interventionism.

Sir John Eccles (1970) has espoused a somewhat similar view. He wants to abandon dualism in favor of a triadic explanation of the mind-body issue. He emphasizes the third-world nature of language and culture. Thus the mind-brain problem becomes the mind-brain-culture (language) problem as set forth in the opening pages of this chapter. As detailed throughout this book, language and culture appear to have unique characteristics which are hard to define as either mental or physical. Is a computer program a physical entity or is it a mental representation? Even our law courts are having difficulty in deciding. Should complex programs which cost large sums to construct, and which are realizable in hardware, be patentable or is society better served by protecting them only with copyrights? Decisions have been made and reversed, and at the time of writing appeal has been made to even higher tribunals for an answer. Eccles would claim, and rightly so, that perhaps some new legislation is in order now that the third world, the world of ideas, has become embodied in this directly useful and palpable mode. The triadic variant of dualism has its merit but has difficulty, as do all variants, explaining the interaction between the worlds (see, for example, the complexity of Fig. 20-1, from Eccles, 1970).

the biologist view—a postcritical approach

Enough of this critical analysis of the mind-body issue. Critical analysis is fun and can be useful, but any single critical analysis is always incomplete. The richness of the whole issue is never truly apprehended, only glimpsed from now one, now another aspect.

I want therefore to propose an alternative to these approaches to the problem: a biological approach is possible, and, in its own fashion, the biological approach can satisfy in a way that the usual approaches cannot. Further, a formally stated "Biologist" view of the mind-body problem will change man's image of himself just as did the Cartesian and identity views, and this change will have profound consequences.

I noted earlier that the Biologist view of the mind-body relationship differs in content and approach from the earlier views. The biologist starts from biological material, from the "real" world of description based on observation and experiment. The data of the Biologist view are derived from descriptive science, while the data of the Cartesian and identity approaches are purely conceptual. From Descartes' "cogito ergo sum" to contemporary academic philosophy, the data to be analyzed have, as a rule, come directly from verbal reports of consciousness whether (in dualism or idealism) from subjective experience or (in physicalism and other forms of identity theory) from highly abstract principles of science (such as uncertainty and indeterminacy) as philosophers have understood them.

One exception must be made. Modern philosophy has recognized behavior as an expression of mind. Behavior has therefore been observed and the observations analyzed. But, paradoxically, the experimental approach of the behaviorist has been rejected as providing only trivia. Elsewhere in science minute observations and detailed experiments hold the key to knowledge. Philosophers seem to believe that in behavioral analysis this route is not, or at least has not been fruitful (or else they would take the behaviorists' experimental data as their starting point for analysis).

The Biologist approach pursued in these chapters does take the behaviorists' contributions seriously. Part III analyzed some of their contributions—and the analysis takes strength, I believe, from setting these contributions into a larger biological context.

There is therefore a basic difference in method between the Cartesian-critical tradition in philosophy and the Biologist view set forth here. This difference in method accounts for a difference in content, in the data subjected to analysis. The data of the biologist stem from science and are largely descriptive, the data of the Cartesian-critical thinkers stem from philosophical tradition and are more obviously subject to convention.

A third difference between the Biologist view and the Cartesian-critical stems from the other two: the aim of the Biologist view of the mind-body problem is what philosophers (e.g., Polanyi, 1960) call post-critical. The biologist's data everywhere show him that structure becomes embodied in a variety of forms through processes and transformations that must be laboriously described. That mental structure (e.g., a phrase of music) can be embodied in brain rhythms, in the score of sheet music, on a long playing record, or on tape does not especially shock him. Every day he views his wife, that strange embodiment he extends to himself to know, only to realize that she can be encoded in a DNA molecule—how else did his daughter turn out to be such an amazing replica? *In the Biologist view, multiple*

*"aspects" turn out to become multiple "realizations," multiple em-
bodiments achieved in what is often a long drawn out stepwise
process.*

Thus the key to the Biologist view of the mind-brain problem is
structure. In a sense the Biologist view is a form of constructional
realism. Biological rather than physicalistic, however, it encompasses
a constructional phenomenology—Images have structure; they are
made by a complex brain process; they are not the givens of
existential awareness. Because the Biologist view is constructional, it
shares the rational approach to epistemology and has therefore a
neo-Kantian flavor (Pribram, 1970; Pribram, 1970b). Because of the
emphasis on the structure of communicative Acts—language and
culture—the Biologist view speaks to the pragmatist with a proposal
for a structural pragmatism (Pribram, 1965).

The Biologist view partakes of all of these critical philosophies yet
transcends them. Going beyond the analytic preoccupations of
philosophy without discarding them, the Biologist view of the
mind-body problem simply accepts it as a biological fact, another
manifestation of the biology the scientist encounters at every turn in
his explorations. The broad aim of the Biologist position on this vital
issue is, therefore, acceptance, and wonder, not critical argument.

To man's view of himself the Biologist position has at least this
much to offer. The mystery of man is biological and shared with
other complex organizations which are never comprehended in their
totality but only in piecemeal. Man's brain is so constructed that
piece by piece he apprehends the whole through the operations of
coding and recoding. Languages, verbal (linguistic) and nonverbal
(cultural), are constituted of these pieces. When, because of linguistic
and cultural affluence, the means-ends reversal occurs, these languages begin to live lives of their own. Thus complexity is compounded and the original organization can easily be lost sight of.
Biological processes have, however, built-in renewal mechanisms.
When the linguistic and cultural structures become too cumbersome
or conflict with each other, they are often degraded, pruned back to
their more essential roots. Clearer vision is then attained of the basic
organization which gave rise to the process originally; historical
comparison can be made between the primitive and the sophisticated
version of the language or culture.

Thus, gradually, wisdom is attained in the regulation of human
affairs. In contrast to the cries of woe that are increasingly heard as
we approach the new millenium, the biologist immersed in the study
of brain process faces social issues hopefully. The power of this
peculiar biological organ, the brain, especially in man, is only

beginning to be fathomed. True, we must get on with the job before some of the cultural-language structures that have suffered the means-ends reversal overwhelm their creators. But the evidence suggests that remedial language-cultures will quickly be formed by those same sorts of brains that initiated the original. Thus wisdom is recurrently achieved. The biological process does not cease. Men's brains, through Image and Act, will create and communicate continuously, constructing languages—the regulators of human affairs.

synopsis

Man's linguistic power is but one manifestation of his brain's proclivity to code and recode whatever is communicated to it. Cultural constructions as a rule are derived from such recoding operations. Successive recoding by generations of genetically related organisms is an aspect of the nature-nurture relationship that leads directly to a consideration of the mind-brain-behavior problem. Contributions made by critical philosophers and Cartesian physiologists, reviewed in the context of the new conceptions that constitute *Languages of the Brain* stimulate the formation of a new post-critical "Biologist" resolution of the problem.

epilogue

The making of this book held many surprises for me. I was not prepared for the fact that the contents of every single chapter would change some cherished view, some dogma that had guided my research efforts and those of my colleagues. Each chapter has therefore become more of an essay than a tight presentation of what is known about a subject. The list of changed views fascinates me even in retrospect. Thus Chapter 1 is the current expression of a long interest in the function of slow potentials in the brain. Ralph Gerard kindled this interest while I was a graduate student—my thesis was to follow through on the Libet and Gerard finding that D.C. shifts could cross a cut in brain tissue. Karl Lashley brought sophistication to this interest, as he did to all my views on brain function. And I began to seriously explore in the laboratory with Wolfgang Köhler the field-theoretic approach to brain function in perception only to become completely disenchanted with it. This disenchantment encompassed Lashley's interference patterns which I did not understand until Sir John Eccles alerted me to his own somewhat ambivalent views on the wave front characteristics of activity at synaptic junctions. Interference patterns came alive for me after this, and the emergence of optical information processing techniques in the form of holography substantiated my interest. But not until the rewriting of chapters began did the slow potential microstructure as a more or less independent brain process coordinate with psychological state take firm root. The microstructure became the focus, and wave mechanical theory a way of looking at the biological fact. I had previously emphasized new approaches to understanding neuron and reflex theory but had not applied myself to understanding perception. The virtue of precipitating fact from the suspension in the original mix also came clear in the writing with the consequence, that the supernatent theory can be discarded whenever it no longer serves the explanatory purpose which engendered it. Thus, gradually the slow potential microstructure emerged real to me.

Chapter 2 has its roots in Lashley's famous search for the engram. Early in the 1960s I predicted that this decade would succeed where Lashley had failed. The slow potential microstructure takes as its anatomical substrate the *neural junction* as unit, not the *neuron*. Thus the long search for modifiability of brain tissue which had invariably come up against the hard fact that neurons are the only cells in the body which do not continue to replicate was circumvented. Neural junctions not only multiply; they are also replete with active chemical processes, any or many of which are candidates for the evanescent, temporary, and long term modification upon which memory must be based.

Chapter 3 also has a history. My serious interest in inhibition began around midnight one evening during the Cuba crisis of 1963. The occasion was a festive farewell party on my last night in Moscow where I had spent six weeks with Professor Alexander Romanovitch Luria studying patients with frontal lobe disease. The party was held at the home of Professor Alexei Nikolaevitch Leontiev. About midnight a quadrilingual discussion (Russian, English, French, and German were necessary since no one language was understood by all) had become heated. I had goaded one of the guests, Professor Peter Khuzmich Anokhin into a long and detailed exposition of the problem of neural and behavioral inhibition. I remember best the drawings made on Mrs. Leontiev's tablecloth which purported to show three levels of inhibition—neuronal, neural system, and behavioral. Less clearly I remember the discussion of Pavlov's distinction between external and internal inhibition—whether the ever flowing vodka or my insistence on operational definitions based on brain facts not behavioral inference clouded the issue, I cannot say. In any case I had been innoculated and began my own foray into theorizing in terms of inhibitory interactions. My initial naivete was abandoned after an incisive discussion with Keffer Hartline and a thorough study of Floyd Ratliff's book, *Mach Bands,* which Emanuel Donchin and I made the sole text for an undergraduate seminar one quarter. Quick on the heels of these exposures came Georg von Bekesy's readable *Sensory Inhibition,* which recalled encounters in the basement of Mem Aud at Harvard where these experiments were initiated and often demonstrated to willing subjects. As has so often been my lot, I did not understand much of what I was exposed to but took it in only to find years later the key piece of the puzzle that clarifies the earlier exposure. Chapter 3 distills these experiences: all decrementing of neural response is not inhibition in the classical neurophysiological sense; hyperpolarization, true neuronal inhibition, is an organizing property of neural function, not just a depressant—from inhibition the slow potential microstructure really derives its *structure.* And the experimental evidence for the importance of the slow potential microstructure is so much greater than I had suspected— witness the fact that retinal organization is *solely* in terms of slow potentials until the ganglion cell layer is reached.

Chapter 4 in one sense extends the Sapir-Whorf hypothesis. Or to paraphrase Wittgenstein, my power to code powers my world. It is critical that the brain sciences keep pace with the second industrial revolution. In 1970 my laboratory has a five-year history of computerization—we now have two general purpose computers and are discussing our need for two more. At the current price of $5000 for a fully capable general purpose machine, this investment is not out of reach for the single investigator. The computer as a stimulus controller, as a response recorder, as a data analyzer, as a simulator of behavioral and brain processes, has proved invaluable. As a source for insight into brain function, the current serial processing computer leaves something to be desired, but it is better than the switchboard that my teachers had to use to make me understand the principles of the brain's mechanisms. I was not prepared at the outset of the search for neural codes for the conclusion that the brain's power lies precisely in its ability to code and recode—to make an infinite variety of languages. Even the brain's capacity for modification—its time binding property—may depend to a large extent on this ability to recode into ever more efficient patterns. And once again, a critical step in the coding operations of the brain appears to be caused by the slow potential, junctional microstructure which makes use of configural designs (analogue mechanisms) to transform one neural pattern into another. In this respect the brain differs radically from present day computers.

Chapter 5 takes the computer analogy to brain function seriously despite these limitations. This chapter therefore sums up parts of an earlier volume, *Plans and the Structure of Behavior* in which George Miller, Eugene Galanter, and I (influenced to a great extent by Jerome Bruner) tore ourselves loose from the restrictive encasement of the narrow behaviorism which we had practiced, to range forth into the world of subjective psychology. Our tool was the computer, our datum the brain's control over its own input. What is new in Chapter 5 is the emphasis on a separate feedforward process which the earlier formulation had not yet dissociated from feedback. The suggested logic which incorporates the feedforward as a parallel processing input, rather than a solely input-outcome informed mechanism is recent and its implications for research remain to be explored. The conception of feedforward in these terms also began during a dinner party, this one at the University of Illinois at the home of Heinz von Foerster. The discussion quickly centered on Ross Ashby's current enthusiasm. He had gained an insight into the feedforward problem after some three years of stewing with it. I did not fully grasp all he expounded at the time, but I would not be at all surprised if my new expanded TOTE (which I am tempted to call the TOTE—TO · BE) were a good fit to his insight.

Part I thus forms a matrix for the remainder of the book. The rows of the matrix describe processes that organize the slow potential junctional microstructure in the brain. The columns describe neural operations that organize feedback and feedforward in the nervous system. Part II applies this matrix to an analysis of the neural processes coordinate with subjective experience—perceptions and feelings.

The surprises in Part II reflect those of the earlier chapters. The subjective behaviorism espoused in *Plans and the Structure of Behavior* is carried to its logical conclusion—Gilbert Ryle's ghosts in the machine are let out of the closet and scrutinized. The formation of Images and Interests is unabashedly discussed in tough-minded operational terms. Here the holographic Image forming characteristics of the slow potential junctional microstructure come into their own, but not at the expense of an experientially modifiable feature filtering process based on TOTE organizations. If someone had suggested in 1960 that I might by 1970 have plausible thoughts relevant to the neurology of perception I would not have believed them. But in 1960 holograms, feature detectors, perceptrons, and the like were in their infancy.

Nor in 1960 did I have a coherent view of the neurology of motivation and emotion. My struggle with this problem took the form of a series of papers and was not resolved until I organized the subject matter under the broader topic of feelings. The fascinating part of this story is that it was the *experimental* neurobehavioral analysis that made it imperative to use concepts such as appetite and affect—this was no solitary armchair decision, nor was it based on philosophical bias. Data forced the community of investigators exploring the core brain mechanisms in motivation and emotion to the subjective behaviorist stance.

Only when the final redrafting was in progress did Chapter 11 take satisfactory shape. I finally realized that the concept Interest covered the problems being addressed. My clinical colleagues in psychiatry and psychology know well what I am referring to—and, of course, so does the lay reader. All other terms such as attitude, arousal, activation, denoting the aspects of motivation and emotion that do not originate directly in the body's physiology have become connotatively contaminated. Thus Part II provides a cybernetic theory of how we take Interest in the world as well as a holographic theory of how we make Images of it.

In Part III I come to terms with my earlier classical behaviorism derived from interaction with Fred Skinner and Charles Ferster. Though the analyses are strictly behavioristic, I was forced into using cognitive and humanistic language by the biological flavor of the neurological data. Biologists and cognitive psychologists think in terms of the structure of process; they speak of competences, they know that transplanted organs as well as organisms can show commitment to achieving effective performance in the face of disruptive influences.

But the real joy in writing this section came from the wealth of neurobehavioral data accumulated in the last five years that clarified earlier puzzling results. The motor cortex story and its Image-of-Achievement is a case in point. The possibility that the cerebellum is a fast-time computer because of the rapid erase feature discovered by Eccles, Ito, and Szentagothai, is another. And the Valenstein-Roberts experiments called to my attention by Stephen Glickman (as well as Glickman's own experimental contributions) in his editorial review of my manuscript, now give these chapters a solid feel; they had a much more speculative flavor when they were initially written some seven years earlier.

Finally, Part IV—the chapters on sign and symbol, and on language. In many ways these chapters have been the most difficult, partly because they, more than any others, encompass the main thrust of my own experimental work. I thus feel at the same time too close to the data to evaluate them in the larger perspective and too far from reaching closure to write about them at all. But no reasonable treatment of neuropsychology can ignore the role of the brain in communicative processes. I decided therefore to state my views baldly so that they could be tested and modified if proved wanting. These views originated in neurosurgical experience and in the approach taken to the problem of language by George Miller and Noam Chomsky. The views were then shaped by long discussions with Alexander Luria, Roman Jakobson, and Jacob Bronowski. Counterpoint was provided by Eberhardt Bay and by Henri Hecaen, and by some challenging disputations with Norman Geschwind. But again, not until the last drafts did the distinction between context-free signs and context-sensitive symbols come completely clear. The realization that most verbs indicated nominalization of actions, not predication, also came late, as did the identification of predication with propositional truth.

In these last chapters I also attempt to chart the immediate future of neurobehavioral and neurophysiological analysis. The Gardners' Washoe and David Premack's Sarah indicate one direction. My brief foray into the neurology of meaning and caring suggests another. And the dipole model of the feature filter can be transcribed into a number of electrophysiological and neurochemical experiments.

Thus, the very subject matter of neuropsychology itself has become redefined in terms of the data forged in the 1960s. I had been teaching the substantive parts of the presentation for a decade at Yale before the book was launched and for another at Stanford while it was being written. My courses centered on the puzzles and paradoxes uncovered by experiment. What was lacking was some overall structure, some coherent set of principles with which to approach these paradoxes—a deficiency also of early unsatisfactory versions of this manuscript. Usually it was not until an early draft of a chapter was written that its structure became at all evident—and so rewriting commenced. The process was repeated when the whole manuscript was finished—only then did chapterization really take hold. Interestingly, however, rarely did the material have to be rearranged—only divisions had to be indicated, headings supplied, and the message of each division more clearly expressed.

This grass roots organization leads me to believe that neuropsychology has come of age. The subject matter of this science is covered in programs and courses variously labeled physiological psychology, behavioral neurophysiology, biopsychology, psychobiology, the biological basis of behavior, and biobehavioral science. Whatever the contents of such endeavors, it is now clear to me that student and teacher alike pursue four different kinds of interest, and that they often encounter cross purposes because these interests are not distinguished and made explicit. Brain mechanisms, psychological functions, behavior modification and control, and communication are all topics in their own right, and each is, to a large extent, served by separate languages. Yet they make good bookmates—interest in any one of them seems to carry over to the others.

The final major surprise to me was the way in which the mind-body issue became resolved. When I began my investigations in this field of inquiry I was sure that biobehavioral research would eliminate mentalism from psychology just as biochemistry had eliminated vitalism from biology. I had not reckoned properly with the brain, however, and its recoding ability. Language became the touchstone of the problem—and what is language, mind or matter? The Biologist resolution of the dilemma was unexpected even when I began to write the last chapter. As with the rest of the book, it just happened.

My worry is that my communicative powers have not portrayed the excitement of this journey of discovery. Much depends on whether I have properly woven a clear pattern out of the threads of evidence. In any case, the manuscript will serve as a journal recording the voyage, a journal I can turn to when making explanations of my interests to my students, colleagues and loved ones. Perhaps it can serve others in this fashion as well.

As we go to press I detect that the yen for exploration is not yet done. A grant proposal is in to the NIMH and experiments are underway to pursue the central-motor (or what in psycholinguistics would be called the "generative") approach to *What Makes Man Human* (Pribram, 1971). On a recent trip I realized a long felt wish to visit the laboratory of Carlo Terzuolo to observe a modern systems approach to the neurophysiology of the reflex (the transformations involved determine, as might be predicted from Chapters 12 and 13, a remarkably linear overall mechanism despite some local nonlinearities; Terzuolo and Popelle, 1968). On the same trip I watched Herbert Jasper (Jasper, 1969; Jasper and Koyama, 1969) perfuse the brain cortex of cats to extract chemical substances released by electrical stimulations of subcortical structures (to realize some of the conjectures of Chapter 15). I also heard with delight (and wrote immediately for a preprint) that David Pollen (1971) has, at Harvard University, demonstrated that "the striate cortex transforms the topographic representation of visual space in the lateral geniculate body into a Fourier transform or spatial frequency representation at the complex cell level via the intermediary simple cell [line sensitive] stage of 'strip integration.' " In short, the brightness distribution falling on adjacent receptive fields is "effectively decomposed into a set of sine wave gratings at all possible position angles and covering a wide range of cycles per degree of visual angle" (fulfilling some of the promise of Fig. 8-12). And within the same week I encountered Robert Shaw and discussed with him ways of testing, by behavioral experiment and computer simulation, the coding of temporal relationships with three dimensional holographic structures. In a more philosophical vein that evening, we were turned on by the similarities between n-dimensional holography and Leibnitz's path from the invention of the integral calculus to his monadology and the similarity of this development with Bertrand Russell's discussion of William James' neutral monism. Indeed, "Truths emerge from facts; but they dip forward into facts again and add to them; which facts again create or reveal new truth. . . and so on indefinitely."

references

Adams, R. The anatomy of memory mechanisms in the human brain. In Talland, G.A., and Waugh, N.C. (eds.) *The Pathology of Memory.* New York: Academic, 1969. Pp. 91-106.

Adey, W.R. Intrinsic organization of cerebral tissue in alerting, orienting, and discriminative responses. In Quarton, G.C., Melnechuk, T., and Schmitt, F.O. (eds.) *The Neurosciences.* New York: The Rockefellar Press, 1967. Pp. 615-33.

Adolph, E.F. *Physiological Regulations.* Lancaster, Pa.: Jacques Cattell Press, 1943. Copyright 1943 by The Ronald Press Company.

Adolph, E.F. Thirst and its inhibition in the stomach. *Amer. J. Physiol.,* 1950, 161: 374-86.

Adrian, E.D., and Matthews, R. The action of light on the eye. Part I. The discharges of impulses in the optic nerve and its relation to the electric change in the retina. *J. Physiol.,* 1927a, 63: 378-414.

Adrian, E.D., and Matthews, R. The action of light on the eye. Part II. The processes involved in retinal excitation. *J. Physiol.,* 1927b, 64: 179-301.

Adrian, E.D., and Zotterman, Y. The impulses produced by sensory nerve-endings. Part II. The response of a single end-organ. *J. Physiol.,* 1926, 61: 151-71.

Agranoff, B.W., Davis, R.E., and Brink, J.J. Memory fixation in the goldfish. *Proc. Nat. Acad. Sci.,* 1965, 54: 788-93.

Albé-Fessard, D. Activities de projection et d'association du neocortex cerebral des mammiferes. *Extrait du Journal de Physiologie,* 1957, 49: 521-88.

Amsel, A. The role of frustrative nonreward in noncontinuous reward situations. *Psychol. Bull.,* 1958, 55: 102-18.

Anand, B.K. Influence of the internal environment on the nervous regulation of alimentary behavior. In Brazier, M.A.B. (ed.) *Brain and Behavior. Vol. II.* Washington, D.C.: American Institute of Biological Sciences, 1963. Pp. 43-116.

Anand, B.K., and Brobeck, J.R. Localization of a "feeding center" in the hypothalamus of the rat. *Proc. Soc. Exp. Biol. Med.*, 1951, 77: 323-24.

Anand, B.K., and Brobeck, J.R. Food intake and spontaneous activity of rats with lesions in the amygdaloid nuclei. *J. Neurophysiol.*, 1952, 15: 421-30.

Andersson, B. The effect of injections of hypertonic NaCl-solution into the different parts of the hypothalamus of goats. *Acta Physiologica Scand.*, 1953, 28: 188-201.

Angevine, J.B., Mancall, E.L., and Yakovlev, P.I. *The Human Cerebellum. An Atlas of Gross Topography in Serial Sections.* Boston: Little, Brown & Company, 1961.

Ashby, W.R. *Design for a Brain: The Origin of Adaptive Behaviour.* 2nd. ed. New York: John Wiley, 1960.

Attneave, F. Some informational aspects of visual perception. *Psychol. Rev.,* 1954, 61: 183-93.

Ayer, A.J. *Language, Truth and Logic.* New York: Dover, 1946.

Bagshaw, M.H., and Benzies, S. Multiple measures of the orienting reaction and their dissociation after amygdalectomy in monkeys. *Exp. Neurol.,* 1968, 20: 175-87.

Bagshaw, M.H., and Coppock, H.W. Galvanic skin response conditioning deficit in amygdalectomized monkeys. *Exp. Neurol.,* 1968, 20: 188-96.

Bagshaw, M.H., Kimble, D.P., and Pribram, K.H. The GSR of monkeys during orienting and habituation and after ablation of the amygdala, hippocampus and inferotemporal cortex. *Neuropsychologia,* 1965, 3: 111-19.

Bagshaw, M.H., Mackworth, N.H., and Pribram, K.H. Method for recording and analyzing visual fixations in the unrestrained monkey. *Perceptual and Motor Skills,* 1970a, 31: 219-22.

Bagshaw, M.H., Mackworth, N.H., and Pribram, K.H. The effect of inferotemporal cortex ablations on eye movements of monkeys during discrimination training. *Int. J. Neuroscience,* 1970b, 1: 153-58.

Bagshaw, M.H., and Pribram, J.D. Effect of amygdalectomy on stimulus threshold of the monkey. *Exp. Neurol.,* 1968, 20: 197-202.

Bagshaw, M.H., and Pribram, K.H. Effect of amygdalectomy on transfer of training in monkeys. *J. comp. physiol. Psychol.,* 1965, 59: 118-21.

Bailey, P. *Intracranial Tumors.* Springfield, Ill.: Charles C Thomas, 1933.

Bailey, P., von Benin, G., and McCulloch, W.S. *The Isocortex of the Chimpanzee.* Urbana: University of Illinois Press, 1950.

Barlow, H.B. Possible principles underlying the transformations of sensory messages. In Rosenblith, W. (ed.) *Sensory Communication.* Cambridge: MIT Press, 1961, Pp. 217-34.

Barrett, T.W. The cortex as interferometer: the transmission of amplitude, frequency and phase in the cerebral cortex. *Neuropsychologia,* 1969a, 7: 135-48.

Barrett, T.W. Studies of the function of the amygdaloid complex in Macaca mulatta. *Neuropsychologia,* 1969b, 7: 1-12.

Batham, E.J., and Pantin, C.F.A. Inherent activity in the sea anemone. *J. Exp. Psychol.,* 1950, 27: 290-301.

Békésy, G. von. *Experiments in Hearing.* New York: McGraw-Hill, 1960.

Békésy, G. von. Interaction of paired sensory stimuli and conduction in peripheral nerves. *Journal of Applied Physiology,* 1963, 18: 1276-84.

Békésy, G. von. *Sensory Inhibition.* Princeton: Princeton University Press, 1967.

Bell, C. *Idea of a New Anatomy of the Brain Submitted for the Observation of His Friends.* London: Strahan and Preston, 1811.

Bennett, E.L., Diamond, I.T., Krech, D., and Rosenzweig, M.R. Chemical and anatomical plasticity of the brain. *Science,* 1964, 46: 610-19.

Bennett, E.L., and Rosenzweig, M.R. Chemical alterations produced in brain by environment and training. In Lajtho, A. (ed.) *Handbook of Neurochemistry.* New York: Plenum Press, 1970. Pp. 173-201.

Bernard, C. *An Introduction to the Study of Experimental Medicine.* New York: Macmillan, 1927 (orig. ed. 1865).

Bernstein, N. *The Co-ordination and Regulation of Movements.* New York: Pergamon Press, 1967.

Beurle, R.L. Properties of a mass of cells capable of regenerating pulses. *Philos. Trans. Royal Soc.,* London, 1956, 240: 55-94.

Bishop, G. Natural history of the nerve impulse. *Physiol. Rev.,* 1956, 36: 376-99.

Bizzi, E. Changes in the orthodromic and antidromic response of optic rapid eye movements of sleep. *J. Neurophysiol.,* 1966a, 29: 861-70.

Bizzi, E. Discharge patterns of single geniculate neurons during the rapid eye movements of sleep. *J. Neurophysiol.,* 1966b, 29: 1087-95.

Blakemore, C., and Campbell, F.W. On the existence of neurones in the human visual system selectively sensitive to the orientation and size of retinal images. *J. Physiol.,* 1969, 203: 237-60.

Block, H.D., and Ginsburg, H. The psychology of robots. In *Readings in Experimental Psychology Today.* Del Mar, Ca.: CRM Books, 1970. Pp. 11-17.

Blout, E.R. Conformations of proteins. In Quarton, G.C., Melnechuk, T., and Schmitt, F.O. (eds.) *The Neurosciences.* New York: The Rockefellar University Press, 1967. Pp. 57-66.

Bodian, David. Neurons, circuits, and neuroglia. In Quarton, G.C., Melnechuk, T., and Schmitt, F.C. (eds.) *The Neurosciences.* New York: The Rockefellar University Press, 1967. Pp. 6-24.

Bogoch, S. *The Biochemistry of Memory.* New York: Oxford University Press, 1968.

Boring, E.G. The physiology of consciousness. *Science,* 1932, 75: 32.

Bower, T.G.R. The visual world of infants. *Scientific American,* 1966, 215: 80-92.

Brady, J.V. The effect of electroconvulsive shock on a conditioned emotional response: the permanence of the effect. *J. comp. physiol. Psychol.,* 1951, 41: 507-11.

Brindley, G.S., and Lewin, W.S. The sensations produced by electrical stimulation of the visual cortex. *J.Physiol.,* 1968, 196: 479-93.

Brindley, G.S., and Merton, P.A. The absence of position sense in the human eye. *J. Physiol.,* 1960, 153: 127-30.

Brobeck, J.R. Review and synthesis. In Brazier, M.A.B. (ed.) *Brain and Behavior, Vol. II.* Washington, D.C.: American Institute of Biological Sciences, 1963. Pp. 389-409.

Broca, P. Remarques sur la siege de la faculte du langage articule, suivies d'une observation d'aphemie (perte de la parole). *Bulletins de la Societe Anatomique de Paris,* Tome VI, 1861, 36: 330-57.

Brodal, A. *The Reticular Formation of the Brain Stem: Anatomical Aspects and Functional Correlations.* Springfield, Ill.: Charles C Thomas, 1958.

Brodie, H.K.H., Murphy, D.L., Goodwin, F.K., and Bunney, W.E., Jr., Catecholamines and mania: the effect of alpha-methyl-para-tyrosine on manic behavior and catecholamine metabolism. *Clinical Pharmacology and Therapeutics,* 1970.

Bronowski, J. Human and animal languages. In *To Honor Roman Jakobson: Essays on the Occasion of His Seventieth Birthday, Vol. I.* Paris: Mouton, 1967. Pp. 374-94.

Brooks, V.B., and Asanuma, H. Pharmacological studies of recurrent cortical inhibition and facilitation. *Amer. J. Physiol.,* 1965, 207: 674-81.

Brown, B.R., and Lohmann, A.W. Complex spatial filtering with binary masks. *Applied Optics,* 1966, 5: 967-69.

Browuer, B. Projection of the retina on the cortex in man. *Assoc. Res. Nerv. & Ment. Dis.,* 1934, 13: 529-34.

Browuer, B., and Zeeman, W.P.C. The projection of the retina in the primary optic neuron in monkeys. *Brain,* 1926, 49: 1-35.

Bruner, J.S. On perceptual readiness. *Psych. Rev.,* 1957, 64: 123-52.

Bullock, T.H. Neuron doctrine and electrophysiology. *Science,* 1959, 129: 997-1002.

Bunney, W.E., Jr., Janowsky, D.S., Goodwin, F.K., Davis, J.M., Brodie, H.K.H., Murphy, D.L., and Chase, T.N. Effect of L-DOPA on depression. *Lancet,* 26 April 1969, 1: 885-86.

Burns, B.D. *The Mammalian Cerebral Cortex.* London: Edward Arnold, 1958.

Burns, B.D. *The Uncertain Nervous System.* London: Edward Arnold, 1968.

Butter, C.M. The effect of discrimination training on pattern equivalence in monkeys with inferotemporal and lateral striate lesions. *Neuropsychologia,* 1968, 6: 27-40.

Cajal. *Histologie du Systeme Nerveux. Vol. 2.* Paris: Maloine, 1911.

Calhoun, J.B. A comparative study of the social behavior of two inbred strains of house mice. *Ecol. Monogr.,* 1956, 26: 81-103.

Calvin, M. Chemical evolution of life and sensibility. In Quarton, G.C., Melnechuk, T., and Schmitt, F.O. (eds.) *The Neurosciences.* New York: The Rockefellar University Press, 1967. Pp. 780-800.

Cannon, W.B. *Bodily Changes in Pain, Horror, Fear and Rage. An Account of Recent Researches into the Function of Emotional Excitement.* New York: Appleton-Century-Crofts, 1929.

Cannon, W.B. The body physiologic and the body politic. *Science,* 1941, 93: 1-10.

Case, T.J. Alpha waves in relation to structures involved in vision. In Cattell, J. (ed.) *Biological Symposia,* VII: 107-16.

Castellucci, V., Pinsker, H., Kupfermann, I., and Kandel, E. Neuronal mechanisms of habituation and dishabituation of the gell withdrawal reflex in aplysia. *Science,* 1970, 167: 1745-48.

Chomsky, N. Formal properties of grammars. In Luce, R.D., Bush, R.R., and Galanter, E.H. (eds.) *Handbook of Mathematical Psychology.* New York: John Wiley, 1963. Pp. 323-418.

Chorover, S.L., and Schiller, P.H. Short-term retrograde amnesia in rats. *J. comp. physiol. Psychol.,* 1965, 59: 73-78.

Chow, K.L. A retrograde cell degeneration study of the cortical projection field of the pulvinar in the monkey. *J. comp. Neurol.,* 1950, 93: 313-39.

Chow, K.L. Bioelectrical activity of isolated cortex—III. Conditioned electrographic responses in chronically isolated cortex. *Neuropsychologia,* 1964, 2: 175-87.

Chow, K.L. Integrative functions of the thalamocortical visual system of cat. In Pribram, K.H., and Broadbent, D. (eds.) *The Biology of Memory.* New York: Academic, 1970. Pp. 273-92.

Chow, K.L., and Dewson, J.H., III. Bioelectrical activity of isolated cortex—I. Responses induced by interaction of low- and high-frequency electrical stimulation. *Neuropsychologia,* 1964, 2: 153-65.

Chow, K.L., and Leiman, A.L. Aspects of the structure and functional organization of the neocortex. In *Neurosciences Bulletin,* 1970, 8: 157-219.

Chow, K.L., and Pribram, K.H. Cortical projection of the thalamic ventrolateral nuclear group in monkeys. *J. comp. Neurol.,* 1956, 104: 57-75.

Clark, R., and Polish, E. Avoidance conditioning and alcohol consumption in Rhesus monkeys. *Science,* 1960, 132: 223-24.

Clark, R., Schuster, C.R., and Brady, J.V. Instrumental conditioning of jugular self-infusion in the Rhesus monkey. *Science,* 1961, 133: 1829-30.

Clemente, C.C., Sterman, M.B., and Wyrwicke, W. Post-reinforcement EEG synchronization during alimentary behavior. *Electroenceph. clin. Neurophysiol.,* 1964, 16: 355-65.

Cohen, Jozef. *Sensation and Perception. I: Vision.* Skokie, Ill.: Rand McNally, 1969.

Conel, J.L. Postnatal development of the human cerebral cortex. Vols. I-VI. Cambridge: Harvard University Press. 1939-1963.

Creutzfeldt, O.D. General physiology of cortical neurons and neuronal information in the visual system. In Brazier, M.A.B. (ed.) *Brain and Behavior.* Washinton: American Institute of Biological Sciences, 1961. Pp. 299-358.

Creutzfeldt, O.D. General physiology of cortical neurons and neuronal information in the visual system. In Brazier, M.A.B. (ed.) *Brain and Behavior.* Washington: American Institute of Biological Sciences, 1961. Pp. 299-358.

Davidson, J.M., Jones, L.E., and Levine, S. Feedback regulation of adrenocorticotropin secretion in "basal" and "stress" conditions: acute and chronic effects of intra-hypothalamic corticoid implantation. *Endocrinology,* 1968, 82: 655-63.

de No, Lorente. In Fulton. *Physiology of Nervous System.* 3rd ed. New York: Oxford University Press, 1949.

Desmedt, J.E. Neurophysiological mechanisms controlling acoustic input. In Rasmussen, G.L., and Windle, W. (eds.) *Neural Mechanisms of Auditory and Vestibular Systems.* Springfield, Ill.: Charles C Thomas, 1960. Pp. 152-64.

Deutsch, J.A., Hamburg, M.D., and Dahl, H. Anticholinesterase-induced amnesia and its temporal aspects. *Science,* 1966, 151: 221-23.

DeValois, R.L. Color vision mechanisms in monkey. *J. gen. Physiol.,* 1960, 43: 115-28.

DeValois, R.L., and Jacobs, G.H. Primate color vision. *Science,* 1968, 162: 533-40.

Dewson, J.H., III. Efferent olivocochlear bundle: some relationships to stimulus discrimination in noise. *J. Neurophysiol.,* 1968, 31: 122-30.

Dewson, J.H. III, Chow, K.L. and Engel, J., Jr. Bi - electrical activity of isolated cortex–II. Steady potentials and induced surface-negative cortical responses. *Neuropsychologia,* 1964. Pp.167-174.

Ditchburn, R.W., and Ginsborg, B.L. Vision with a stabilized retinal image. *Nature,* 1952, 170: 36.

Dodwell, P.C. *Visual Pattern Recognition.* New York: Holt, Rinehart & Winston, 1970.

Donchin, E., Otto, D., Gerbrant, L.K., and Pribram, K.H. While a monkey waits: electrocortical events recorded during the foreperiod of a reaction time study. *Electroenceph. clin. Neurophysiol.,* 1971.

Douglas, R.J. Transposition, novelty, and limbic lesions. *J. comp. physiol. Psychol.,* 1966, 62: 354-57.

Douglas, R.J. The hippocampus and behavior. *Psychol. Bull.,* 1967, 67: 416-42.

Douglas, R.J., Barrett, T.W., Pribram, K.H., and Cerny, M.C. Limbic lesions and error reduction. *J. comp. physiol. Psychol.,* 1969, 68: 437-41.

Douglas, R.J., and Pribram, K.H. Learning and limbic lesions. *Neuropsychologia,* 1966, 4: 197-220.

Dowling, J.E. Site of visual adaptation. *Science,* 1967, 155: 273.

Dowling, J.E., and Boycott, B.B. Neural connections of the retina: fine structure of the inner plexiform layer. *Quant. Biol.,* 1965, 30: 393-402.

Dowling, J.E., and Boycott, B.B. Organization of the primate retina: electron microscopy. *Proc. Roy. Soc. B.,* 1966, 166: 80-11.

Eccles, J.C. *The Neurophysiological Basis of Mind.*

Eccles, J.C. The physiology of imagination. *Scientific American,* 1958, 199: 135-46.

Eccles, J.C. *The Physiology of Synapses.* Berlin: Springer Verlag, 1964.

Eccles, J.C. Postsynaptic inhibition in the central nervous system. In Quarton, G.C., Melnechuk, T., and Schmitt, F.O. (eds.) *The Neurosciences.* New York: The Rockefellar University Press, 1967. Pp. 408-27.

Eccles, J.C. *Facing Reality*. New York, Heidelberg, Berlin: Springer-Verlag, 1970.

Eccles, J.C., Ito, M., and Szentagothai, J. *The Cerebellum as a Neuronal Machine*. New York: Springer-Verlag, 1967.

Echline, F.A., Arnett, V., and Zoll, J. Paroxysmal high voltage discharge from isolated and partially isolated human and animal cortex. *Electroenceph. clin. Neurophysiol.*, 1952, 4: 147-64.

Eddington, A. *The Nature of the Physical World*. Ann Arbor: University of Michigan Press, 1958.

Edds, M.V., Jr. Neuronal specificity in neurogenesis. In Quarton, G.C., Melnechuk, T., and Schmitt, F.O. (eds.) *The Neurosciences*. New York: The Rockefellar University Press, 1967. Pp. 230-40.

Elul, R., and Adey, W.R. Nonlinear relationship of spike and waves in cortical neurons. *The Physiologist*, 1966, 8: 98-104.

Engstrom, D.K., London, P., and Hart, J.T. EEG alpha feedback training and hypnotic susceptibility. *Nature* (in press).

Estes, W.K. The statistical approach to learning theory. In Koch, S. (ed.) *Psychology: A Study of a Science II*. New York: McGraw-Hill, 1959. Pp. 380-491.

Evans, D.C. Computer logic and memory. *Scientific American*, 1966, 215: 74-87.

Evarts, E.V. Effect of ablation of prestriate cortex on auditory-visual association in monkey. *J. Neurophysiol.*, 1952, 15: 191-200.

Evarts, E.V. Representation of movements and muscles by pyramidal tract neurons of the precentral motor cortex. In Yahr, M.D., and Purpura, D.P. (eds.) *Neurophysiological Basis of Normal and Abnormal Motor Activities*. Hewlett, N.Y.: Raven Press, 1967. Pp. 215-54.

Evarts, E.V. Relation of pyramidal tract activity to force exerted during voluntary movement. *J. Neurophysiol.*, 1968, 31: 14-27.

Festinger, L., Burnham, C.A., Ono, H., and Bamber, D. Efference and the conscious experience. *J. Exp. Psychol.*, 1967, 74: 1-36.

Flechsig, P. *Die localisation der geistigen vorgänge insbesondere der sinnesempfindungen des menschen*. Leipsig, 1896.

Fox, S.S., Liebeskinde, J.C., O'Brien, J.H., and Dingle, R.D.G. Mechanisms for limbic modification of cerebellar and cortical afferent information. In Adey, W.R., and Tokizane, T. (eds.) *Progress in Brain Research Vol. 27*. Amsterdam: Elsevier Publishing Co., 1967. Pp. 254-80.

Fox, S.S., and O'Brien, J.H. Duplication of evoked potential waveform by curve of probability of firing a single cell. *Science*, 1965, 147: 888-90.

Freud, S. *On aphasia: A Critical Study* (1891). New York: International Universities Press, 1953. In Pribram, K.H. (ed.) *Brain and Behavior: Adaptation*. Baltimore: Penguin Books, 1969.

Freud, S. Project for a scientific psychology. Appendix In *The Origins of Psycho-Analysis, Letters to Wilheim Fliess, Draft and Notes 1887-1902*. New York: Basic Books, Inc., 1954.

Fritsch, G., and Hitzig, E. On the electrical excitability of the cerebrum. In Pribram, K.H. (ed.) *Brain and Behaviour, Vol. 2. Perception and Action*. Baltimore: Penguin, 1969. Pp. 353-64 (orig. Pub. 1870).

Frohlich, F.W. *Die Empfindungszeit*. Gustav Fischer, Jena, 1929.

Fugita, Y., and Sato, T. Intracellular records from hippocampal pyramidal cells in rabbit during theta rhythm activity. *J. Neurophysiol.*, 1964, 27: 1011-25.

Fuortes, M.G.F., and Hodgkin, A.L. Changes in time scale and sensitivity in the ommatidia of limulus. *J. Physiol.*, 1964, 172: 239.

Fuxe, E., Hamberger, B., and Hokfelt, T. Distribution of noradrenaline nerve terminals in cortical areas of the rat. *Brain Res.*, 1968, 8: 125-31.

Gabor, D. Microscopy by reconstructed wave fronts. *Proc. Roy. Soc.,* 1949, A197: 454-87.

Gabor, D. Microscopy by reconstructed wave fronts, II. *Proc. Roy. Soc.,* 1961, B64: 449-69.

Galambos, R. Suppression of auditory nerve activity by stimulation of efferent fibers to cochlea. *J. Neurophysiol.,* 1956, 19: 424-37.

Galambos, R., Norton, T.T., and Frommer, C.P. Optic tract lesions sparing pattern vision in cats. *Exp. Neurol.,* 1967, 18: 8-25.

Galbraith, G., London, P., Leibovitz, M.P., Cooper, C., and Hart, J.T. An electroencephlographic study of hypnotic susceptibility. *J. comp. physiol. Psychol.,* 1970.

Ganz, L. Sensory deprivation and visual discrimination. In Teuber, H.L. (ed.) *Handbook of Sensory Physiology, Vol. 8.* New York: Springer-Verlag, 1971.

Gardner, R.A., and Gardner, B.T. Teaching sign language to a chimpanzee. *Science,* 1969, 165: 664-72.

Gerard, R.W., and Young, J.Z. Electrical activity of the central nervous system of the frog. *Proc. Roy. Soc. B.,* 1937, 122: 343-52.

Gerbrandt, L., Bures, J. and Buresova, O. Investigations of plasticity in single units in the mamallian brain. In Pribram, K.H., and Broadbent, D.E. (eds.) *The Biology of Memory.* New York: Academic Press, 1970. Pp.223-35.

Gesteland, R.C., Lettvin, J.Y., Pitts, W.H., and Chung S-H. A code in the nose. In Oestreicher, H.L., and Moore, D.R. (eds.) *Cybernetic Problems in Bionics.* New York: Gordon and Breach, 1968. Pp. 313-22.

Gibson, J.J. *The Senses Considered as Perceptual Systems.* Boston: Houghton Mifflin, 1966.

Glassman, E. *Molecular Approaches to Psychobiology.* Belmont, Calif.: Dickenson Publishing Co., 1967.

Glickman, S.E., and Feldman, S.M. Habituation of the arousal response to direct stimulation of the brainstem. *Electroenceph. clin. Neurophysiol.,* 1961, 13: 703-9.

Glickman, S.E., and Schiff, B.B. A biological theory of reinforcement. *Psych. Rev.,* 1967, 74: 81-109.

Goldman, P.S., Lodge, A., Hammer, L.R., Semmes, J., and Mishkin, M. Critical flicker frequency after unilateral temporal lobectomy in man. *Neuropsychologia,* 1968, 6: 355-63.

Grandstaff, N.W. Frequency analysis of EEG during milk drinking. *Electroenceph. clin. Neurophysiol.,* 1969, 27: 55-57.

Grandstaff, N., and Pribram, K.H. Habituation: electrical changes with visual stimulation (in prep.).

Granit, R. Stimulus intensity in relation to excitation and pre- and post-excitatory inhibition in isolated elements of mammalian retinae. *J. Physiol.,* 1944, 103: 103-18.

Granit, R. Centrifugal and antidromic effects on ganglion cells of retina. *J. Neurophysiol.,* 1955, 18: 388-411.

Granit, R., and Kellerth, J.O. The effects of stretch receptors on motoneurons. In Yahr, M.D., and Purpura, D.P. (eds.) *Neurophysiological Basis of Normal and Abnormal Motor Activities.* Hewlett, N.Y.: Raven Press, 1967. Pp. 3-28.

Gray, J.A.B., and Lal, S. Effects of mechanical and thermal stimulation of cats' pads on the excitability of dorsal horn neurones. *J. Physiol.,* 1965, 179: 154-62.

Grossman, S.P. Direct adrenergic and cholinergic stimulation of hypothalamic mechanisms. *Amer. J. Physiol.,* 1962, 202: 872-82.

Grossman, S.P. The VMH: A center for affective reaction, satiety, or both? *Physiology and Behavior,* 1966, 1:10.

Groves, P.M., and Thompson, R.F. Habituation: A dual-process theory. *Psych. Rev.,* 1970, 77: 419-50.

Grueninger, W.E., Kimble, D.P., Grueninger, J., and Levine, S. GSR and corticosteroid response in monkeys with frontal ablations. *Neuropsychologia,* 1965, 3: 205-16.

Grueninger, W.E., and Pribram, K.H. Effects of spatial and nonspatial distractors on performance latency of monkeys with frontal lesions. *J. comp. Physiol. Psych.*, 1969, 68: 203-9.

Grundfest, H. Synaptic and ephaptic transmission. In Quarton, G.C., Melnechuk, T., and Schmitt, F.O. (eds.) *The Neurosciences.* New York: The Rockefellar University Press, 1967. Pp. 353-72.

Grusser, O.J., and Grutzner, A. Reaktionen einzelner neurone des optischen cortex der katze nach elektrischen reizserien des nervus opticus. *Arch. Psychiat. Nervenkr.*, 1958, 197: 405-32.

Gumnit, R.J. D.C. potential changes from auditory cortex of cat. *J. Neurophysiol.*, 1960, 23: 667-75.

Gumnit, R.J. The distribution of direct current responses evoked by sounds in the auditory cortex of the cat. *Electroenceph. clin. Neurophysiol.*, 1961, 13: 889-95.

Guthrie, E.R. Conditioning: a theory of learning in terms of stimulus, response, and association. In *National Society for the Study of Education, The Forty-First Yearbook.* Bloomington: Public School Publishing Co., 1942.

Hagbarth, K.E., and Kerr, D.I.B. Central influences on spinal afferent conduction. *J. Neurophysiol.*, 1954, 17: 295-307.

Hamburger, V. Experimental embryology. *Encyclopedia Britannica,* 1961, 8: 973-80.

Hearst, E., and Pribram, K.H. Appetitive and aversive generalization gradients in amygdalectomized monkeys. *J. comp. physiol. Psychol.*, 1964a, 58: 296-98.

Hearst, E., and Pribram, K.H. Facilitation of avoidance behavior by unavoidable shocks in normal and amygdalectomized monkeys. *Psych. Reports.*, 1964b, 14: 39-42.

Hebb, D.O. *The Organization of Behavior. A Neuropsychological Theory.* New York: John Wiley, 1949.

Hebb, D.O. Drives and the CNS (conceptual nervous system). *Psych. Rev.*, 1955, 62: 243-54.

Hecht, S. In Murchison, C. (ed.) *Handbook of General Experimental Psychology.* Worcester: Clark University Press, 1934. Pp. 704-828.

Hein, A. Recovering spatial motor coordination after visual cortex lesions. In *Perception and Its Disorders.* Res. Publ. A.R.N.M.D., XLVIII, 1970, 163-75.

Held, R. Action contingent development of vision in neonatal animals. In Kimble, D.P. (ed.) *Experience and Capacity.* New York: New York Academy of Sciences, 1968. Pp. 31-111.

Henry, C.E., and Scoville, W.B. Suppression-burst activity from isolated cerebral cortex in man. *Electroenceph. clin. Neurophysiol.*, 1952, 4: 1-22.

Hering, E. *Outlines of a Theory of Light Sense.* Trans. Hurvich, L.M. and Jameson, D. Cambridge: Harvard University Press, 1964.

Hernandez-Peon, R., and Scherer, H. Central mechanisms controlling conduction along central sensory pathways. *Acta Neurol. Latino Americana,* 1955, I: 256-64.

Hilgard, E. *Introduction to Psychology.* New York: Harcourt, Brace & Jovanovich, 1962.

House, E.L., and Pansky, B. *Neuroanatomy.* New York: McGraw-Hill, 1960.

Howard, I.P., Craske, B., and Templeton, W.B. Visuomotor adaptation to discordant ex-afferent stimulation. *J.Exp. Psychol.*, 1965, 70: 181-91.

Hubel, D.H., and Wiesel, T.N. Receptive fields, binocular interaction and functional architecture in the cat's visual cortex. *J. Physiol.*, 1962, 160: 106-54.

Hunter, W.S. The delayed reaction in animals and children. *Animal Behav. Mono.*, 1913, 2: 1-86.

Hurvich, L.M., and Jameson, D. Perceived color, induction effects, and opponent-response mechanisms. *J. Genl. Physiol.*, 1960, 43: 63-80.

Huttenlocher, P.R. Evoked and spontaneous activity in single units of medial brain stem during natural sleep and waking. *J. Neurophysiol.*, 1961, 24: 451-68.

Hydén, H. The neuron. In Brachet, J., and Mirsky, A.F. (eds.) *The Cell, Vol. IV.* New York and London: Academic, 1961. Pp. 215-323.

Hydén, H. Activation of nuclear RNA in neurons and glia in learning. In Kimble, D.P. (ed.) *The Anatomy of Memory.* Palo Alto, Calif: Science and Behavior Books, 1965. Pp. 178-239.

Hydén, H. Biochemical aspects of learning and memory. In Pribram, K.H. (ed.) *On the Biology of Learning.* New York: Harcourt, Brace & Jovanovich, 1969. Pp. 95-125.

Ingvar, D.N. Electrical activity of isolated cortex in the unanaesthetized cat with intact brain stem. *Acta physiol. Scand.,* 1955, 33: 151-68.

Jacobsen, C.F. Recent experiments on the function of the frontal lobes. *Psychol. Bull.,* 1928, 25: 1-11.

Jacobsen, C.F. Studies of cerebral function in primates. I. The function of the frontal association areas in monkeys. *Comp. Psychol. Monogr.,* 1936, 13: 3-60.

Jacobsen, C.F., Wolfe, J.B., and Jackson, J.A. An experimental analysis of the functions of the frontal association areas in primates. *J. nerv. ment. Dis.,* 1935, 82: 1-14.

Jakobson, R. Two aspects of language and two types of aphasic disturbances. Part II. In Jakobson, R., and Halle, M. (eds.) *Fundamentals of Language.* The Hague: Mouton, 1956. Pp. 53-82.

Jakobson, R. Towards a linguistic typology of aphasic impairments. In de Reuch, A.V.S., and O'Connor, M. (eds.) *Disorders of Language.* Boston: Little, Brown, 1964. Pp. 21-42.

Jakobson, R. Linguistic types of aphasia. In Carterette, E.C. (ed.) *Brain Function Vol. III, Speech, Language and Communication.* Berkeley and Los Angeles: University of California Press, 1966. Pp. 67-91.

James, W. *Pragmatism—A New Name for Some Old Ways of Thinking.* New York: Longmans Green and Co., 1931 (1st ed. 1907).

Jansen, J., and Brodal, A. Das kleinhirn. In Mollendorff, W. von (ed.) *Handbuch der Mikroskopischen Anatomie des Menschen, Vol. 3.* Berlin: Julius Springer, 1958.

Jasper, H.H. (ed.) *Reticular Formation of the Brain.* Boston: Little, Brown, 1958.

Jasper, H.H. Neurochemical mediators of specific and non-specific cortical activation. In Evans, C.R., and Mulholland, T.B. (eds.) *Attention in Neurophysiology.* London: Butterworths, 1969. Pp. 377-95.

Jasper, H.H., and Koyama, I. Rate of release of amino acids from the cerebral cortex in the cat as affected by brainstem and thalamic stimulation. *Canadian Journal of Physiology and Pharmacology,* 1959, 47: 889-905.

John, E.R. *Mechanisms of Memory.* New York: Academic, 1967.

John, E.R., Herrington, R.N., and Sutton, S. Effects of visual form on the evoked response. *Science,* 1967, 155: 1439-42.

John, E.R., and Morgades, P.P. The pattern and anatomical distribution of evoked potentials and multiple unit activity elicited by conditioned stimuli in trained cats. *Communications in Behavioral Biology, Part A., Vol. 3, No. 4.* New York: Academic, 1969. Pp. 181-207.

Journal of Applied Physiology. Interaction of paired sensory stimuli and conduction in peripheral nerves by G. von Békésy, 1963, 18: 1276-84.

Jouvet, M. The states of sleep. *Scientific American,* 1967, 216: 62-72.

Jung, R. Korrelationen von neuronentatigkeit und sehen. In Jung, R., and Kornhuber, H. (eds.) *Neurophysiologie and Psychophysik des visuellen Systems.* Symposium Freiburg, Springer, Berlin, Gottingen, Heidelberg, 1961. Pp. 410-34.

Jung, R. Neuronal integration in the visual cortex and its significance for visual information. In Rosenblith, W. (ed.) *Sensory Communication.* New York: John Wiley, 1961. Pp. 627-74.

Jung, R. Neuronal integration in the visual cortex and its significance for visual information. As excerpted in Pribram, K.H. (ed.) *Brain and Behavior 2: Perception and Action.* Baltimore: Penguin, 1969. Pp. 14-46.

Kamiya, J. Conscious control of brain waves. *Psychology Today,* 1968, 1: 56-60. In *Readings in Experimental Psychology Today.* Del Mar, Ca.: CRM Books, 1970. Pp. 51-55.

Kant, E. *Critique of Pure Reason* (N. Kemp Smith, trans.). New York: Macmillon, 1963.

Kappers, C.U.A., Huber, G.C., and Crosby, E.C. *The Comparative Anatomy of the Nervous System of Vertebrates, Including Man.* New York: Macmillan, 1936.

Katz, J.J., and Halstead, W.C. Protein organization and mental function. *Comp. Psychol. Monogr.,* 1950, 20: 1-38.

Kelly, C.R. *Manual and Automatic Control.* New York: John Wiley, 1968.

Kemp, J.M., and Powell, T.P.S. The cortico-striate projection in the monkey. *Brain,* 1970, 93: 525-46.

Kennard, M.A. Alterations in response to visual stimuli following lesions of frontal lobe in monkeys. *Arch. Neurol. Psychiat.,* 1939, 41: 1153-65.

Kerr, D.I.B., and Hagbarth, K.E. An investigation of olfactory centrifugal fiber system. *J. Neurophysiol.,* 1955, 18: 362-74.

Kimble, D.P. Possible inhibitory function of the hippocampus. *Neuropsychologia,* 1969, 7: 235-44.

Kimble, D.P., Bagshaw, M.H., and Pribram, K.H. The GSR of monkeys during orienting and habituation after selective partial ablations of the cingulate and frontal cortex. *Neuropsychologia,* 1965, 3: 121-28.

King, M.B., and Hoebel, B.G. Killing elicited by brain stimulation in rats. *Domm. Behav. Biol.,* Part A, 1968, 2: 173-77.

Köhler. W. The present situation in brain physiology. *Am. Psychologist,* 1958, 13: 150.

Konorski, J. *Integrative Activity of the Brain. An Interdisciplinary Approach.* Chicago: University of Chicago Press, 1967.

Konrad, K.W., and Bagshaw, M.H. Effect of novel stimuli on cats reared in a restricted environment. *J. comp. physiol. Psychol.,* 1970, 70: 157-64.

Kraft, M.S., Obrist, W.D., and Pribram, K.H. The effect of irritative lesions of the striate cortex on learning of visual discriminations in monkeys. *J. comp. physiol. Psychol.,* 1960, 53: 17-22.

Krasne, F.B. General disruption resulting from electrical stimulation of ventro-medial hypothalamus. *Science,* 1962, 138: 822-23.

Kretch, D., and Crutchfield, R.S. *Elements of Psychology.* New York: Knopf, 1962.

Krieg, W.J.S. *Functional Neuroanatomy. 3rd ed.* Evanston, Ill.: Brain Books, 1966.

Kruger, L. Morphological alterations of the cerebral cortex and their possible role in the loss and acquisition of information. In Kimble, D.P. (ed.) *The Anatomy of Memory.* Palo Alto: Science and Behavior Books, 1965. Pp. 88-139.

Kuffler, S.W., and Hunt, C.C. The mammalian small-nerve fibers: a system for efferent nervous regulation of muscle spindle discharge. *Res. Publ. Ass. Nerv. Ment. Dis.,* 1952, 30: 24-47.

Kupfermann, I., Castellucci, V., Pinsker, H., and Kandel, K. Neuronal correlates of habituation and dishabituation of the gell withdrawal reflex in aplysia. *Science,* 1970, 167: 1743-45.

Lacey, J.I., Kagan, J., Lacey, B.C., and Moss, H.A. The visceral level: situational determinants and behavioral correlates of autonomic response patterns. In Knapp, P.H. (ed.) *Expression of the Emotions in Man.* New York: International Universities Press, 1963. Pp. 161-208.

Lacey, J.I., and Lacey, B.C. The relationship of resting autonomic cyclic activity to motor impulsivity. In Solomon, C., Cobb, S., and Penfield, W. (eds.) *The Brain and Human Behavior.* Baltimore: Williams & Wilkins, 1958. Pp. 144-209.

Langer, S.K. *Philosophy in a New Key: A Study in the Symbolism of Reason, Rite, and Art.* New York: Mentor Books, 1951.

Larsell, O. *Anatomy of the Nervous System. 2nd ed.* New York: Appleton-Century-Crofts, 1951.

Lashley, K.S. *Brain Mechanisms and Intelligence.* Chicago: University of Chicago Press, 1929.

Lashley, K.S. The problem of cerebral organization in vision. In *Biological Symposia, Vol. VII, Visual Mechanisms.* Lancaster: Jaques Cattell Press, 1942. Pp. 301-22.

Lashley, K.S. In search of the engram. In Society for Experimental Biology (Grt. Britain) *Physiological Mechanisms in Animal Behavior.* New York: Academic, 1950. Pp. 454-82.

Lashley, K.S. The problem of serial order in behavior. In Jeffress, L.A. (ed.) *Cerebral Mechanisms in Behavior, The Hixon Symposium.* New York: John Wiley, 1951. Pp. 112-46.

Lashley, K.S. In Beach, F.A., Hebb, D.O., Morgan, C.T., and Nissen, H.W. (eds.) *The Neuropsychology of Lashley.* New York: McGraw-Hill, 1960.

Lashley, K.S., Chow, K.L., and Semmes, J. An examination of the electrical field theory of cerebral integration. *Psych. Rev.,* 1951, 58: 123-36.

Lawrence, D.H., and Festinger, L. *Deterrents and Reinforcement: The Psychology of Insufficient Reward.* Stanford: Stanford University Press, 1962.

Le Gros Clark, W.E., Beattie, J., Riddoch, G., and Dott, N.M. *The Hypothalamus.* Edinburgh: Oliver & Boyd, 1938.

Leith, E.N. and Upatnicks, J. *J. Opt. Soc. Am.* 54: 1295. Nov. 1964.

Leith, E.N. and Upatnicks, J. Photography by laser. *Scientific American,* 1965, 212: 24-35.

Leskell, L. *Acta Physiol. Scand.,* 1945, 10 (Suppl. 31): 1-84.

Lewis, E.R. Neural subsystems: goals, concepts and tools. In Quarton, G.C., Melnechuk, T. and Adelman, G. (eds.) *The Neurosciences* (Second Study). New York: The Rockefellar University Press, 1970. Pp. 384-95.

Li, C.L., Cullen, C., and Jasper, H.H. Laminar microelectrode analysis of cortical unspecific recruiting responses and spontaneous rhythms. *J. Neurophysiol.,* 1956, 19: 131-43.

Libet, B. Brain stimulation and conscious experience. In Eccles, J.C. (ed.) *Brain and Conscious Experience.* New York: Springer-Verlag, 1966. Pp. 165-81.

Lilly, J.C. A 25-channel potential field recorder. In *Second Annual IRE-AIEE Conference on Electronic Instrumentation in Nucleonics and Medicine.* New York: Institute of Radio Engineers, 1949.

Lindsley, D. Average evoked potentials for achievements, failures and prospects. In Donchin, E., and Lindsley, D. (eds.) *Average Evoked Potentials.* NASA, 1969. Pp. 1-43.

Lindsley, D.B. Emotion. In Stevens, S.S. (ed.) *Handbook of Experimental Psychology.* New York: John Wiley, 1951. Pp. 473-516.

Lindsley, D.B. The reticular activation system and perceptual integration. In Sheer, D.E. (ed.) *Electrical Stimulation of the Brain.* Austin: University of Texas Press, 1961. Pp. 331-49.

Livanov, M.N., and Ananiev, V.M. Electrophysiological investigation of spatial distribution of activity of the rabbit cortex. *Fizol. Z.* (Mosk.), 1955, 41: 461-69.

Livingston, R.B. Some brain stem mechanisms relating to psychosomatic functions. *Psychosom. Med.,* 1955, 17: 347-54.

Lloyd, D.P.C. Spinal mechanisms involved in somatic activities. In Field, J., Magoun, H.W., and Hall, V.E. (eds.) *Handbook of Physiology, Neurophysiology II.* Washington: American Physiological Society, 1959. Pp. 929-49.

London, P., and Hart, J.T. EEG alpha rhythms and hypnotic susceptibility. *Nature*, 1968, 219: 71-72.

Lorenz, K. Innate bases of learning. In Pribram, K.H. (ed.) *On the Biology of Learning.* New York: Harcourt, Brace & Jovanovich, 1969. Pp. 13-94.

Luckhardt, A.B., and Carlson, A. J. Contributions to the physiology of the stomach. XVIII: On the chemical control of the gastric hunger mechanism. *Amer. J. Physiol.*, 1915, 36: 37.

Luria, A.R. *The Nature of Human Conflicts.* New York: Evergreen Press, 1960.

Luria, A.R. Factors and forms of aphasia. In de Reuch, A.V.S., and O'Connor, M. (eds.) *Disorders of Language.* Boston: Little, Brown, 1964. Pp. 143-61.

Luria, A.R., Pribram, K.H., and Homskaya, E.D. An experimental analysis of the behavioral disturbance produced by a left frontal arachnoidal endothelloma (meningioma). *Neuropsychologia*, 1964, 2: 257-80.

Mace, G.A. Psychology and aesthetics. *Brit. J. Aesthetics*, 1962, 2: 3-16.

MacKay, D.M. Cerebral organization and the conscious control of action. In Eccles, J.C. (ed.) *Brain and Conscious Experience.* New York: Springer-Verlag, 1966. Pp. 422-45.

MacLean, P.D., and Pribram, K.H. A neuronographic analysis of the medial and basal cerebral cortex. I. Cat. *J. Neurophysiol.*, 1953, 16: 312-23.

McConnel, J.V., Shigehisa, T. and Salive, H. Attempts to transfer approach and avoidance responses by RNA injections in rats. In Pribram, K.H. and Broadbent, D.E. (eds.) *The Biology of Memory.* New York: Academic Press, 1970. Pp. 129-135.

Magendie, F. Experiences sur les fonctions des racines des nerfs rachidiens.   exp., 1822, 2: 276-79.

Magoun, H.W. Caudal and cepalic influences of the brain stem reticular formation. *Physiol. Rev.*, 1950, 30: 459-74.

Magoun, H.W. *The Waking Brain.* Springfield: Charles C Thomas, 1958.

Malis, L.I., Pribram, K.H., and Kruger, L. Action potentials in "motor" cortex evoked by peripheral nerve stimulation. *J. Neurophysiol.*, 1953, 16: 161-67.

Marg, E., and Adams, J.E. Evidence for a neurological zoom system in vision from angular changes in some receptive fields of single neurons with changes in fixation distance in the human visual cortex. *Experientia*, 1970, 26: 270-71.

Marshall, W.H. and Talbot, S.A. Recent evidence for neural mechanisms in vision leading to a general theory of sensory acuity. In Cattell, J. (ed.) *Biological Symposia.* Lancaster: The Jacques Cattell Press, 1942. Pp.117-164.

Matthews, P.B.C. Muscle spindles and their motor control. *Physiol. Rev.*, 1964, 44: 219-88.

Maturana, H.R., Lettvin, J.Y., McCulloch, W.S., and Pitts, W.H. Anatomy and physiology of vision in the frog (Rana pipiens). *J. gen. Physiol.*, 1960, 43 (Suppl.): 129-75.

Mayér, J. Regulatory and metabolic experimental obesities. In Brazier, M.A.B. (ed.) *Brain and Behavior, Vol. II.* Washington: American Institute of Biological Sciences, 1963. Pp. 273-318.

McCleary, R.A. Response specificity in the behavioral effects of limbic lesions in the cat. *J. comp. physiol. Psychol.*, 1961, 54: 605-13.

McCulloch, W.S. *Embodiments of Mind.* Cambridge: MIT Press, 1965.

McCullough, C. Color adaptation of edge-detectors in the human visual system. *Science*, 1965, 149: 1115-1116.

McGaugh, J.L. and Petrinovich, L. The effect of strychnine sulphate on maze-learning. *Amer. J. Psychol.*, 1959, 72: 99-102.

Merton, P.A. Speculations on the servo-control of movement. In Malcolm, J.L., and Gray, J.A.B. (eds.) *The Spinal Cord.* London: J. & A. Churchill, Ltd., 1953. Pp. 247-60.

Mettler, F.A. Cortical subcortical relations in abnormal motor functions. In Yahr, M.D., and Purpura, D.P. (eds.) *Neurophysiological Basis of Normal and Abnormal Motor Activities.* Hewlett, N.Y.: Raven Press, 1967. Pp. 445-97.

Meyer, J.S. Studies of cerebral circulation in brain injury. IV: Ischemia and hypoxemia of the brain stem and respiratory center. *Electroenceph. clin. Neurophysiol.*, 1957, 9: 83-100.

Meynert, T. Der Bau der Grosshirnrinde und seine ortlichen Verschiedenheiten, nebst einer pathologisch-anatomischen Corollarium. *Viertel jahrschr. Psychiat.*, 1867-1868, 1: 77-93, 125-27.

Michael, R.P. Estrogen-sensitive neurons and sexual behavior in female cats. *Science*, 1962, 136: 322.

Miller, G.A. On turning psychology over to the unwashed. *Psychology Today*, 1969, 3: 67-68.

Miller, G.A., Galanter, E.H., and Pribram, K.H. *Plans and the Structure of Behavior.* New York: Holt, Rinehart & Winston, 1960.

Miller, N.E., Bailey, C.J., and Stevenson, J.A. Decreased "hunger" but increased food intake resulting from hypothalamic lesions. *Science*, 1950, 112: 256-59.

Milner, B. Intellectual function of the temporal lobes. *Psychol. Bull.*, 1954, 51: 52-62.

Milner, B. Psychological defects produced by temporal lobe excision. In *The Brain and Human Behavior* (ARNMD Vol. XXXVI). Baltimore: Williams & Wilkins, 1958. Pp. 244-57.

Milner, B. The memory defect in bilateral hippocampal lesions. *Psychiatric Research Reports*, 1959, 11: 43-52.

Milner, P.M. *Physiological Psychology.* New York: Holt, Rinehart and Winston, 1970.

Mishkin, M., and Hall, M. Discriminations along a size continuum following ablation of the inferior temporal convexity in monkeys. *J. comp. physiol. Psychol.*, 1955, 48: 97-101.

Mishkin, M., and Pribram, K.H. Visual discrimination performance following partial ablations of the temporal lobe: I. Ventral vs. lateral. *J. comp. physiol. Psychol.*, 1954, 47: 14-20.

Mishkin, M., and Weiskrantz, L. Effects of cortical lesions in monkey on critical flicker frequency. *J. comp. physiol. Psychol.*, 1959, 52: 660-66.

Mittelstaedt, H. Discussion. In Kimble, D.P. (ed.) *Experience and Capacity.* New York: The New York Academy of Sciences, 1968. Pp. 46-49.

Morin, F., Schwartz, H.G., and O'Leary, J.L. Experimental study of the spinothalamic and related tracts. *Acta Psychiat. et Neurologica Scandinavia*, 1951, XXVI: 3-4.

Morrell, F. Effect of anodal polarization on the firing pattern of single cortical cells. In Furness, F.N. (ed.) *Pavlovian Conference on Higher Nervous Activity.* Ann. N.Y. Acad. Sci., 1961a. Pp. 813-1198.

Morrell, F. Electrophysiological contributions to the neural basis of learning. *Physiol. Rev.*, 1961b, 41: 443-94.

Morrell, F. Lasting changes in synaptic organization produced by continuous neuronal bombardment. In Delafresnaye, J.F., Fessard, A., and Konorski, J. (eds.) *Symposium on Brain Mechanisms and Learning.* Oxford: Blackwell Scientific Publications, 1961c. Pp. 375-92.

Morrell, F. Information storage in nerve cells. In Fields, W.S., and Abbott, W. (eds.) *Information Storage and Neural Control.* Springfield: Charles C Thomas, 1963. Pp. 189-229.

Morrell, F. Modification of RNA as a result of neural activity. In Brazier, M.A.B. (ed.) *Brain Function. II: RNA and Brain Function; Memory and Learning.* UCLA Forum Med. Sci. No. 2. Los Angeles: Univ. of California Press, 1964. Pp. 183-202.

Morrell, F. Electrical signs of sensory coding. In Quarton, G.C., Melnechuk, T., and Schmitt, F.O. (eds.) *The Neurosciences: A Study Program.* New York: The Rockefellar University Press, 1967. Pp. 452-69.

Morris, C. *Signs, Language and Behavior.* New York: Braziller, 1946.

Mountcastle, V.B. Modality and topographic properties of single neurons of cat's somatic sensory cortex. *J. Neurophysiol.*, 1957, 20: 408-34.

Murray, R.L., and Cobb, G.C. *Physics: Concepts and Consequences.* Englewood Cliffs, N.J.: Prentice-Hall, 1970.

Niu, M.C. Current evidency concerning chemical inducers. In *Evolution of Nervous Control from Primitive Organisms to Man.* Washington: American Association for the Advancement of Science, Pub. No. 52, 1959. Pp. 7-30.

Nobel, K.W., and Dewson, J.H., III. A corticofugal projection from insular and temporal cortex to the homolateral inferior colliculus in cat. *J. Aud. Research,* 1966, 6: 67-75.

Olds, J. Physiological mechanisms of reward. In Jones, M.R. (ed.) *Nebraska Symposium on Motivation.* Lincoln: University of Nebraska Press, 1955. Pp. 73-138.

Olds, J. Differential effects of drives and drugs on self-stimulation at different brain sites. In Sheer, D.E. (ed.) *Electrical Stimulation of the Brain.* Austin: University of Texas Press, 1961. Pp. 350-66.

Olds, J., and Milner, P. Positive reinforcement produced by electrical stimulation of septal area and other regions of rat brain. *J. comp. physiol. Psychol.,* 1954, 47: 419-27.

Ornstein, R.E. *On the Experience of Time.* Hammondsworth, England: Penguin Education, 1969.

Penfield, W. Consciousness, memory and man's conditioned reflexes. In Pribram, K.H. (ed.) *On the Biology of Learning.* New York: Harcourt, Brace & Jovanovich, 1969. Pp. 127-68.

Penfield, W., and Boldrey, E. Somatic motor sensory representation in the cerebral cortex of man as studied by electrical stimulation. *Brain,* 1937, 60: 389-443.

Perkel, D.H., and Bullock, T.H. Neural coding. *Neurosciences Res. Prog. Bull.,* 1968, 6: 221-348.

Perkins, C.C., Jr. An analysis of the concept of reinforcement. *Psych. Rev.,* 1968, 75: 155-72.

Phillips, C.G. Changing concepts of the precentral motor area. In Eccles, J.C. (ed.) *Brain and Conscious Experience.* New York: Springer-Verlag, 1965. Pp. 389-421.

Pinsker, H., Kupfermann, I., Castellucci, V., and Kandel, E. Habituation and dishabituation of the gell withdrawal reflex in aplysia. *Science,* 1970, 167: 1740-42.

Pittendrigh, C.S. Circadian rhythms and the circadian organization of living systems. *Quart. Biol.,* 1960, 25: 159-73.

Polanyi, M. *Personal Knowledge, Towards a Post-Critical Philosophy.* Chicago: University of Chicago Press, 1960.

Polyak, S.L. *The Retina: Structure of the Retina and the Visual Perception of Space.* Chicago: University of Chicago Press, 1941.

Pomerat, C.M. *Dynamic Aspects of Tissue Culture.* Los Angeles: Wexler Film Productions, 1964.

Pool, J.L., Collins, L.M., Kessler, E., Vernon, L.J., and Feiring, E. Surgical procedure. In Mettler, F.A. (ed.) *Selective Partial Ablation of the Frontal Cortex.* New York: Paul B. Hoeber, Inc., Medical Book Dept. of Harper & Brothers, 1949. Pp. 34-47.

Poppen, R., Pribram, K.H., and Robinson, R.S. The effects of frontal lobotomy in man on performance of a multiple choice task. *Exp. Neurol.,* 1965, 11: 217-29.

Premack, D. Toward empirical behavior laws. 1. Positive reinforcement. *Psychol. Rev.,* 1959, 66: 219-33.

Premack, D. Reversibility of the reinforcement relation. *Science,* 1962, 136: 255-57.

Premack, D. Reinforcement theory. In Levine, D. (ed.) *Nebraska Symposium on Motivation.* Lincoln: University of Nebraska Press, 1965. Pp. 123-88.

Premack, D. The education of Sarah: a chimp learns the language. *Psychology Today,* 1970, 4: 55-58.

Premack, D., and Collier, G. Analysis of nonreinforcement variables affecting response probability. In Munn, N.L. (ed.) *Psychological Monographs, General and Applied, Vol. 76.* Washington: American Psychological Association, 1962. Pp. 524-44.

Pribram, K.H. Comparative neurology and the evolution of behavior. In Simpson, G.G. (ed.) *Evolution and Behavior.* New Haven: Yale University Press, 1958. Pp. 140-64.

Pribram, K.H. Discussion. In Brazier, M.A.B. (ed.) *Brain and Behavior.* Washington, D.C.: American Institute of Biological Sciences, 1961. Pp. 57-58.

Pribram, K.H. On the neurology of thinking. *Behav. Sci.,* 1959, 4: 265-87.

Pribram, K.H. A review of theory in physiological psychology. In *Annual Review of Psychology, Vol. 11.* Palo Alto: Annual Reviews, Inc., 1960a. Pp. 1-40.

Pribram, K.H. The intrinsic systems of the forebrain. In Field, J., Magoun, H.W., and Hall, V.E. (eds.) *Handbook of Physiology, Neurophysiology II.* Washington: American Physiological Society, 1960b. Pp. 1323-44.

Pribram, K.H. Implications for systematic studies of behavior. In Sheer, E. (ed.) *Electrical Stimulation of the Brain.* Austin: University of Texas Press, 1961. Pp. 563-74.

Pribram, K.H. Interrelations of psychology and the neurological disciplines. In Koch, S. (ed.) *Psychology: A Study of a Science. Vol. 4, Biologically Oriented Fields: Their Place in Psychology and in Biological Sciences.* New York: McGraw-Hill, 1962. Pp. 119-57.

Pribram, K.H. Control systems and behavior. In Brazier, M.A.B. (ed.) *Brain and Behavior. Vol. II: Internal Environment and Alimentary Behavior.* Washington, D.C.: American Institute of Biological Sciences, 1963. Pp. 371-87.

Pribram, K.H. Discussion. In Kimble, D.P. (ed.) *The Anatomy of Memory.* Palo Alto: Science and Behavior Books, 1965. Pp. 140-76.

Pribram, K.H. Proposal for a structural pragmatism: some neuropsychological considerations of problems in philosophy. In Wolman, B., and Nagle, E. (eds.) *Scientific Psychology: Principles and Approaches.* New York: Basic Books, 1965. Pp. 426-59.

Pribram, K.H. Some dimensions of remembering: steps toward a neuropsychological model of memory. In Gaito, J. (ed.) *Macromolecules and Behavior.* New York: Academic, 1966. Pp. 165-87.

Pribram, K.H. The limbic systems, efferent control of neural inhibition and behavior. In Adey, W.R., and Tokizane, T. (eds.) *Progress in Brain Research, Vol. 27.* Amsterdam: Elsevier Publishing Co., 1967. Pp. 318-36.

Pribram, K.H. The amnestic syndromes: disturbances in coding? In Talland, G.A., and Waugh, N.C. (eds.) *Psychopathology of Memory.* New York: Academic, 1969a. Pp. 127-57.

Pribram, K.H. Four R's of remembering. In Pribram, K.H. (ed.) *On the Biology of Learning.* New York: Harcourt, Brace & Jovanovich, 1969b. Pp. 193-225.

Pribram, K.H. The primate frontal cortex. In Pribram, K.H. (ed.) Inhibition in Neuropsychology (A Symposium). *Neuropsychologia,* 1969c, 7: 257-66.

Pribram, K.H. The neurophysiology of remembering. *Scientific American,* Jan. 1969d, 73-86.

Pribram, K.H. The biology of mind: Neurobehavioral Foundations. In Gilgen, A. (ed.) *Scientific Psychology: Some Perspectives.* New York: Academic, 1970a. Pp. 45-70.

Pribram, K.H. The primate brain and human learning. In Linhart, J. (ed.) *Proceedings of the International Conference on Psychology of Human Learning. Vol. I.* Prague, Czechoslovak Academy of Sciences, 1970b. Pp. 27-61.

Pribram, K.H. Neurological notes on knowing. In Royce, J.R., and Rozeboom, W.W. *The Psychology of Knowing.* New York: Simon and Breach (in press).

Pribram, K.H., and Bagshaw, M.H. Further analysis of the temporal lobe syndrome utilizing frontotemporal ablations in monkeys. *J. comp. Neurol.,* 1953, 99: 347-75.

Pribram, K.H., Blehert, S.R., and Spinelli, D.N. Effects on visual discrimination of crosshatching and undercutting the inferotemporal cortex of monkeys. *J. comp. physiol. Psychol.,* 1966, 62: 358-64.

Pribram, K.H., Chow, K.L., and Semmes, J. Limit and organization of the cortical projection from the medial thalamic nucleus in monkeys. *J. comp. Neurol.,* 1953, 98: 433-48.

Pribram, K.H., Douglas, R.J., and Pribram, B.J. The nature of nonlimbic learning. *J. comp. physiol. Psychol.,* 1969, 69: 765-72.

Pribram, K.H., and Fulton, J.F. An experimental critique of the effects of anterior cingulate ablations in monkeys. *Brain,* 1954, 77: 34-44.

Pribram, K.H., and Kruger, L. Functions of the "olfactory brain." *Ann. N.Y. Acad. Sci.,* 1954, 58: 109-38.

Pribram, K.H., Kruger, L., Robinson, R., and Berman, A.J. The effects of precentral lesions on the behavior of monkeys. *Yale J. Biol. & Med.,* 1955-56, 28: 428-43.

Pribram, K.H., Lim, H., Poppen, R., and Bagshaw, M.H. Limbic lesions and the temporal structure of redundancy. *J. comp. physiol. Psychol.,* 1966, 61: 368-73.

Pribram, K.H., and MacLean, P.D. A neuronographic analysis of the medial and basal cerebral cortex: II. Monkey. *J. Neurophysiol.,* 1953, 16: 324-40.

Pribram, K.H., Mishkin, M., Rosvold, H.E., and Kaplan, S.J. Effects on delayed-response performance of lesions of dorsolateral and ventromedial frontal cortex of baboons. *J. comp. physiol. Psychol.,* 1952, 45: 565-75.

Pribram, K.H., Spinelli, D.N., and Kamback, M.C. Electrocortical correlates of stimulus response and reinforcement. *Science,* 1967, 157: 94-96.

Pribram, K.H., Spinelli, D.N., and Reitz, S.L. Effects of radical disconnexion of occipital and temporal cortex on visual behaviour of monkeys. *Brain,* 1969, 92: 301-12.

Pribram, K.H., and Tubbs, W.E. Short-term memory, parsing and the primate frontal cortex. *Science,* 1967, 156: 1765-67.

Pribram, K.H., Wilson, W.A., and Connors, J. The effects of lesions of the medial forebrain on alternation behavior of rhesus monkeys. *Exp. Neurol.,* 1962, 6: 36-47.

Psychology Today. Del Mar, Ca.: CRM Books, 1970.

Purpura, D.P. Discussion. In Brazier, M.A.B. (ed.) *The Central Nervous System and Behavior.* New York: Josiah Macy, Jr. Foundation, 1958.

Purpura, D.P. Discussion. In Brazier, M.A.B. (ed.) *Brain and Behavior, Vol. II.* Washington: American Institute of Biological Sciences, 1962.

Purpura, D.P. Comparative physiology of dendrites. In Quarton, G.C., Melnechuk, T., and Schmitt, F.O. (eds.) *The Neurosciences.* New York: The Rockefellar University Press, 1967. Pp. 372-93.

Quilliam, T.A. Some characteristics of myelinated fibre populations. *J. Anat.,* 1956, 90: 172-87.

Quillian, M.R. Word concepts: a theory simulation of some basic semantic capabilities. *Behav. Sci.,* 1967, 12: 410-30.

Quine, W.V. *Word and Object.* Cambridge: MIT Press, 1960.

Rall, T., and Gilman, A.G. The role of cyclic AMP in the nervous system. *Neurosciences Research Program Bulletin,* 1970, 8: 221-323.

Ralston, H.J., III. Evidence for presynaptic dendrites and a proposal for their mechanism of action. *Nature,* April, 1971.

Ranson, S.W., and Clark, S.L. *The Anatomy of the Nervous System.* Philadelphia: Saunders, 1959.

Ranson, S.W., Fisher, C., and Ingram, W.R. Hypothalamic regulation of temperature in the monkey. *A.M.A. Arch. Neurol. Psychiat.,* 1937, 38: 445-66.

Rasmussen, G.L. The olivary feduncle and other fiber projections of the superior complex. *J. comp. Neurol.,* 1946, 83: 141.

Ratliff, F. *Mach Bands.* San Francisco: Holden Day, 1965.

Reitz, S.L., and Pribram, K.H. Some subcortical connections of the inferotemporal gyrus of monkey. *Exp. Neurol.,* 1969, 26: 632-45.

Rémond, A. Integrated and topological analysis of the EEG. In Brazier, M.A.B. (ed.) *Computer Techniques in EEG Analysis.* Supplement 20 to "The EEG Journal," 1961. Pp. 64-67.

Richter, C.P. Experimental production of cycles in behavior and physiology in animals. *Acta med. Scand.,* 1955, 152, Sup. 307: 36-37.

Riggs, L.A., Ratliff, F., Cornsweet, J.C., and Cornsweet, T.N. The disappearance of steadily fixated test objects. *J. Opt. Soc. Amer.,* 1953, 43: 495-501.

Roberts, L. Activation and interference of cortical functions. In Sheer, D.E. (ed.) *Electrical Stimulation of the Brain.* Austin: University of Texas Press, 1961. Pp. 533-53.

Roberts, W.W. Are hypothalamic motivational mechanisms functionally and anatomically specific? *Brain, Behavior and Evolution,* 1969, 2: 317-42.

Robinson, B.W. Forebrain alimentary responses: some organizational principles. In Wayner, M.J. (ed.) *Thirst, First International Symposium on Thirst in the Regulation of Body Water.* New York: Pergamon Press, 1964.

Rock, I. Perception from the standpoint of psychology. In *Perception and Its Disorders.* Res. Publ. A.R.N.M.D. Vol. XLVIII, 1970. Pp. 1-11.

Rodieck, R.W. Quantitative analysis of cat retinal ganglion cell response to visual stimuli. *Vision Research,* 1965, 5: 583-601.

Rose, J.E., Malis, L.I., and Baker, C.P. Neural growth in the cerebral cortex after lesions produced by monoenergetic denterous. In Rosenblith, W.A. (ed.) *Sensory Communication.* New York: John Wiley, 1961. Pp. 279-301.

Rose, J.E., and Woolsey, C.N. The relations of thalamic connections, cellular structure and evocable electrical activity in the auditory region of the cat. *J. comp. Neurol.,* 1949, 91: 441-66.

Rothblat, L., and Pribram, K.H. Selective attention: Input filter or response selection? An electro-physiological analysis. *Brain Research,* 1972.

Ruch, T.C. Motor systems. In Stevens, S.S. (ed.) *Handbook of Experimental Psychology.* New York: John Wiley, 1951. Pp. 154-208.

Rushton, W.A.H. Increment threshold and dark adaptation. *J. Opt. Soc. Amer.,* 1963, 53: 104-9.

Russell, R.W., Singer, G., Flanagan, F., Stone, M., and Russell, J.W. Quantitative relations in amygdala modulation of drinking. *Physiology and Behavior,* 1968, 3: 871-75.

Ryle, G. *The Concept of Mind.* New York: Barnes & Noble, 1949.

Schachter, S. Cognitive effects on bodily functioning: studies of obesity and eating. In Glass, D. (ed.) *Neurophysiology and Emotion.* New York: The Rockefeller University Press and Russell Sage Foundation, 1967. Pp.117-144.

Schachter, S., and Singer, T.E. Cognitive social and physiological determinants of emotional state. *Psychol. Rev.,* 1962, 69: 379-97.

Schapiro, S., and Vukovich, K.R. Early experience effects upon cortical dendrites: a proposed model for development. *Science,* 1970, 167: 292-94.

Scheibel, M.E., and Scheibel, A.B. Structural substrates for integrative patterns in the brain stem reticular core. In Jasper, H.H. (ed.) *Reticular Formation of the Brain.* Boston: Little, Brown, 1958. Pp. 31-38.

Scheibel, M.E., and Scheibel, A.B. Anatomical basis of attention mechanisms in vertebrate brains. In Quarton, G.C., Melnechuk, T., and Schmitt, F.O. (eds.) *The Neurosciences.* New York: The Rockefeller University Press, 1967a. Pp. 577-602.

Scheibel, M.E., and Scheibel, A.B. Structural organization of nonspecific thalamic nuclei and their projection toward cortex. *Brain Res.,* 1967b, 6: 60-94.

Schwartzbaum, J.S., and Pribram, K.H. The effects of amygdalectomy in monkeys on transposition along a brightness continuum. *J. comp. physiol. Psychol.,* 1960, 53: 396-99.

Sharpless, S.K. The effect of use and disuse on the efficacy of neurohumoral excitatory processes. *Proc. 75th Annual Convention of the American Psychological Association.* Washington, D.C., 1967.

Sharpless, S.K. Isolated and deafferented neurons: disuse supersensitivity. In Jasper, Ward, and Pope (eds.) *Basic Mechanisms of the Epilepsies.* Boston: Little, Brown, 1969. Pp. 329-48.

Sharpless, S., and Jasper, H. Habituation of the arousal reaction. *Brain,* 1956, 79: 655-80.

Sherrington, C. *The Integrative Action of the Nervous System.* New Haven: Yale University Press, 1947 (first published 1906).

Sholl, D.A. *The Organization of the Cerebral Cortex.* New York: John Wiley, 1956.

Sjöstrand, F.S. The molecular structure of membranes. In Bogoch, S. (ed.) *The Future of the Brain Sciences.* New York: Plenum Press, 1969. Pp. 117-57.

Skinner, B.F. *The Behavior of Organisms: An Experimental Analysis.* New York: Appleton-Century-Crofts, 1938.

Skinner, B.F. *Contingencies of Reinforcement: A Theoretical Analysis.* New York: Appleton-Century-Crofts, 1969.

Sokolov, E.N. Neuronal models and the orienting reflex. In Brazier, M.A.B. (ed.) *The Central Nervous System and Behavior.* New York: Josiah Macy, Jr. Foundation, 1960. Pp. 187-276.

Sokolov, E.N. *Perception and the Conditioned Reflex.* New York: Macmillan, 1963.

Sokolov, E.N., Pakula, A., and Arakelov, G.G. The after effects due to an intracellular electric stimulation of the giant neuron A in the left parietal ganglion of the mollusk Limnaea Stagnalis. In Pribram, K.H., and Broadbent, D. (eds.) *The Biology of Memory.* New York: Academic, 1970. Pp. 175-90.

Spence, K.W. *Behavior Theory and Conditioning* (Silliman Lectures, 1955). New Haven: Yale University Press, 1956.

Sperry, R.W. Neurology and the mind-brain problem. *American Scientist,* 1952, 40: 291-312.

Sperry, R.W. A modified concept of consciousness. *Psych. Rev.,* 1969, 76: 532-536.

Sperry, R.W. Perception in the absence of the neocortical commissures. In *Perception and Its Disorders.* Res. Publ. A.R.N.M.D., XLVIII, 1970, 123-38.

Sperry, R.W., Gazzaniga, M.S., and Bogen, J.E. Interhemispheric relationships: the neocortical commissures: syndromes of hemisphere deconnection. In Vinken, P.J., and Bruyn, G.W. (eds.) *Handbook of Clinical Neurology. Vol. 4.* Amsterdam: North Holland Publishing Co., 1969. Pp. 273-90.

Sperry, R.W., Miner, N., and Meyers, R.E. Visual pattern perception following subpial slicing and tantalum wire implantations in the visual cortex. *J. comp. physiol. Psychol.,* 1955, 48: 50-58.

Spinelli, D.N. OCCAM: A content addressable memory model for the brain. In Pribram, K.H., and Broadbent, D. (eds.) *The Biology of Memory.* New York: Academic, 1970. Pp. 273-306.

Spinelli, D.N., and Pribram, K.H. Changes in visual recovery functions produced by temporal lobe stimulation in monkeys. *Electroenceph. clin. Neurophysiol.,* 1966, 20: 44-49.

Spinelli, D.N., and Pribram, K.H. Changes in visual recovery function and unit activity produced by frontal cortex stimulation. *Electroenceph. clin. Neurophysiol.,* 1967, 22: 143-49.

Spinelli, D.N., Pribram, K.H. and Bridgeman, B. Visual receptive field organization of single units in the visual cortex of monkey. *Intern. J. Neuroscience,* 1970. Pp. 67-74.

Spinelli, D.N., Pribram, K.H., and Weingarten, M. Centrifugal optic nerve responses evoked by auditory and somatic stimulation. *Exp. Neurol.,* 1965, 12: 303-19.

Spinelli, D.N., Starr, A., and Barrett, T. Auditory specificity in unit recording from cat's visual cortex. *Exp. Neurol.,* 1968, 22: 75-84.

Spinelli, D.N., and Weingarten, M. Afferent and efferent activity in single units of the cat's optic nerve. *Exp. Neurol.,* 1966, 3: 347-61.

Sprague, J.M. Interaction of cortex and superior colliculus in mediation of visually guided behavior in the cat. *Science,* 1966, 153: 1544-47.

Stamm, J.S. Electrical stimulation of frontal cortex in monkeys during learning of an alternation task. *J. Neurophysiol.,* 1961, 24: 414-26.

Stamm, J.S., and Knight, M. Learning of visual tasks by monkeys with epileptogenic implants in temporal cortex. *J. comp. physiol. Psychol.*, 1963, 56: 254-60.

Stamm, J.S., and Pribram, K.H. Effects of epileptogenic lesions of inferotemporal cortex on learning and retention in monkeys. *J. comp. physiol. Psychol.*, 1961, 54: 614-18.

Stamm, J.S., and Warren, A. Learning and retention by monkeys with epileptogenic implants in posterior parietal cortex. *Epilepsia*, 1961, 2: 229-42.

Starzl, T.E., Taylor, C.W., and Magoun, H.W. Collateral afferent excitation of reticular formation of brain stem. *J. Neurophysiol.*, 1951, 14: 479-96.

Stein, L. Chemistry of reward and punishment. In Efron, D.H. (ed.) *Psychopharmacology. A Review of Progress, 1957-1967.* Washington, D.C.: U.S. Government Printing Office, Pub. Ser. Publ. No. 1836, 1968, 105-35.

Stroke, G.W. *An Introduction to Coherent Optics and Holography.* 2nd ed. New York: Academic, 1969.

Strong, O.S., and Elwyn, A. *Human Neuroanatomy.* Baltimore: Williams & Wilkins, 1943.

Strumwasser, F. Neurophysiological aspects of rhythms. In Quarton, G.C., Melnechuk, T., and Schmitt, F.O. (eds.) *The Neurosciences.* New York: The Rockefellar University Press, 1967. Pp. 516-28.

Stumpf, W.E. Estrogen-neurons and estrogen-neuron systems in the peri-ventricular brain. *The American Journal of Anatomy,* 129, No. 2, 1970. ©The Wistar Institute Press 1970. Pp. 207-18.

Sutin, J. The periventricular stratum of the hypothalamus. In Pfeiffer, C.C., and Smythies, J.R. (eds.) *International Review of Neurobiology.* New York and London: Academic, 1966. Pp. 263-300.

Svaetichin, G. Horizontal and amaercne cells of retina-properties and mechanisms of their control upon bipolar and ganglion cells. *Act. Cient. U.S.,* 1967, 18: 254.

Szentagothai, J. Architecture of the cerebral cortex. In Jaspar, H.H., Ward, A.A., Jr., and Pope, A. (eds.) *Basic Mechanisms of the Epilepsies.* Boston: Little, Brown, 1969. Pp. 13-28.

Talbot, S.A., and Marshall, U.H. Physiological studies on neural mechanisms of visual localization and discrimination. *Amer. J. Ophthal.,* 1941, 24: 1255-64.

Taub, E., Bacon, R.C., and Berman, A.J. Acquisition of a trace-conditioned avoidance response after deafferentiation of the responding limb. *J. comp. physiol. Psychol.,* 1965, 59: 275-79.

Teitelbaum, P. Sensory control of hypothalamic hyperphagia. *J. comp. physiol. Psychol.,* 1955, 48: 156-63.

Teitelbaum, P. Random and food directed activity in hyperphagic and normal rats. *J. comp. physiol. Psychol.,* 50: 486-90.

Terzuolo, C.A., and Poppele, R.E. Myotatic reflex: its input-output relation. *Science,* 1968, 159: 743-45.

Teuber, H.L. Perception. In Field, J., Magoun, H.W., and Hall, V.E. (eds.) *Handbook of Physiology, Neurophysiology III.* Washington: American Physiological Society, 1960. Pp. 1595-668.

Teuber, H.L. The riddle of frontal lobe function in man. In Warren, J.M., and Akert, K. (eds.) *The Frontal Granular Cortex and Behavior.* New York: McGraw-Hill, 1964. Pp. 410-45.

Teuber, H.L., Battersby, W., and Bender, M. *Visual Field Defects After Penetrating Missile Wounds of the Brain.* Cambridge: Harvard University Press, 1960.

Teuber, H.L., and Bender, M.B. Neuro-ophthalmology: the oculo-motor systems. *Progress in Neurology and Psychiatry,* 1951, 6: 148-78.

Thomas, P.K. Growth changes in the diameter of peripheral nerve fibres in fishes. *J. Anat.,* 1956, 90: 5-14.

Thompson, R.F. *Foundations of Physiological Psychology.* New York: Harper & Row, 1967.

Thompson, R.F. and Spencer, W.A. Habituation: a model phenomenon for the study of neuronal substrates of behavior. *Psych. Rev.,* 1966, 173: 16-43.

Tolman, E.C. *Purposive Behavior in Animals and Men.* New York: Appleton-Century-Crofts, 1932.

Trabasso, T., and Bower, G.H. *Attention in Learning Theory and Research.* New York: John Wiley, 1968.

Truex, R.C. and Carpenter, M.B. *Human Neuroanatomy,* 6th ed. Baltimore: Williams & Wilkins, 1969.

Tulving, E. Short term and long term memory: different retrieval mechanisms. In Pribram, K.H., and Broadbent, D. (eds.) *The Biology of Memory.* New York: Academic, 1970. Pp. 7-9.

Ukhtomski, A.A. Concerning the condition of excitation in dominance. *Novoe y refteksologie i fiziologii nervoisystemry,* 1926, 2: 3-15. Abstract in *Psychol. Abstr.,* 1927, 2388.

Valenstein, E.S. Stability and plasticity of motivation systems. In Quarton, G.C., Melnechuk, T., and Adelman, G. (eds.) *The Neurosciences* (Second Study). New York: The Rockefeller University Press, 1970. Pp. 207-17.

Valenstein, E.S., Cox, V.C., and Kakolewski, J.W. The hypothalamus and motivated behavior. In Tapp, J.T. (ed.) *Reinforcement and Behavior.* New York: Academic, 1969. Pp. 242-85.

van Heerden, P.J. *The Foundation of Empirical Knowledge.* N.V. Uitgeverij Wistik-Wassenaar, The Netherlands, 1968.

van Heerden, P.J. Models for the brain. *Nature,* January 10, 1970, 225: 177-78

van Heerden, P.J. Models for the brain. *Nature,* July 25, 1970, 227: 410-11.

Verzeano, M., Laufer, M., Spear, P., and McDonald, S. The activity of neuronal networks in the thalamus of the monkey. In Pribram, K.H., and Broadbent, D.E. (eds.) *Biology of Memory.* New York: Academic, 1970. Pp. 239-71.

Verzeano, M., and Negishi, K. Neuronal activity in cortical thalamic networks: a study with multiple microelectrodes. *J. Gen. Physiol.,* 1960, 43: 177-95.

von Bonin, G., and Bailey, P. *The Neocortex of Macaca Mulatta.* Urbana: University of Illinois Press, 1947.

Voss, J.F. In Voss, J.F. (ed.) *Approaches to Thought.* Columbus: Charles E. Meredith, 1969.

Walker, A.E. *The Primate Thalamus.* Chicago: University of Chicago Press, 1938.

Walter, W.G. *The Living Brain.* New York: Norton, 1953.

Walter, W.G. Electrical signs of association expectancy, and decision in the human brain. *Electroenceph. clin. Neurophysiol.,* 1967, Suppl. 25: 258-63.

Walter, W.G., Cooper, R., Aldridge, V.J., McCallum, W.C., and Winter, A.L. Contingent negative variation: an electric sign of sensorimotor association and expectancy in the human brain. *Nature,* 1964, 23: 380-84.

Walter, W.G., and Shipton, H.W. A new toposcopic display system. *Electroenceph. clin. Neurophysiol.,* 1951, 3: 281-92.

Wegener, J.C. The effect of cortical lesions on auditory and visual discrimination behavior in monkeys. *Cortex,* 1968, IV: 203-32.

Weingarten, M., and Spinelli, D.N. Changes in retinal perceptive field organization with the presentation of auditory and somatic stimulation. *Exp. Neurol.,* 1966, 15: 363-76.

Weiskrantz, L. Central nervous system and the organization of behavior. In Kimble, D.P. (ed.) *The Organization of Recall.* New York: The New York Academy of Sciences, 1967. Pp. 234-93.

Weiss, P. Experimental analysis of coordination by the disarrangement of central-peripheral relations. *Symposia of the Soc. for Exp. Biol.,* 1950, IV, Animal Behavior, 92-109.

Weiss, P. $1 + 1 \neq 2$. In Quarton, G.C., Melnechuk, T., and Schmitt, F.O. (eds.) *The Neurosciences*. New York: The Rockefellar University Press, 1967. Pp. 801-21.

Welt, C., Aschoff, J.C., Kameda, K., and Brooks, V.B. Intracortical organization of cat's motorsensory neurons. In Yahr, M.D., and Purpura, D.P. (eds.) *Neurophysiological Basis of Normal and Abnormal Motor Activities*. Hewlett, N.Y.: Raven Press, 1967. Pp. 255-94.

Werblin, F.S., and Dowling, J.E. Organization of the retina of the mudpuppy, Necturus maculosus. II. Intracellular recording. *J. Neurophysiol.,* 1969, 32: 339-55.

Werner, G. The topology of the body representation in the somatic afferent pathway. In Quarton, G.S., Melnechuk, T.M., and Schmitt, F.O. *The Neurosciences, Vol. II.* New York: The Rockefeller University Press, 1970. Pp. 605-16.

Whalen, R.E. Effects of mounting without intromission and intromission without ejaculation on sexual behavior and maze learning. *J. comp. physiol. Psychol.,* 1961, 54: 409-15.

White, R.W. Competence and the psychosexual stages of development. In Jones, M.R. (ed.) *Nebraska Symposium on Motivation*. Lincoln: University of Nebraska Press, 1960. Pp. 97-140.

Whitlock, D.G., and Nauta, W.J. Subcortical projections from the temporal neocortex in Macaca Mulatta. *J. comp. Neurol.,* 1956, 106: 183-212.

Whyte, L.L. A hypothesis regarding the brain modifications underlying memory. *Brain,* 1954, 77: 158-65.

Willshaw, D.J., Buneman, O.P., and Longuet-Higgens, H.C. Non-holographic associative memory. *Nature,* 1969, 222: 960-62.

Willshaw, D.J., Longuet-Higgins, H.C., and Buneman, O.P. Discussion. *Nature,* January 10, 1970, 225: 178.

Wilson, W.A., Jr., and Mishkin, M. Comparison of the effects of inferotemporal and lateral occipital lesions on visually guided behavior in monkeys. *J. comp. physiol. Psychol.,* 1959, 2: 10-17.

Wittgenstein, L. *Tractatus Logico-Philosophicus.* London: Routledge & Kegan Paul, 1922.

Woolsey, C.N., and Chang, T.H. Activation of the cerebral cortex by antidromic volleys in the pyramidal tract. *Res. Publ. Ass. Nerv. Ment. Dis.,* 1948, 27: 146.

Young, J.Z. *The Life of Mammals.* New York: Oxford University Press, 1957.

Zimbardo, P.G. *The Cognitive Control of Motivation.* Glenview, Ill.: Scott, Foresman, 1969.

index

authors' index

subject index

A- and b-waves of the electro-retinogram, 56
Abstractive process, 67
Accommodation (Piagetian), 302
Acetylcholine (ACh). *See* Cholinergic mechanisms
Achievement, 215, 241-43, 251, 266, 290-91, 298-305, 376, 390
Act(s), Action, 11, 208-13, 217, 220, 226, 230, 238-52, 256, 263, 266, 273, 292-93, 296, 301-2, 305, 309, 312, 327, 332, 337-38, 344, 352, 365-69, 376, 379, 385; communicative property of, 302, 305, 309, 328, 331, 369, 374, 378, 384; interrupted, 212; learning from, 255, 256, 379; scotomata of, 241; sensory cortex for, 301; skilled, 217; valuing, 293; *see also* Bias, Feedforward, TOTE; voluntary, willed, 100, 229, 233
Action system(s), 367, 379
Activation, 77, 206, 207, 264, 280, 346, 350, 390
Activity, 229, 236, 248, 271, 296
Actor, 348, 379
Actualization, 302, 327
Acuity, 317
Adaptation, 54-59, 64, 65, 87, 94, 131, 161, 250, 326. *See also* Habituation
Addiction, 292, 293, 302
Address, 157, 326, 349. *See also* Content addressable memory mechanism
Adjective(s), 367
Adjustment, internal, 211. *See also* Coping mechanisms
Adjustment, postural, 228
Adrenaline (epinephrine). *See* Aminergic mechanisms
Adverb(s), 367
Adypsia, 188. *See also* Drinking; Satiety; Thirst
Affect(s), 195-97, 200, 206, 212-13, 266, 272-74, 293, 300, 308, 338, 373, 390; signal aspect of, 213. *See also* Emotions; "Stop" mechanism
Afferent fibers (channel), 84, 85, 87, 91, 176, 177, 209-11, 222, 226, 321-23, 327
Affluence, 295, 297
After-image, 109, 133
Aggressiveness, Agonistic behavior, 183, 266
Agnosia(s), 359
Agraphia, 355, 360. *See also* Aphasia
Alerting, 176, 183, 300, 346
Alexia, 358
All-or-none law of nerve impulse, 25
Alpha (α) motoneurons, 86, 221, 222, 228
Alpha rhythm (waves), 106, 207

Alternation behavior, 205, 333, 342, 343, 345
Aluminum hydroxide (alumina) cream, 45-46, 110-11, 122-24. *See also* Irritative lesion
Amacrine cells of the retina, 19, 57, 59, 64
American sign language, 309
Aminergic mechanisms, 180-83, 192-98, 208, 273-84, 290. *See also* Synaptic vesicles, transmitters
Amnesia, retrograde, 44
Amphetamine, 275
Amputation (phantom limb), 168
Amygdala, Amygdalectomy, 173, 179, 187-89, 192-93, 200-202, 205, 211, 280, 284-88, 308, 318, 340-46
Analogue cross-correlation mechanism, 105, 152, 388
Anand-Brobeck center, 190. *See also* Far-lateral hypo-thalamic feeding mecha-nism; Feeding behavior
"And" functions (logic), 68-72
Androgens, 173
Anesthesia, anesthetics, 45, 85, 229
Angular gyrus, 369
Anisotropic ordering(s) of macromolecules, 157
Anodal polarization, 78
Antegrade amnesia, 281
Anterior lobe of cerebellum, 227, 228, 229, 232, 233, 242
Anterior frontal (prefrontal) cortex, 211, 281, 287, 308, 334, 338-51, 355-57; electrical stimulation of, 347, 349; fronto-limbic forebrain, 308, 344, 350, 371; interaction with motor mechanisms, 351; lesions, 334, 337, 342-47, 359, 371-72; lobotomy (leukotomy), 337-41, 356; site of recording, 282
Anticipatory responses, 246, 250, 285. *See also* Fast-time computations; Motor cortex; Neocerebellar system
Antidepressant drugs, 183. *See also* Catechol amines; DOPA
Antidromic conduction of nerve impulse, 78, 249
Antimetabolites, 38, 40
Ape communication, 366
Aphagia, 188
Aphasia, 355-59, 365; Broca's (expressive; motor), 353, 354; Wernicke's (receptive; sensory), 354
Apical dendrites, 30, 78, 275, 281
Aplesia Californica (sea slug), 19, 52
Appetite(s); appetitive be-havior, 175, 180, 195-200, 206, 212, 213, 266, 272, 274, 293, 300, 308, 338,

Appetite(s) (cont'd)
373, 390. *See also* "Go" mechanism; motivation
Approach, 280, 337
Aqueduct of Sylvius, 281
Arboreal habits, 233
Arborization (branching) of nerve fibers, 16, 27, 64
Archicerebellum, 232
Arrival patterns of nerve im-pulses, 105, 112-14, 152, 162, 270. *See also* Depar-ture patterns; Junctional slow potential micro-structure
Arousal, 206-8, 264, 292, 390. *See also* Activation; Electroencephalogram (EEG)
Articulatory disturbances of language (dysarthria), 355
Assertiveness, 167, 183, 300
Assimilation (Piagetian), 302
Association cortex, 130, 162, 209, 308, 312-22, 331, 338, 341, 344, 345, 362, 368
Association, processes of, 312, 314, 318, 360-70
Associative connections, 9, 10, 353, 362, 365
Associative memory, 153. *See also* Hologram
Associative net, 154, 156, 338
Associative recall, 162, 362
Astereognosis, 245
Atrophy of disuse, 159
Attention, 88, 100, 207, 273, 312, 321-29; focusing of, 331, 350; selective, 138, 298, 299, 312, 324, 331, 350
Attitude, 390
Auditory mechanism(s), 87, 88, 108, 117, 145, 163, 164, 192, 314, 321, 369
Automata, 101, 103
Autonomic lability and stability, 208
Averaging circuit(s), 158
Aversion; avoidance, 44, 280, 292, 337
Awareness, 104, 105, 106, 108, 136, 152, 346, 384
Axodendritic coupling, 275
Axon(s), 6, 8, 12, 13, 25, 36, 40, 53, 166, 275, 277, 279. *See also* Nerve fibers; Nerve impulse; collaterals, 89; terminals, branched, 6, 19, 40, 275
Axonal growth (cones), 27, 28, 31, 35, 43-46

"Bahnung." *See* Facilitation.
Basal dendrites, 32, 127
Basal ganglia, 187, 225-40, 248, 250, 281, 318, 320, 337, 368
Basilar membrane of the cochlea, 168
Behavior: appetitive, *see* Appetite(s); biasing of, 294, 297, 300; con-sequences of, 244, 264, 265, 292; context-depen-

"Cognito ergo sum" (cont'd)
See also Cartesian dualism;
Mind-brain-behavior
problem
Cognitive process(es), 100-
104, 254, 255, 352, 374,
380, 390
Coherence plot, 24
Coherent light, 145-50. *See
also* Laser; Physical hologram
Colliculus, superior and inferior, 320, 321. *See also*
Auditory; Visual
Color vision, 126, 316,
321, 324
Columnar structure of cortex,
126-30, 152, 158, 235, 325
Commissure, cerebral. *See*
Corpus callosum
Commisurotomy, 363, 364
Commitment, 215, 287, 290-
94, 298-302, 395
Communication, 1, 213, 250,
302, 305, 309, 331, 334,
336, 351, 352, 358, 360,
366, 369, 373-79, 385,
391; chimpanzee, 334, 366;
emotional, 351; nonverbal,
369; propositional, 374;
social, 377, 378
Communicative act(s), 305,
309, 331, 369, 378, 384
Communicative aspects of
language, 358
Comparator, 93, 235, 236.
See also Consonance; Correlation; match-mismatch;
dissonance
Competence, 215, 260-66,
271, 273, 290, 298-302;
cholinergic, 284; genetic,
263, 266; modification of,
263, 290; tissue, 258, 269,
270, 279
Competing responses, 266,
267, 292
Compulsion neurosis, 344
Computations, fast-time, 237.
See also Cerebellum;
Fourier transforms; Motor
cortex
Computer(s), 67, 82, 87, 110,
127, 144, 220, 283, 329,
371, 388-90; programs,
127, 128, 150, 325,
376, 382
Concurrence (simultaneity) in
linguistics, 359
Conditional behavior, 79, 265,
272, 273, 279
Conditioned emotional re-
sponse, 44
Conditioning, operant, 204,
284, 295, 296, 297
Conduction, nerve impulse,
8, 15, 16, 112, 114, 115,
230, 261
Cone(s) of the retina, 4, 57
Configural (configurational)
representation, 66, 140,
370, 388. *See* Holograms;
Junctional slow potential
microstructure; Match and
mismatch; Neuroelectric
response
Conformational change(s) of
macromolecules, 39, 43,
66, 157, 206, 325, 326

Conscious experience, 109,
170, 383
Consciousness-expanding
drug(s), 212
Consequence(s) of behavior,
236, 244, 263, 264, 273,
292, 294, 297-302, 331
Consolidation processes in
memory, 44-47, 349
Consonance, 286-90, 294,
297. *See also* Coping mechanisms; Correlation process;
Dissonance; Incongruence
Constancy, perceptual, 110,
123, 132, 133, 159, 170,
246, 256, 312, 326, 379
Construction(s): cultural,
375, 385; linguistic, 380;
mental, intervention of,
380, *see also* mind-brain-
behavior problem; phenom-
enal, 380, 384; "reality" as
a, 377-80
Constructional realism, 384
Content addressable memory
mechanism, 157, 326, 349
Context, 66, 252, 255, 262,
273, 284, 290, 308, 309,
331, 337, 344, 345, 351;
dependency, sensitivity,
308, 331, 337, 338, 344-51,
367, 391, *see also* Symbols;
-free construction(s), 309,
344, 347, 365, *see also*
Sign(s); Significance
Contiguity theory of reinforcement, 255, 256, 262, 263,
270, 273
Contingencies of reinforcement, 152, 253, 270, 281,
300. *See also* Operant
conditioning
Contour, 61, 126, 138, 163
Contraction(s), muscle, 221,
222, 225, 226, 229, 237,
246, 301
Contraction(s), of the
stomach, 185, 272
Contrast enhancement, 64,
65, 89, 95, 286, 322. *See
also* Lateral inhibition;
Mach bands.
Contrast, temporal, 65
Control (servo) mechanisms,
83, 140, 213-15, 221, 223,
280, 293, 369, 373
Control of muscle contractions, 223, 226, 237
Control, verbal, 359, 369
Control, selective, 299, 321,
350. *See also* Input control;
Modification of behavior
Convergence, 21, 70, 125,
176, 177, 248
Convergent series (of trans-
formations), 170, 236
Convolutional integrals, 142-
44, 149, 152. *See also*
Coding; Fourier transforms;
Holograms; Reversible
transformations
Convulsion(s), electroconvul-
sive shock, 44, 45
Coordination, spatial, 10, 228
Coping mechanisms (internal
control), 208-13
Core brain mechanisms, 175-
83, 186, 213, 264, 266,
270, 275, 280, 281, 300,

Core brain mechanisms
(cont'd)
305-7, 390. *See also* Hypothalamus; Reticular formation; homeostats, 180, 197,
199, 272, 293, *see also*
"Go" mechanisms, "Stop"
mechanisms, Thermostats;
receptor mechanism(s),
171, 178, 180, 183, 196,
213, *see also* Drinking,
Eating, Respiration, Sexual
activity, Temperature
regulation; stimulation,
176, 264
Corollary discharge, 90, 93,
312. *See also* Bias; Feedforward mechanism(s)
Corpus callosum, 47, 179,
362, 365
Corpus striatum. *See* Basal
ganglia; Caudate nucleus;
Putamen
Correct performance,
290, 379
Correlation process(es), "cor-
relograms," 93, 105, 153-
57, 165, 370, 373. *See also*
Associative processes; Holographic process(es)
Cortex, 8, 10, 13, 21, 30, 34,
40, 63, 114-16, 119, 122,
139, 206, 211, 226, 235,
236, 241, 242, 248, 275,
284, 360, *see also* specific
organ, e.g., Cerebellar cortex, Cerebral cortex,
Inferior temporal cortex;
synaptic domains in, 21,
78; thickening of, due to
stimulation, 32, 279
Cortical columns, 126-30,
152, 158, 235, 325
Cortical control over input
processes, 209, 248, 280,
287, 300, 318, 338, 347,
368, 374
Cortico-cortical association,
360, 365, 367
"Critical periods," in development of embryos, 47. *See
also* Sensitive periods
Critical philosophies, 377,
382, 384, 385. *See also*
Linguistic processes; Post-
critical philosophy
Cross-correlation, 152, 349,
370. *See also* Holography
Cross-hatches of cortex, 111,
122, 315
Culture, 375, 376, 382-85
Curiosity, 199
Currents, negative (cathodal)
and positive (anodal), 284
"Cybernetic" theory of motivation and emotion, 214,
300-301, 390
Cyclic adenine monophos-
phate (cyclic AMP),
275, 279

D.C. fields, 110-12, 386
De-afferentation of limbs,
230
Decimal system of coding, 71
Decision theory, 371
Decoding, 67-82, 149, 220,
261, 359

426

We would like to thank the following for permission to reprint artwork: Page 27, courtesy of Altman, 1967. Page 29, courtesy of C. M. Pomerat, et. al., Pasadena Foundation for Medical Research, from the film, "Dynamic Aspects of the Neuron in Tissue Culture." Page 31, Kruger, Lawrence, "Morphological Alterations of the Cerebral Cortex and Their Possible Role in the Loss and Acquisition of Information," in Daniel P. Kimble (Ed.), The Anatomy of Memory. Palo Alto, California: Science and Behavior Books, 1965. Page 36, courtesy of Drs. M. B. Bunge and R. P. Bunge. Page 37, Hyden, Holgar, "Activation of Nuclear RNA of Neurons and Glia in Learning," in Daniel P. Kimble (Ed.), The Anatomy of Memory. Palo Alto, California: Science and Behavior Books, 1965. Page 46, originally published by the University of California Press; reprinted by permission of The Regents of the University of California. Page 93, from Visual Pattern Recognition by Peter C. Dodwell. Copyright © 1970 by Holt, Rinehart and Winston, Inc. Reprinted by permission of Holt, Rinehart and Winston, Inc. Page 102, Gerald Duckworth & Co. Ltd. Page 144, from Sensory Inhibition by Georg von Bekesy (copyright © 1967 by Princeton University Press). Page 181, O. S. Strong and A. Elwyn, Human Neuroanatomy © 1943 The Williams & Wilkins Co., Baltimore, Md. Page 182, by H. K. H. Brodie, D. C. Murphy, F. K. Goodwin, and W. E. Bunney, Jr. Page 224, R. F. Thompson, Foundations of Physiological Psychology, Harper & Row, 1967. Page 247, from Physiological Psychology by Peter M. Milner. Copyright © 1970 by Holt, Rinehart and Winston, Inc. Reprinted by permission of Holt, Rinehart and Winston, Inc. Page 359, J. & A. Churchill, Publishers. The charts on pages 62, 73, 106, 194, 199, 287, 317, 346, and 359 were redrawn from the original sources noted on legends.